T0226886

Psychosis in Children and Adolescents: A Guide for Clinicians

Editors

ELLEN M. HOUSE
JOHN W. TYSON Jr

CHILD AND ADOLESCENT PSYCHIATRIC CLINICS OF NORTH AMERICA

www.childpsych.theclinics.com

Consulting Editor
TODD E. PETERS

January 2020 • Volume 29 • Number 1

ELSEVIER

1600 John F. Kennedy Boulevard • Suite 1800 • Philadelphia, Pennsylvania, 19103-2899

http://www.theclinics.com

CHILD AND ADOLESCENT PSYCHIATRIC CLINICS OF NORTH AMERICA Volume 29, Number 1
January 2020 ISSN 1056–4993, ISBN-13: 978-0-323-71119-7

Editor: Lauren Boyle
Developmental Editor: Kristen Helm

Child and Adolescent Psychiatric Clinics of North America (ISSN 1056-4993) is published quarterly by Elsevier Inc., 360 Park Avenue South, New York, NY 10010-1710. Months of issue are January, April, July, and October. Business and Editorial Offices: 1600 John F. Kennedy Boulevard, Suite 1800, Philadelphia, PA 19103-2899. Periodicals postage paid at New York, NY and additional mailing offices. Subscription prices are $338.00 per year (US individuals), $661.00 per year (US institutions), $100.00 per year (US & Canadian students), $388.00 per year (Canadian individuals), $804.00 per year (Canadian institutions), $446.00 per year (international individuals), $804.00 per year (international institutions), and $200.00 per year (international students). International air speed delivery is included in all *Clinics* subscription prices. All prices are subject to change without notice. **POSTMASTER:** Send address changes to *Child and Adolescent Psychiatric Clinics of North America*, Elsevier Health Sciences Division, Subscription Customer Service, 3251 Riverport Lane, Maryland Heights, MO 63043. **Customer Service: 1-800-654-2452 (U.S. and Canada); 314-447-8871 (outside U.S. and Canada). Fax: 314-447-8029. E-mail:** JournalsCustomer Service-usa@elsevier.com **(for print support) or** journalsonlinesupport-usa@elsevier.com **(for online support).**

Reprints. For copies of 100 or more of articles in this publication, please contact the Commercial Reprints Department, Elsevier Inc., 360 Park Avenue South, New York, New York 10010-1710 Tel.: 212-633-3874; Fax: 212-633-3820, E-mail: reprints@elsevier.com.

Child and Adolescent Psychiatric Clinics of North America is covered in *MEDLINE/PubMed (Index Medicus), ISI, SSCI, Research Alert, Social Search, Current Contents,* and *EMBASE/Excerpta Medica.*

Contributors

CONSULTING EDITOR

TODD E. PETERS, MD, FAPA
Medical Director, Child and Adolescent Services, Chief Medical Information Officer (CMIO), Sheppard Pratt Health System, Sheppard Pratt Physicians PA Clinical Operations Liaison, Baltimore, Maryland, USA

EDITORS

ELLEN M. HOUSE, MD
Clinical Assistant Professor of Psychiatry, Augusta University/University of Georgia Medical Partnership, Health Science Campus, Athens, Georgia, USA

JOHN W. TYSON Jr, MD
Staff Child and Adolescent Psychiatrist, First Episode and Early Psychosis Program, Assistant Psychiatrist, Acute Psychiatry Service, Instructor of Psychiatry, Massachusetts General Hospital, Boston, Massachusetts, USA

AUTHORS

JOSE ALBERTO ARRIOLA, MD, MPH
Assistant Professor, Department of Psychiatry and Behavioral Sciences, Consult-Liaison Psychiatry, Vanderbilt University Medical Center, Nashville, Tennessee, USA

ROBERT F. ASARNOW, PhD
Department of Psychiatry & Biobehavioral Sciences, University of California, Los Angeles, Department of Psychology, University of California, Los Angeles, Brain Research Institute, University of California, Los Angeles, California, USA

DAVID BECKMANN, MD, MPH
Addiction Recovery Management Service, First Episode and Early Psychosis Program, Department of Psychiatry, Massachusetts General Hospital, Harvard Medical School, Boston, Massachusetts, USA

JULIA BROWNE, PhD
Massachusetts General Hospital, Center of Excellence in Psychosocial and Systemic Research, Harvard Medical School, Boston, Massachusetts, USA

GABRIELLE A. CARLSON, MD
Professor of Psychiatry and Pediatrics, Director, Child and Adolescent Psychiatry, Stony Brook University School of Medicine, Stony Brook, New York, USA

CORINNE CATHER, PhD
Massachusetts General Hospital, Center of Excellence in Psychosocial and Systemic Research, Harvard Medical School, Boston, Massachusetts, USA

TARA CHANDRASEKHAR, MD
Assistant Professor, Department of Psychiatry and Behavioral Sciences, Duke University School of Medicine, Durham, North Carolina, USA

DREW C. COMAN, PhD
Clinical Psychologist, Massachusetts General Hospital, Harvard Medical School, Boston, Massachusetts, USA

JOHN NATHAN COPELAND, MD
Medical Instructor, Department of Psychiatry and Behavioral Sciences, Duke University School of Medicine, Durham, North Carolina, USA

ALLYSON WITTERS CUNDIFF, MD
Assistant Professor, Department of Psychiatry, Child and Adolescent Psychiatry, Vanderbilt University Medical Center, Nashville, Tennessee, USA

BRIAN DENIETOLIS, PsyD
Department of Psychiatry, University of Massachusetts Medical School, Worcester, Massachusetts, USA

ABIGAIL L. DONOVAN, MD
Director, First Episode and Early Psychosis Program, Associate Director, Acute Psychiatry Service, Associate Psychiatrist, Massachusetts General Hospital, Assistant Professor of Psychiatry, Boston, Massachusetts, USA

DAVID I. DRIVER, MD
Child Psychiatry Branch, National Institute of Mental Health, National Institutes of Health, Bethesda, Maryland, USA

YAEL DVIR, MD
Department of Psychiatry, University of Massachusetts Medical School, Worcester, Massachusetts, USA

ANNE EDEN EVINS, MD, MPH
Massachusetts General Hospital, Center for Addiction Medicine; Harvard Medical School, Boston, Massachusetts, USA

ROBERT L. FINDLING, MD, MBA
Division of Child and Adolescent Psychiatry, Department of Psychiatry and Behavioral Sciences, Johns Hopkins University School of Medicine, Baltimore, Maryland, USA

JENNIFER K. FORSYTH, PhD
Department of Psychiatry & Biobehavioral Sciences, University of California, Los Angeles, Los Angeles, California, USA

CATHERINE FUCHS, MD, DFAACAP
Professor, Department of Psychiatry, Child and Adolescent Psychiatry, Vanderbilt University Medical Center, Nashville, Tennessee, USA

JODIE GILMAN, PhD
Massachusetts General Hospital, Center for Addiction Medicine, Harvard Medical School, Boston, Massachusetts, USA

NITIN GOGTAY, MD
Child Psychiatry Branch, National Institute of Mental Health, National Institutes of Health, Bethesda, Maryland, USA

BRIEN J. GOODWIN, MS
Department of Psychological and Brain Sciences, University of Massachusetts Amherst, Amherst, Massachusetts, USA

PHILIP D. HARVEY, PhD
Leonard M. Miller Professor, Department of Psychiatry and Behavioral Sciences, University of Miami Miller School of Medicine, Research Service, Bruce W. Carter VA Medical Center, Miami, Florida, USA

SAMANTHA HINES, BA
Supported Employment and Education Specialist, Department of Psychiatry, Massachusetts General Hospital, Harvard Medical School, Boston, Massachusetts, USA

ELLEN M. HOUSE, MD
Clinical Assistant Professor of Psychiatry, Augusta University/University of Georgia Medical Partnership, Health Science Campus, Athens, Georgia, USA

ELIZABETH C. ISNER, BS
Medical Student, University of Miami Miller School of Medicine, Miami, Florida, USA

HAL KRONSBERG, MD
Division of Child and Adolescent Psychiatry, Department of Psychiatry and Behavioral Sciences, Johns Hopkins University School of Medicine, Baltimore, Maryland, USA

ESTHER S. LEE, MD
Division of Child and Adolescent Psychiatry, Department of Psychiatry and Behavioral Sciences, Johns Hopkins University School of Medicine, Baltimore, Maryland, USA

KELSEY LEIGH LOWMAN, AB
Department of Psychiatry, Massachusetts General Hospital, Boston, Massachusetts, USA

ANNE B. McBRIDE, MD
Assistant Professor of Clinical Psychiatry, Program Director of the UC Davis Child and Adolescent Psychiatry Residency, Department of Psychiatry and Behavioral Sciences, University of California, Davis Medical Center, Sacramento, California, USA

PATRICK McGORRY, PhD, MD
Professor, Orygen, The National Centre of Excellence in Youth Mental Health, Centre for Youth Mental Health, The University of Melbourne, Parkville, Victoria, Australia

JAMES McKOWEN, PhD
Addiction Recovery Management Service, Department of Psychiatry, Massachusetts General Hospital, Harvard Medical School, Boston, Massachusetts, USA

JESSICA MERRITT, MD
Child and Adolescent Fellow, Department of Psychiatry, Child and Adolescent Psychiatry, Vanderbilt University Medical Center, Nashville, Tennessee, USA

KIM T. MUESER, PhD
Massachusetts General Hospital Center of Excellence in Psychosocial and Systemic Research, Center for Psychiatric Rehabilitation, Boston University, Boston, Massachusetts, USA

JESSICA NARGISO, PhD
Addiction Recovery Management Service, Department of Psychiatry, Massachusetts General Hospital, Harvard Medical School, Boston, Massachusetts, USA

BARNABY NELSON, PhD
Professor, Orygen, The National Centre of Excellence in Youth Mental Health, Centre for Youth Mental Health, The University of Melbourne, Parkville, Victoria, Australia

CAROLY PATAKI, MD
Health Sciences Clinical Professor of Psychiatry and Biobehavioral Sciences, David Geffen School of Medicine, University of California, Los Angeles, Los Angeles, California, USA

PAMELA RAKHSHAN ROUHAKHTAR, MA
Department of Psychology, University of Maryland, Baltimore County, Baltimore, Maryland, USA

JUDITH L. RAPOPORT, MD
Child Psychiatry Branch, National Institute of Mental Health, National Institutes of Health, Bethesda, Maryland, USA

JASON SCHIFFMAN, PhD
Professor, Department of Psychology, University of Maryland, Baltimore County, Baltimore, Maryland, USA

CHARLES L. SCOTT, MD
Professor of Clinical Psychiatry, Chief of the Division of Psychiatry and the Law, Training Director of the UC Davis Forensic Fellowship Training Program, Department of Psychiatry and Behavioral Sciences, University of California, Davis Medical Center, Sacramento, California, USA

LINMARIE SIKICH, MD
Associate Professor, Department of Psychiatry and Behavioral Sciences, Duke University School of Medicine, Durham, North Carolina, USA

MAJA SKIKIC, MD
Assistant Professor, Department of Psychiatry and Behavioral Sciences, Vanderbilt University Medical Center, Nashville, Tennessee, USA

MARINA SPANOS, PhD
Faculty Research Associate, Department of Psychiatry and Behavioral Sciences, Duke University, Durham, North Carolina, USA

KATE J. STANTON, MD
Department of Psychiatry, University of Massachusetts Medical School, Worcester, Massachusetts, USA

YASAS TANGUTURI, MBBS, MPH
Assistant Professor, Department of Psychiatry, Child and Adolescent Psychiatry, Vanderbilt University Medical Center, Nashville, Tennessee, USA

SHARI THOMAS, MD
Healthy Foundations Group, Bethesda, Maryland, USA

JOHN W. TYSON Jr, MD
Staff Child and Adolescent Psychiatrist, First Episode and Early Psychosis Program, Assistant Psychiatrist, Acute Psychiatry Service, Instructor of Psychiatry, Massachusetts General Hospital, Boston, Massachusetts, USA

LISA WATT, MSN
Addiction Recovery Management Service, Department of Psychiatry, Massachusetts
General Hospital, Boston, Massachusetts, USA

ABIGAIL WRIGHT, PhD
Massachusetts General Hospital, Center of Excellence in Psychosocial and Systemic
Research, Harvard Medical School, Boston, Massachusetts, USA

AMY M. YULE, MD
Addiction Recovery Management Service, Department of Psychiatry, Massachusetts
General Hospital, Harvard Medical School, Boston, Massachusetts, USA

Contents

> Psychotic experiences may be part of normal development or indicate a wide range of mental disorders. This article shows how a systematic, domain-based, phenomenological approach to assessing psychotic symptoms in youth facilitates the gathering of the nuanced clinical information necessary to understand a child's specific experience. Mapping this information onto a narrative timeline, while understanding the evolution and developmental context of psychotic experiences, is essential in making an accurate diagnostic formulation and appropriate treatment plan for youth presenting with psychotic experiences.

> Evaluating the patient with first episode psychosis (FEP) requires a careful assessment that includes a thorough history, examination, and workup. This begins with a thoughtful consideration of the differential diagnoses and is followed and supported by laboratory, encephalographic, and imaging studies where appropriate. This article presents some of the diagnostic considerations for a patient presenting with psychosis with an emphasis on the secondary causes and proposes a tiered approach to the workup of FEP that is clinically guided.

> This is an updated review of child and adolescent somatic disorders associated with psychosis/psychotic symptoms, organized into neurologic, infectious, genetic, inborn errors of metabolism, autoimmune, rheumatologic, endocrine, nutritional, metabolic, and iatrogenic categories. When possible clinical manifestations or types of psychotic symptoms and proposed neuropathogenesis causing the neuropsychiatric symptoms are included. In some cases, the psychiatric symptoms may be the first presentation of the disease. The authors hope that this review will aid child and adolescent psychiatrists in considering alternative etiologies of youth presenting with psychosis and encourage appropriate physical examination, history, and further work-up when suspected.

Psychosis is a unique and significant risk factor associated with violent and suicidal behavior and warrants special consideration. This article presents a careful review of the literature on violence risk and psychosis and suicide risk and psychosis as it pertains to youth or those who have been newly diagnosed with or are at high risk for psychotic disorders. Each topic is covered in reference to general considerations and specific psychotic symptoms (eg, hallucinations, delusions, paranoia). The reader can refer to practical boxes to assist in identifying relevant risk factors and examples of questions to ask the patient and family.

Twenty-five years ago "at risk" for psychosis criteria were introduced to the field. Prediction studies have identified a range of risk factors involved in transition from "at risk" status to first episode psychotic illness, with recent interest in dynamic and multimodal prediction models. Treatment studies have indicated that risk of transition to psychotic disorder can at least be delayed in this clinical population. Although the strongest evidence to date is for cognitive behavioral therapy, the optimal type and sequence of treatment remains an active area of research.

The clinical severity, impact on development, and poor prognosis of childhood-onset schizophrenia may represent a more homogeneous group. Positive symptoms in children are necessary for the diagnosis, and hallucinations are more often multimodal. In healthy children and children with a variety of other psychiatric illnesses, hallucinations are not uncommon and diagnosis should not be based on these alone. Childhood-onset schizophrenia is an extraordinarily rare illness that is poorly understood but seems continuous with the adult-onset disorder. Once a diagnosis is confirmed, aggressive medication treatment combined with family education and individual counseling may prevent further deterioration.

Mood disorders, including major depression and mania, can present with psychotic features. In youth psychotic-like phenomena such as "seeing faces in the dark" or "hearing noises" are fairly common. Rates of lifetime psychotic symptoms are much higher than rates of psychosis during a "current" episode of mania or depression in youth. Psychotic phenomena can be mood congruent or incongruent. A detailed mental status examination and clinical history include questioning to ensure the informants understand the questions being asked. There are interviews that structure how questions are asked, and rating scales that help anchor severity and quality of the mood episode.

Autism spectrum disorders (ASDs) and schizophrenia spectrum disorders co-occur at elevated rates. Although these conditions are diagnostically distinct, they share multiple clinical features and genetic risk factors. This article describes the epidemiologic features and clinical manifestations of psychosis in individuals with ASDs, while also discussing shared genetic risk factors and affected brain regions. Components of a diagnostic assessment, including a thorough developmental, behavioral, medical, and psychiatric history, will be reviewed. The authors highlight the manifestations of catatonia in this population and note the shared features between catatonia and ASDs. Finally, treatment approaches and areas for future study are suggested.

There is growing evidence to support the link between childhood trauma and psychosis. Childhood trauma increases the risk for psychosis and affects severity and type of psychotic symptoms, and frequency of comorbid conditions, including depression and substance use. Childhood trauma is linked to more severe functional impairment in individuals with psychosis. There is evidence to support gender differences in the influence of childhood trauma on the course of psychotic illnesses, appearing to be more profound in girls and women. Other biological markers that may explain the link between childhood trauma and psychosis include brain-derived neurotrophic factor and other inflammatory markers.

Youth experiencing psychosis also frequently misuse substances, making it clinically challenging to differentiate substance-induced psychosis (SIP) from a primary psychotic disorder (PPD), which has important implications for management and prognosis. This article presents practical considerations related to differentiating SIP from PPD, including information on substances associated with symptoms of psychosis. Recommendations for management of SIP are also reviewed, including screening for and treating comorbid substance use disorders and using evidence-based medication and psychosocial interventions.

The rapidly changing landscape of cannabis in terms of availability, potency, and routes of administration, as well as the decrease in risk perception and changing norms, have contributed to an increase in the popularity of cannabis. Cannabis use is associated with a poorer recovery from a psychotic disorder, increasing the risk of relapse, rehospitalization, and lower social functioning. Data are mixed regarding cannabis use as a component cause of psychosis in people at risk for psychotic disorder. Care providers, parents, and schools must educate youth and adolescents about the risks of cannabis use.

Neurobiology of Psychosis in Youth

The genetic architecture of schizophrenia is complex and highly polygenic. This article discusses key findings from genetic studies of childhood-onset schizophrenia (COS) and the more common adult-onset schizophrenia (AOS), including studies of familial aggregation and common, rare, and copy number variants. Extant literature suggests that COS is a rare variant of AOS involving greater familial aggregation of schizophrenia spectrum disorders and a potentially higher occurrence of pathogenic copy number variants. The direct utility of genetics to clinical practice for COS is currently limited; however, identifying common pathways through which risk genes affect brain function offers promise for novel interventions.

Cognitive impairments are a central feature of schizophrenia. These impairments are present across the course of the illness, from prodromal to more chronic patients. Social cognitive deficits, now known to be related to social outcomes in the real world, are also impaired in cases with early-onset psychosis. Similarly, disability in everyday functions is present and is correlated with impairments in performance on measures of the ability to perform everyday functional and social skills. This constellation of impairments leads to wide-ranging social and functional deficits. Treatments offered for adult-onset cases should be offered to early-onset cases as well.

Management and Interventions for Psychosis in Youth

An increasing number of antipsychotic medications have demonstrated efficacy in randomized placebo-controlled trials in the treatment of children and adolescents with schizophrenia. This review summarizes and synthesizes relevant antipsychotic medication studies, with particular emphasis on second-generation agents, and discusses other clinical considerations that may influence medication selection. With the exception of clozapine demonstrating superior efficacy in the improvement of psychotic symptoms in treatment-resistant patients, many antipsychotic agents have been shown to be similarly efficacious, including first-generation medications. Consideration of the side-effect profile, which can differ substantially from medication to medication, is essential when choosing treatment options.

Coordinated specialty care (CSC) first-episode models are an evidence-based practice in the treatment of first-episode psychosis. Group, individual, and family therapies in CSC aim to help the client and family understand and cope with the experience of psychosis, promote symptomatic and functional recovery and improve quality of life, and support the pursuit of personally meaningful goals of the client. Common elements to these interventions include building a therapeutic alliance, recovery orientation, education, and skills training, which can be directed to a range of targets, including problem-solving, communication, social skills, and social cognition.

Recovery-oriented treatment for youth with psychosis goes beyond a symptom and deficit-amelioration model, promoting engagement and functioning within the community. Given the challenges young people with psychosis face, early psychosis treatment programs often integrate rehabilitative components targeting functional outcomes. The current article reviews 4 community rehabilitation programs in early psychosis: care coordination, cognitive rehabilitation, supported education and employment, and peer support. For each of these rehabilitative intervention programs, we discuss challenges faced by youth with psychosis, clinical intervention practices, the current state of evidence, and clinical and/or research considerations.

A major recovery milestone for youth affected by psychosis is reintegration back into a school setting, an important, attainable, treatment goal. The emergence of psychosis often results in either an onset or exacerbation of prior neurocognitive and learning challenges for affected students. Gold standard practice in clinical care for psychosis comprises comprehensive supportive educational services explicitly focused on successful academic reintegration and achievement. This article discusses how providers can guide school teams and their institutions to identify psychosis in their student populations along with a delineation of key educational programming that helps youth reintegrate back into school and achieve academic success.

CHILD AND ADOLESCENT PSYCHIATRIC CLINICS

FORTHCOMING ISSUES

April 2020
Autism Spectrum Disorder Across the Lifespan: Part I
Thomas Flis, Scott R. Pekrul, Robert Schloesser, and Robert W. Wisner-Carlson, *Editors*

July 2020
Autism Spectrum Disorder Across the Lifespan: Part II
Thomas Flis, Scott R. Pekrul, Robert Schloesser, and Robert W. Wisner-Carlson, *Editors*

October 2020
Measurement-Based Care in Child and Adolescent Psychiatry
Jessica Jeffrey, Eugene Grudnikoff, Barry Sarvet, and Rajeev Krishna, *Editors*

RECENT ISSUES

October 2019
Eating Disorders in Child and Adolescent Psychiatry
James Lock and Jennifer Derenne, *Editors*

July 2019
Depression in Special Populations
Warren Y.K. Ng and Karen Dineen Wagner, *Editors*

April 2019
The Science of Well-Being: Integration into Clinical Child Psychiatry
David Rettew, Matthew Biel, and Jeff Bostic, *Editors*

ISSUE OF RELATED INTEREST

Psychiatric Clinics of North America
https://www.psych.theclinics.com/
Pediatric Clinics of North America
https://www.pediatric.theclinics.com/
Neurologic Clinics
https://www.neurologic.theclinics.com/

AACAP Members: Please go to www.jaacap.org for information on access to the Child and Adolescent Psychiatric Clinics. *Resident* Members of AACAP: Special access information is available at www.childpsych.theclinics.com.

THE CLINICS ARE AVAILABLE ONLINE!
Access your subscription at:
www.theclinics.com

Preface

Psychosis in Children and Adolescents: A Guide for Clinicians

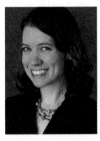 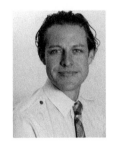

Ellen M. House, MD   John W. Tyson Jr, MD
Editors

Children and adolescents presenting with psychosis create challenging diagnostic and treatment dilemmas for mental health clinicians. Psychotic experiences (PEs) in youth lie on a continuum from developmentally appropriate, nonpathologic phenomena; to schizophrenia spectrum disorders; to markers of other mental health conditions. Despite the diagnostic complexity of youth with PEs, these are relatively frequent phenomena in children and adolescents, with almost 10% of youth in community samples reporting PEs.[1] Appropriate evaluation and diagnosis are keys to creating an effective, risk-minimizing, and recovery-oriented treatment plan for these children and their families. In this issue of the *Child and Adolescent Psychiatric Clinics of North America*, we hope to provide clinicians with the knowledge and evidenced-based tools necessary to effectively evaluate, diagnose, and treat children who present with PEs.

The issue is divided into 3 sections: (1) evaluation and differential diagnosis, (2) neurobiology, and (3) management and interventions. In the first section, we focus on the evaluation of PEs in children and adolescents, starting with guidance on how to conduct the diagnostic interview, followed by a discussion of the role of the physical examination and a review of the strength of evidence for laboratory testing and neuroimaging in youth with PEs. This is followed by an article detailing medical causes of secondary psychosis in youth. The issue then focuses on the risk assessment for youth with psychosis, a necessary discussion given the stigmatization of youth with psychotic symptoms, one which assumes violent behavior in these individuals despite low incidence rates of violence toward others.

The first section continues with a deeper dive into the various diagnostic considerations for PEs in children and adolescents. Prodrome, childhood-onset schizophrenia, affective disorders, autism spectrum disorders, trauma, and substance-induced

Child Adolesc Psychiatric Clin N Am 29 (2020) xv–xvi
https://doi.org/10.1016/j.chc.2019.09.001
1056-4993/20/© 2019 Published by Elsevier Inc.

psychosis are all covered in detail. Last, given the rapidly changing cultural and legal landscape regarding cannabis use and its impact on youth, we have included an article dedicated specifically to the interplay between cannabis and psychosis.

The second section provides an update for clinicians on the ever-evolving neurobiological research in children and youth with PEs. The issue provides an update on the genetics of childhood-onset schizophrenia, followed by an article detailing the neurocognitive impact of psychosis in youth, with specific commentary on social cognition and functional impact in children with early-onset schizophrenia.

The final section focuses on evidence-based management recommendations. Starting with a review of the psychopharmacologic approaches to youth with psychosis, including the management of antipsychotic side effects, we then progress through reviews of psychotherapies for individuals and their families, community-based rehabilitative programming, and, finally, school-based interventions for children and adolescents with psychosis.

Our great hope for this issue of the *Child and Adolescent Psychiatric Clinics of North America* is that it will provide clinicians with the necessary tools and knowledge to effectively assess and care for these challenging and rewarding children and families. We deeply appreciate all of the authors' contributions in creating such a rich issue focused on the care of this vulnerable population.

Ellen M. House, MD
Augusta University/
University of Georgia Medical Partnership
Health Sciences Campus, Russell Hall
1425 Prince Avenue
Athens, GA 30602, USA

John W. Tyson Jr, MD
First Episode and Early Psychosis Program
Massachusetts General Hospital
32 Fruit Street, Yawkey 6A
Boston, MA 02114, USA

E-mail addresses:
Ellen.house@uga.edu (E.M. House)
Jtyson2@partners.org (J.W. Tyson)

REFERENCE

1. Healy C, Brannigan R, Dooley N, et al. Childhood and adolescent psychotic experiences and risk of mental disorder: a systematic review and meta-analysis. Psychol Med 2019;49(10):1589–99.

Evaluation and Differential Diagnosis of Psychosis in Youth

Assessing Youth with Psychotic Experiences: A Phenomenological Approach

John W. Tyson Jr, MD[a],*, Ellen M. House, MD[b],
Abigail L. Donovan, MD[a]

KEYWORDS

- Psychosis • Schizophrenia • Phenomenology • Diagnosis • Assessment
- Hallucinations • Delusions

KEY POINTS

- Psychotic experiences (PEs) lie on a continuum from developmentally appropriate, non-pathologic phenomena to schizophrenia spectrum disorders, to markers of other mental health conditions.
- PEs can manifest in multiple symptom domains: perceptual, thought, behavioral, affective, cognitive, and motor.
- Acquiring the historical data along a narrative developmental timeline using a systematic, domain-based, phenomenological approach facilitates the creation of an accurate diagnostic formulation and treatment plan.

Few chief complaints induce greater panic in child mental health clinicians than psychosis. The complexity of these presentations and the lack of standardized training and clear diagnostic pathways can make accurate assessments daunting. This article argues that using a systematic, domain-based approach to youth presenting with psychotic symptoms allows a thorough and thoughtful differential formulation and thus the development of an effective, evolvable treatment plan.

The use of the term psychosis can be traced back to German physician Karl Canstatt in 1841.[1] Although this term has evolved considerably, modern clinicians define psychosis broadly as a brain disturbance that impairs a person's ability to discern reality. Psychosis is a state rather than a single illness entity. Psychotic experiences (PEs) lie on a continuum from developmentally appropriate,

Conflicts of Interest: The authors have no financial or commercial conflicts of interest to disclose.
[a] First Episode and Early Psychosis Program, Massachusetts General Hospital, 32 Fruit Street, Yawkey 6A, Boston, MA 02114, USA; [b] Augusta University/University of Georgia Medical Partnership, Health Science Campus, Russell Hall, 1425 Prince Avenue, Athens, GA 30602, USA
* Corresponding author.
E-mail address: Jtyson2@partners.org

nonpathologic phenomena, to schizophrenia spectrum disorders (SSDs), to markers of other mental health conditions. PEs are common in childhood. A recent meta-analysis of almost 30,000 youth from community samples found that 9.8% of participants reported PEs.[2] PEs can manifest in multiple symptom domains: perceptual, thought, behavioral, affective, cognitive, and motor.[3] By evaluating psychosis through these domains and using a phenomenological approach, clinicians are able to gather the relevant historical data necessary to create an informed formulation and treatment plan.

The Diagnostic and Statistical Manual of Mental Disorders (DSM-5) provides a framework for conceptualizing psychotic disorders but fails to capture their phenomenological nuances, especially in children and adolescents.[4] Thus clinicians must avoid being complacent in the assessment. Do not just "check the boxes" to arrive at a diagnosis of schizophrenia and start an antipsychotic, because this may cause unnecessary harm to the child. Clinicians should note that PEs are more prevalent in youth than in adults, many PEs are nonpathologic, and most PEs do not denote an underlying psychotic disorder.[5] Nonpathologic PEs are typically transient,[6] often perceived as positive, nonthreatening and nondistressing,[7] usually experienced as less dangerous and more controllable,[8] and by definition are not associated with functional impairment. However, the presence of PEs in childhood, even among non–help-seeking, community samples, is associated with a 3-fold risk of any mental health disorder and 4-fold risk of a psychotic disorder.[2] Thus, clinicians must fully comprehend the child's experience, and how the symptoms fit into the child's developmental trajectory, to determine whether the symptoms represent mental disorder and, if so, what disorder.

The history is critical. The goal is to craft a cohesive narrative of the child's life. PEs must be understood in the context of the child's development, family and social circumstances, culture, and cognition. Start the narrative timeline at the first signs of any behavioral, emotional, or cognitive difficulties. Primary psychotic disorders, such as schizophrenia, are neurodevelopmental processes, and thus have premorbid manifestations. Tracking the trajectory of such early manifestations allows clinicians to follow the evolution of symptoms, which is essential to understanding the phenomenology. Interview the child separately and gather information from all relevant caregivers. Additional collateral is often necessary, including information from teachers, pediatricians, friends, coaches, or others. Genetic family history; prenatal/natal/postnatal history; medical history; substance use history; and early development, including physical, emotional, and social milestone acquisition, are all essential. Review current and prior functioning in academic, social, and familial domains. Children with PE, whether or not they meet criteria for a psychiatric disorder, are more likely than their peers to experience known schizophrenia risk factors, including birth seasonality, lower birth weight, theory of mind deficits, lower intelligence quotient, trauma, family dysfunction, and urbanicity,[9,10] and an in-depth history should cover these domains.

For example, a 15-year-old boy presents to the office with a chief complaint of hearing voices for 2 months. Although the clinician will eventually delve deeper into his experience of hearing voices, exploring the early history reveals that the boy had behavioral issues beginning in kindergarten, displayed early attentional deficits, developed obsessive-compulsive symptoms in elementary school, and later developed depression and a decline in social and cognitive functioning in high school. Following this timeline allows the clinician to understand the trajectory of illness, putting it into a more salient developmental context. If the interview starts when the voices begin, the rich narrative details and clues to the neurodevelopmental progression of disease, essential in diagnosing schizophrenia, are lost. This article explores how to assess the domains of psychosis and use the information to craft a formulation and treatment plan for youth.

PERCEPTUAL DISTURBANCES

Perceptual disturbances in a child may represent normal development, an SSD, or another primary mental health disorder[11] and thus require nuanced interpretation. Start with open-ended questioning to avoid leading the child, then proceed to more direct, detail-oriented questions for each sensory domain: hearing, vision, smell, taste, and touch. Ask about the full range of anomalous perceptual experiences, illusions, and hallucinations, as well as associated symptoms (**Box 1**).

Perceptual disturbances often prompt clinicians to question the presence of an underlying psychotic disorder. However, like other PEs, perceptual disturbances in children lie on a continuum from healthy to pathologic states. Hallucinations can occur as early as age 5 years,[12] are frequently reported in nonclinical samples,[2,13,14] and are often transient.[15-17] Prevalence rates of perceptual disturbances are higher in children and adolescents than in adults (12.7% and 12.4% respectively, compared with 5.8% in adults),[15] giving credence to the notion that PEs are more common in childhood, are often self-limiting, and can even be part of typical development.[15,18] However, even if nonpathologic, perceptual disturbances are often distressing[19] and are associated with poorer global functioning into adulthood.[20]

Pathologic perceptual disturbances are present in many mental health conditions in youth, including disorders of mood, anxiety, trauma, personality, neurodevelopment, substance use, and conduct. Their presence in childhood indicates a generally increased risk of diverse mental disorders later in life.[21,22] In community samples, most adolescents who report hallucinations meet criteria for at least 1 (nonpsychotic) DSM-IV disorder[23] and become more closely associated with mental disorder the older the age of presentation.[24] Auditory hallucinations can be correlated with an increased risk for depression,[21] suicidal ideation and suicide attempts,[25] disruptive behavior disorders,[26] a 5-fold to 16-fold increased risk of an SSD,[27] and a variety of

---

Box 1
Assessing perceptual disturbances

Have you ever heard/seen/felt/smelled/tasted things no one else could?

Can you tell me about them?

How do you experience them? How vivid are they?

Do they sound like my voice talking to you? Or something else?

How often are these experiences happening? For how long do they last?

Where do they happen? Do they occur at a specific time of day?

Where do you think the experiences are coming from?

How do you explain why this is happening?

Does it seem real to you?

Does anything make them better or worse? Can you control them?

Do your emotions influence them? Are they better or worse when you are angry, happy, sad?

Do they bother you?

Do they ever instruct you to do things? Do you listen to them? Why (not)?

other psychiatric and medical disorders. Children experiencing perceptual abnormalities are a diagnostically heterogeneous group and those driven to seek treatment are likely to experience functional decline and emotional distress.[12]

THOUGHT DISTURBANCES

Thought disturbances are another common presenting symptom. These disturbances can consist of abnormalities of content, such as delusions, or of form, such as disorganized speech. Delusions are beliefs that are fixed, not culturally normative, and inflexible to change despite conflicting evidence, and can present in a variety of themes, such as persecutory, referential, influence, somatic, religious, and grandiose. The assessment of thought content should start with open-ended curiosity about the child's ideas. Wonder with the youth about the origin of these beliefs, when they started, and how they came to be. Consider whether these beliefs could be rational and appropriate, recognizing that many children live in situations that are, in reality, unstable or dangerous. When assessing for self-referential content, it may help to give a relevant example from current social media, music, or television; distinguishing personal reference from identification with a theme (ie, a person being able to relate to a song's lyrics vs the lyrics actually being written about that person). The assessment for aberrant thought content should start broadly and screen for additional content beyond what is readily offered (**Box 2**).

Box 2
Assessing thought disturbances

Have you had any thoughts that have been bothering you, or seem new or different for you?

Can you describe them to me?

Have your thoughts seemed faster, slower, or harder to follow?

How do you experience the thoughts? Where do they come from?

Do they seem like your own thoughts, or is something else influencing them?

Do you ever feel like thoughts are being put into your head or taken out?

Do you ever feel like your mind or body is not under your control?

Do you ever feel like others around you can know exactly what you are thinking, like your thoughts can be heard out loud?

Do you ever worry you are being watched or followed? By whom? Why would this happen?

Do you worry about something serious happening in your body?

Do things around you seem to be happening for a special reason?

Are you getting special messages only you can understand?

Do you ever feel you have special talents? Or that God has a special role for you?

How do you explain why these thoughts are happening? Do they seem real to you?

How often are these experiences happening? For how long do they last?

Do they occur at a specific time of day?

Do your emotions influence them?

Does anything make them better or worse? Can you control them?

Do they bother you?

Delusions are a core symptom of psychotic disorders. They can occur in children, but are generally less frequent than in adults, are typically vague in early and middle childhood, and often accompany hallucinations.[11] Delusions of persecution (eg, "The government is monitoring me") are the most common type of delusion in youth with a first episode of psychosis, but delusions of influence (eg, "My teacher can control my thoughts") correlate with severity of hallucinations and negative symptom burden.[28] Of note, adolescents with religious delusions are also likely to have longer durations of untreated psychosis compared with adolescents with other delusions.[29]

Delusions are not specific to SSDs and occur across the spectrum of mental health diagnoses in children. Persecutory delusions can be associated with depression[30] and are more likely to be mood congruent. Youth with cannabis-related or stimulant-related psychosis have more delusions of influence, guilt, sin, or jealousy compared with youth with primary psychoses.[28] Children with autism spectrum disorders (ASDs) also experience delusions. Youth with high-functioning pervasive developmental disorders have a higher likelihood of delusions than their matched peers (62.2% vs 25.5%) and these are associated with higher rates of anxiety and depression.[31]

Disorder of the flow or form of thought (formal thought disorder), most commonly observed through speech abnormalities, is a cardinal feature of schizophrenia and must be evaluated on mental status examination. Note any pauses, perseveration, poverty of thought, tangentiality, circumstantiality, neologisms, and derailment. Feedback from family about ineffective communication, vagueness, and illogicality is important, particularly in determining onset and progression.

Abnormalities of thought process are common in childhood-onset schizophrenia and are also predictive of subsequent psychosis in clinically high-risk adolescents.[32] However, disorganization of speech and thought is not pathognomonic for a SSD. Youth with ASD also experience increased rates of speech and thought abnormalities[33] and can show formal thought disorders, including poverty of thought, illogicality, loosening of association, and derailment at rates higher than their typically developing peers.[33,34] In ASD, thought disorder symptoms are often time limited, with rapid onset and resolution,[35] and correlate with stress or anxiety.[34] Thus, careful assessment of how these symptoms occur within the overall developmental history is essential to clarify the presence of an SSD.

BEHAVIORAL DISTURBANCES

Disorganized behavior may manifest as an inability to sustain goal-directed behavior (such as self-care), or bizarre, nonpurposeful, nonsensical, or unpredictable acts. Clinicians must first attempt to understand the child's thought process and content before attempting to understand the behavior. For instance, a behavior may be clearly nonsensical, bizarre, or unpredictable in its origin; or it may be a logical reaction to illogical thinking. For instance, a teenager who begins to cover up her windows in response to a belief that she is being surveilled would be an example of logical behavior stemming from illogical persecutory thinking and would be classified as disorganized to the outside observer. Behavioral disorganization can be observed during the mental status examination or inferred from information provided by collateral contacts. Again, the timeline and developmental trajectory of the behavior (whether it represents a change or is part of a long-standing pattern) and, whether it is correlated with other PEs is critical. Children with developmental disorders, including ASD, may show disorganized behavior in the form repetitive actions or responses to idiosyncratic thinking. Youth with obsessive-compulsive disorder (OCD) may perform compulsive rituals that can appear disorganized to the outside observer. Patients with catatonia (secondary to a variety of psychiatric or nonpsychiatric causes) may show nonpurposeful behaviors, and multiple items on the widely used Bush-Francis Catatonia Rating Scale could be classified as disorganized (combativeness, excitement, impulsivity) but also overlap heavily with the motor domain of psychosis.[36]

AFFECTIVE SYMPTOMS

Anxiety and mood disorders are common in children, with more than 8% of children between the ages of 6 and 17 years carrying a diagnosis, and rates have been increasing over time.[37] Affective and anxiety symptoms and PEs co-occur, and there is a bidirectionality of experience: psychotic disorders can present initially with mood or anxiety symptoms; mood and anxiety disorders can cause PEs; and youth that go on to develop psychotic disorders can have comorbid, distinct anxiety, and mood diagnoses.

PEs can occur in major depressive disorder, bipolar disorder, trauma disorders, OCD, severe anxiety disorders, as well as personality disorders. The presence of psychotic symptoms in youth with diagnoses of mood or anxiety disorders is associated with worse long-term outcomes compared with those without PE.[38] Most youth at clinical high risk for the development of a psychotic disorder experience anxiety and/or depression,[39,40] and often report that anxiety symptoms are more distressing than subthreshold PEs.[41]

Clinical assessment should include screening for any mood abnormalities, including symptoms of depression, mania/hypomania, and anxiety. Developing a deep understanding of the timeline and relationship between symptoms is essential, as well as obtaining reliable collateral information to provide context for a child's presentation. Assess whether the PEs are solely in the context of mood symptoms or whether they exist outside of mood episodes. Screen for past trauma leading to hypervigilance that could be perceived as paranoia, and dissociation or flashbacks that can be confused with PEs. Ask the youth and family whether there are any recurrent thoughts, rituals, or compulsions. The disorganized behavior or delusions might be rituals or obsessions from OCD. If paranoid thinking only occurs in the context of significant emotional dysregulation, screen for other symptoms of borderline personality disorder.

In addition to a comprehensive history, a thorough mental status examination is essential, exploring both mood and affect, the internal experience and the outward manifestation of emotional states. Parents are often essential in recognizing mood and anxiety symptoms in young children; however, parents of teenagers can miss and under-report mood symptoms[42]; make sure to ask parents and children separately about the presence of mood or anxiety symptoms. Ask children or adolescents how they have been feeling over the past weeks to months and watch for concordance with affect. Use the history to determine whether the observed flat affect is caused by depression, lack of eye-to-eye gaze and emotional reciprocity from an ASD, or diminished emotional expression and avolition caused by negative symptoms of schizophrenia. Observe for signs of mania such as psychomotor agitation, pressured speech, euphoria, flight of ideas, and distractibility. Comorbidity is common in psychiatric illnesses, and although anxiety, mood, and psychotic disorders co-occur, a deep understanding of symptom interplay and the developmental timeline, as well as what is most distressing to the child, is essential in determining a differential diagnosis and treatment plan.

COGNITIVE DYSFUNCTION

Cognitive dysfunction is increasingly recognized as a core feature of SSDs,[43] and the presence of cognitive impairments is correlated with poor long-term functional outcomes.[44–46] Epidemiologic studies have consistently shown that cognitive impairments precede the development of frank psychotic symptoms in youth who subsequently develop psychotic disorders.[47,48]

Cognitive deficits in schizophrenia are heterogeneous, ranging from discrete to global, but cognitive functioning can be up to 2 standard deviations less than age-matched healthy controls.[48,49] The affected areas of cognition can include attention, executive function, memory, processing speed, and social cognition.[50] In multiple models predicting conversion to a psychotic disorder, disorganized communication, poor social functioning, and poor verbal memory were predictive factors in illness development and functional outcome,[46,51–53] making these essential areas to explore in an assessment (**Box 3**).

Cognitive deficits can be present in many other disorders as well (such as attention-deficit/hyperactivity disorder [ADHD], depression, anxiety disorders, substance use), but with different characteristics, associated symptoms, timing of onset, and chronicity. Cognitive decline occurring in adolescence, after grossly normal functioning, with subsequent chronic cognitive impairment, is unique to SSD, and thus important for differential diagnosis.[54] A careful history, with attention to the development and timeline of symptoms, can aid in differential diagnosis. For instance, an adolescent presenting with so-called attention problems is generally more likely to have ADHD than schizophrenia, but an underlying psychotic disorder may rise on the differential if cognitive symptoms were not present earlier in childhood or if other PEs are reported.

MOTOR SYMPTOMS

Motor symptoms are commonly observed and assessed in the context of neuroleptic treatment, but motor abnormalities can exist in antipsychotic-naive individuals with schizophrenia, including youth. Phenomenologically, abnormal motor functioning can be described in terms of increased activity (restlessness, excitement, tremors,

---

Box 3
Assessing cognitive dysfunction

Have your child's recent grades been consistent, or has there been a decline?

Have you noticed a change in the child's cognitive abilities (such as memory, reading, or information processing)?

Have your child's social abilities changed? Has the child struggled recently to make and keep friends? Or has this always been the case?

Is this the same child you have always known, or has something fundamental changed?

Have elementary school teachers or coaches noted issues with attention, focus, and distractibility in the past, or are these new concerns?

Does your child seem to think more slowly, struggle to communicate thoughts, or take longer to answer?

Has your child had trouble remembering things more than before?

Has your child struggled to learn specific subjects or with learning in general? Has this always been the case or is it a recent change?

agitation, motor impulsiveness, tics, choreiform movements, and so forth) or decreased activity (psychomotor retardation, poverty of movement, stupor, motor blocking, last-minute responses, and ambitendency).[55] Motor symptoms are routinely broken down in the schizophrenia literature into 3 categories: neurologic soft signs (eg, motor coordination, sensory integration, balance, and sequencing of complex motor acts), abnormal involuntary movements (eg, dyskinesia, repetitive and involuntary choreiform movements, akathisia, hyperkinesia, dystonia, and spontaneous parkinsonism), and catatonic signs (eg, stupor, mutism, waxy flexibility, rigidity, posturing, mannerism, negativism, and stereotypy).[55]

Motor symptoms can provide information about underlying brain dysfunction, including evidence of specific affective and motor neural network aberrations visible on neuroimaging.[55] Furthermore, the presence of abnormal motor symptoms such as neurologic soft signs and extrapyramidal signs can correlate with cognitive impairment.[56] Catatonic signs and dyskinesia in drug-naive states are significantly associated with poorer long-term psychosocial functioning in patients with first-episode psychosis.[57] Moreover, higher levels of parkinsonism, akathisia, neurologic soft signs, and catatonic symptoms 6 months after a first psychotic episode have significant associations with poor long-term psychosocial functioning.[57]

It is important to assess for abnormal motor signs on mental status examination and to evaluate further via physical and neurologic examination if indicated. Caregivers should be asked about their observations, because many children do not readily report these symptoms or are not aware of their presence. In addition, motor symptoms are not unique to schizophrenia. Stereotyped or repetitive motor movements are symptoms of ASD, psychomotor slowing can be observed in depression, and psychomotor agitation can be seen in mania. The timeline, onset, and associated symptoms can help distinguish these entities.

FORMULATION AND DIFFERENTIAL DIAGNOSIS

Once the clinician has gathered the relevant history and the developmental timeline of a child's symptomatic evolution, this information should be coherently synthesized into a diagnostic formulation. Even in child and adolescent mental health, in which co-morbidity is often the rule rather than the exception, diagnostic parsimony should be attempted. At times, determining a diagnosis is straightforward, but, often, information is lacking, significant discrepancies in the history exist, or the symptoms are consistent with several diagnoses, and a clear conclusion cannot be reached. Formulation and diagnoses can, and should be, revised over time, as the youth develops and matures, and symptoms either continue, resolve, or emerge, with the simple passage of time often leading to diagnostic clarity (**Box 4**).

TREATMENT PLANNING

Once a clinician has determined the causal nature of a child's symptoms, or a leading hypothesis has been developed, a comprehensive treatment plan should be created. Elements can include psychoeducation (for the patient and family), additional medical evaluations or testing, psychotherapy (individual, group, family), school/employment accommodations, rehabilitative interventions, and psychopharmacology.

First, clinicians should summarize their findings with the patient and caregivers to provide a conceptualization of the child's symptoms and explain how a diagnostic determination has been made. Second, patients and caregivers should be given accurate and culturally sensitive psychoeducation regarding the symptoms and/or diagnosis. In cases in which a child's psychotic symptoms are determined to be benign

Box 4
Differential diagnostic considerations for youth with psychotic phenomena
SSD: schizophrenia, schizophreniform, schizoaffective, brief psychotic disorder
Major depressive disorder with psychotic features
Bipolar I disorder with psychotic features (depressed, mixed, or manic)
Substance-induced psychotic disorder
OCD
Posttraumatic stress disorder/trauma-related disorder
Anxiety disorder
Autism spectrum disorder
Disruptive behavior disorder
Personality disorder
Adjustment disorder
Bereavement disorder
Other developmental, intellectual, or genetic disorder
Medical illness
Benign, developmentally normative symptom presentations

or a normative developmental phenomenon, providing an explanatory model for understanding the symptoms is valuable, as well as offering reassurance and next steps for further monitoring.[18] In situations in which a child's symptoms are determined to be part of an active or developing mental health condition, treatment recommendations should follow accepted guidelines for that specific condition. PEs, per se, are not an indication for the use of antipsychotic medication; rather, antipsychotic medication should be used judiciously, in accordance with research evidence and accepted protocols for the specific diagnosis. For youth with a first episode of psychosis (primary or affective), a referral to a coordinated specialty care program should be strongly considered, given evidence of superior outcomes compared with traditional community care.[58] In these cases, antipsychotic medication should be started promptly to reduce the duration of untreated psychosis and improve long-term outcomes.[59] In addition, it is critical to monitor the evolution of the child's symptoms over time to help refine or alter the diagnostic formulation and resultant treatment plan if needed.[60]

SUMMARY

PEs may be part of normal development or indicate a wide range of mental disorder. Using a systematic, domain-based, phenomenological approach to assessing psychotic symptoms in youth facilitates the gathering of the nuanced clinical information necessary to understand a child's specific experience. Mapping this information onto a narrative timeline, while understanding the evolution and developmental context of PEs, is essential in making an accurate diagnostic formulation and appropriate treatment plan for youth presenting with PEs.

REFERENCES

1. Burgy M. The concept of psychosis: historical and phenomenological aspects. Schizophr Bull 2008;34(6):1200–10.

2. Healy C, Brannigan R, Dooley N, et al. Childhood and adolescent psychotic experiences and risk of mental disorder: a systematic review and meta-analysis. Psychol Med 2019;49(10):1589–99.
3. Freudenreich O. Schizophrenia? Target 6 symptom clusters. Curr Psych 2009;(6):74.
4. American Psychiatric Association. Diagnostic and statistical manual of mental disorders. 5th edition. Washington, DC: American Psychiatric Press; 2013.
5. Stevens JR, Prince JB, Prager LM, et al. Psychotic disorders in children and adolescents: a primer on contemporary evaluation and management. Prim Care Companion CNS Disord 2014;16(2) [pii:PCC.13f01514].
6. van Os J, Linscott RJ, Myin-Germeys I, et al. A systematic review and meta-analysis of the psychosis continuum: evidence for a psychosis proneness-persistence-impairment model of psychotic disorder. Psychol Med 2009;39: 179–95.
7. Stip E, Letourneau G. Psychotic symptoms as a continuum between normality and pathology. Can J Psychiatry 2009;54(3):140–51.
8. Peters E, Ward T, Jackson M, et al. Clinical relevance of appraisals of persistent psychotic experiences in people with and without need for care: an experimental study. Lancet 2017;4(12):927–36.
9. Polanczyk G, Moffitt T, Arseneault L, et al. Etiological and clinical features of childhood psychotic symptoms: results from a birth cohort. Arch Gen Psychiatry 2010; 67(4):328–38.
10. Tochigi M, Nishida A, Shimodera S, et al. Season of birth effect on psychotic-like experiences in Japanese adolescents. Eur Child Adolesc Psychiatry 2013;22(2): 89–93.
11. Sikich L. Diagnosis and evaluation of hallucinations and other psychotic symptoms in children and adolescents. Child Adolesc Psychiatr Clin N Am 2013; 22(4):655–73.
12. Maijer K, Palmen S, Sommer I. Children seeking help for auditory verbal hallucinations; who are they? Schizophr Res 2017;183:31–5.
13. Laurens K, Hobbs M, Sunderland M, et al. Psychotic-like experiences in a community sample of 80000 children aged 9 to 11 years: an item response theory analysis. Psychol Med 2012;42(7):133–49.
14. Kelleher I, Connor D, Clarke M, et al. Prevalence of psychotic symptoms in childhood and adolescence: a systematic review and meta-analysis of population based studies. Psychol Med 2012;42:1857–63.
15. Maijer K, Begemann M, Palmen S, et al. Auditory hallucinations across the lifespan: a systematic review and meta-analysis. Psychol Med 2017;48:879–88.
16. Bartels-Velthuis A, van de Willige G, van Os J, et al. Course of auditory vocal hallucinations in childhood: 5 year follow-up study. Br J Psychiatry 2011;299(4): 296–302.
17. Bartels-Velthuis A, Wigman J, Jenner J, et al. Course of auditory vocal hallucinations in childhood: 11-year follow up study. Acta Psychiatr Scand 2016; 134(1):6–15.
18. Maijer K, Hayward M, Fernyhough C, et al. Hallucinations in children and adolescents: an updated review and practical recommendations for clinicians. Schizophr Bull 2019;45(Supplement_1):S5–23.
19. Bartels-Velthuis A, Jenner J, van de Willige G, et al. Prevalence and correlates of auditory vocal hallucinations in middle childhood. Br J Psychiatry 2010; 196(1):41–6.

20. Healy C, Campbell D, Coughlan H, et al. Childhood psychotic experiences are associated with poorer global functioning throughout adolescence and into early adulthood. Acta Psychiatr Scand 2018;138:26–34.
21. Dhossche D, Ferdinand R, Van der Ende J, et al. Diagnostic outcome of self-reported hallucinations in a community sample of adolescents. Psychol Med 2002;32(4):619–27.
22. Fisher H, Caspi A, Poulton R, et al. Specificity of childhood psychotic symptoms for predicting schizophrenia by 38 years of age: a birth cohort study. Psychol Med 2013;43(10):2077–86.
23. Kelleher I, Keeley H, Corcoran P, et al. Clinicopathological significance of psychotic experiences in non-psychotic young people: evidence from four population based studies. Br J Psychiatry 2012;201(1):1495–506.
24. Schimmelmann B, Michael C, Martz-Irngartinger A, et al. Age matters in the prevalence and clinical significance of ultra-high-risk for psychosis symptoms and criteria in the general population: findings from the BEAR and BEARS-kid studies. World Psychiatry 2015;14:189–97.
25. Fujita J, Takahashi Y, Nishida A, et al. Auditory verbal hallucinations increase the risk for suicide attempts in adolescents with suicidal ideation. Schizophr Res 2015;168:209–12.
26. Edelsohn GA, Rabinovich H, Portney R. Hallucinations in non-psychotic children: findings from a psychiatric emergency service. Ann N Y Acad Sci 2003;1008:261–4.
27. Poulton R, Caspi A, Moffit T, et al. Children's self reported psychotic symptoms and adult schizophreniform disorder. A 15 year longitudinal study. Arch Gen Psychiatry 2000;57:1053–8.
28. Paolini E, Moretti P, Compton M. Delusions in first-episode psychosis: principal component analysis of twelve types of delusions and demographic and clinical correlates of resulting domains. Psychiatry Res 2016;243:5–13.
29. Kaleda V, Popovich U, Romanenko N, et al. Endogenous episodes of juvenile psychosis with religious delusions. Zh Nevrol Psikhiatr Im S S Korsakova 2017;117(12):13–20.
30. Hartley S, Barrowclough C, Haddock G. Anxiety and depression in psychosis: a systematic review of associations with positive psychotic symptoms. Acta Psychiatr Scand 2013;128:327–46.
31. Goto A, Miyawaki D, Kusaka H, et al. High prevalence of non-psychotic delusions in children with high-functioning pervasive developmental disorder. Osaka City Med J 2015;61(2):73–80.
32. Bearden CE, Wu KN, Caplan R, et al. Thought disorder and communication deviance as predictors of outcome in youth at clinical high risk for psychosis. J Am Acad Child Adolesc Psychiatry 2011;50(7):669–80.
33. Ziermans T, Swaab H, Stockmann A, et al. Formal thought disorder and executive functioning in children and adolescents with autism spectrum disorder: old leads and new avenues. J Autism Dev Disord 2017;47(6):1756–68.
34. Solomon M, Ozonoff S, Carter C, et al. Formal thought disorder and the autism spectrum: relationship with symptoms, executive control, and anxiety. J Autism Dev Disord 2008;38(8):1474–84.
35. Tantam D, Girgis S. Recognition and treatment of Asperger syndrome in the community. Br Med Bull 2009;89:41–62.
36. Bush G, Fink M, Petrides G, et al. Catatonia. I. Rating scale and standardized examination. Acta Psychiatr Scand 1996;93(2):129–36.

37. Bitsko RH, Holbrook JR, Ghandour RM, et al. Epidemiology and impact of health-care provider diagnosed anxiety and depression among US children. J Dev Behav Pediatr 2018;39(5):395–403.

38. Wigman JT, van Nierop M, Vollebergh WA, et al. Evidence that psychotic symptoms are prevalent in disorders of anxiety and depression, impacting on illness onset, risk, and severity–implications for diagnosis and ultra-high risk research. Schizophr Bull 2012;38(2):247–57.

39. McAusland L, Buchy L, Cadenhead KS, et al. Anxiety in youth at clinical risk for psychosis. Early Interv Psychiatry 2017;11(6):480–7.

40. Woods SW, Addington J, Cadenhead KS, et al. Validity of the prodromal risk syndrome for first psychosis: findings from the North American Prodrome Longitudinal Study. Schizophr Bull 2009;35(5):894–908.

41. Fusar-Poli P, Nelson B, Valmaggia L, et al. Comorbid depressive and anxiety disorders in 509 individuals with an at-risk mental state: impact on psychopathology and transition to psychosis. Schizophr Bull 2014;40(1):120–31.

42. Eg J, Bilenberg N, Costello E, et al. Self-and parent-reported depressive symptoms rated by the mood and feelings questionnaire. Psychiatry Res 2018;268: 419–25.

43. Keefe RSE, Harvey PD. Cognitive impairment in schizophrenia. Handb Exp Pharmacol 2012;213:11–37.

44. Heinrichs RW, Zakzanis KK. Neurocognitive deficit in schizophrenia: a quantitative review of the evidence. Neuropsychology 1998;12:426–45.

45. Fett AJ, Viechtbauer W, Dominguez M, et al. The relationship between neurocognition and social cognition with functional outcomes in schizophrenia: a meta-analysis. Neurosci Biobehav Rev 2011;35:573–88.

46. Bolt LK, Amminger GP, Farhall J, et al. Neurocognition as a predictor of transition to psychotic disorder and functional outcomes in ultra-high risk participants: findings from the NEURAPRO randomized clinical trial. Schizophr Res 2019;206: 67–74.

47. Woodberry KA, Giuliano AJ, Seidman LJ. Premorbid IQ in schizophrenia: a meta-analytic review. Am J Psychiatry 2008;165(5):579.

48. Mesholam-Gately RI, Giuliano AJ, Goff KP, et al. Neurocognition in first-episode schizophrenia: a meta-analytic review. Neuropsychology 2009;23:315–36.

49. Brewer WJ, Wood SJ, Phillips LJ, et al. Generalized and specific cognitive performance in clinical high-risk cohorts: a review highlighting potential vulnerability markers for psychosis. Schizophr Bull 2006;32(3):538–55.

50. Nuechterlein KH, Barch DM, Gold JM, et al. Identification of separable cognitive factors in schizophrenia. Schizophr Res 2004;72(1):29–39.

51. Addington J, Farris M, Stowkowy J, et al. Predictors of transition to psychosis in individuals at clinical high risk. Curr Psychiatry Rep 2019;21(6):39.

52. Addington J, Liu L, Perkins DO, et al. The role of cognition and social functioning as predictors in the transition to psychosis for youth with attenuated psychotic symptoms. Schizophr Bull 2017;43(1):57–63.

53. Cornblatt BA, Carrion RE, Auther A, et al. Psychosis prevention: a modified clinical high risk perspective from the Recognition and Prevention (RAP) Program. Am J Psychiatry 2015;172:986–94.

54. Meier MH, Caspi A, Reichenberg A, et al. Neuropsychological decline in schizophrenia from the premorbid to the postonset period: evidence from a population-representative longitudinal study. Am J Psychiatry 2014;171:91–101.

55. Hirjak D, Kubera K, Thomann P, et al. Motor dysfunction as an intermediate phenotype across schizophrenia and other psychotic disorders: progress and perspectives. Schizophr Res 2018;200:104–11.
56. Cuesta M, Moreno-Izco L, Ribeiro M, et al. Motor abnormalities and cognitive impairment in first-episode psychosis patients, their unaffected siblings and healthy controls. Schizophr Res 2018;200:50–5.
57. Cuesta M, Garcia de Jalon E, Sol Campos M, et al. Motor abnormalities in first-episode psychosis patients and long-term psychosocial functioning. Schizophr Res 2018;200:97–103.
58. Kane JM, Robinson DG, Schooler NR, et al. Comprehensive versus usual community care for first-episode psychosis: 2-year outcomes from the NIMH RAISE early treatment program. Am J Psychiatry 2016;173:362–72.
59. Thomson A, Griffiths H, Fisher R, et al. Treatment outcomes and associations in an adolescent-specific early intervention for psychosis service. Early Interv Psychiatry 2019;13(3):707–14.
60. Bromet EJ, Kotov L, Fochtmann LJ, et al. Diagnostic shifts during the decade following first admission for psychosis. Am J Psychiatry 2012;168:1186–94.

First Episode Psychosis Medical Workup

Evidence-Informed Recommendations and Introduction to a Clinically Guided Approach

Maja Skikic, MD[a],*, Jose Alberto Arriola, MD, MPH[b]

KEYWORDS

- First episode psychosis • Secondary psychosis • Psychosis workup
- Medical etiologies • Psychosis laboratories

KEY POINTS

- First episode psychosis has several causes, including primary psychiatric disorders as well as nonpsychiatric medical conditions that cause secondary psychosis.
- Evaluating the patient with first episode psychosis requires a careful assessment that includes a thorough history, examination, and workup. This begins with a thoughtful consideration of the differential diagnoses and is followed and supported by laboratory, encephalographic, and imaging studies where appropriate.
- Without a clear guide, determining which additional tests to order can quickly become daunting and may result in underdiagnosis of secondary causes of psychosis.
- Testing for all secondary causes of psychosis is not practical, cost-effective, or recommended in common practice.

INTRODUCTION

Evaluating the patient with first episode psychosis (FEP) requires a careful assessment that includes a thorough history, examination, and workup. This begins with a thoughtful consideration of the differential diagnoses and is followed and supported by laboratory, encephalographic, and imaging studies where appropriate. Because indiscriminate testing of all possible causes of FEP is neither practical nor cost-effective, it is essential that the provider know which clinical findings and elements

Disclosure Statement: The authors have nothing to disclose.
[a] Department of Psychiatry and Behavioral Sciences, Vanderbilt University Medical Center, 1601 23rd Avenue South, Nashville, TN 37212, USA; [b] Department of Psychiatry and Behavioral Sciences, Consult-Liaison Psychiatry, Vanderbilt University Medical Center, 1601 23rd Avenue South, Nashville, TN 37212, USA
* Corresponding author.
E-mail address: maja.skikic@vumc.org

Child Adolesc Psychiatric Clin N Am 29 (2020) 15–28
https://doi.org/10.1016/j.chc.2019.08.010
1056-4993/20/© 2019 Elsevier Inc. All rights reserved.

childpsych.theclinics.com

of the history would warrant additional testing. This document presents some of the diagnostic considerations for a patient presenting with psychosis with an emphasis on the secondary causes and proposes a tiered approach to the workup of FEP that is clinically guided.

In the latter part of the article, a guide is presented providing specific elements of the history, review of symptoms, and examination that aims at supporting pretest probability for further second-tier testing and aids the provider in deciding which additional tests to order. It is worth mentioning that this guide, although broad, does not represent all possible causes of secondary psychosis, and clinical judgment remains chief in informing further evaluation.

DIFFERENTIAL DIAGNOSIS OF FIRST EPISODE PSYCHOSIS
Primary Psychoses and Other Psychiatric Disorders

- Schizophrenia
- Other schizophrenia spectrum disorders: attenuated psychotic disorder, brief psychotic disorder, schizophreniform disorder
- Delusional disorder
- Schizoaffective disorder
- Mood disorders: bipolar disorder, major depressive disorder with psychotic features
- Posttraumatic stress disorder
- Dissociative identity disorder
- Personality disorders: paranoid, schizotypal, schizoid, borderline personality disorders
- Eating disorders: anorexia nervosa
- Delirium/altered mental status

Secondary Psychoses

- *Substance-induced psychosis*: most commonly cannabis, stimulants, hallucinogens, synthetic agents, corticosteroids, anticholinergics, alcohol, and sedative/hypnotics
- *Psychotic disorder due to another medical condition*: see **Boxes 1** and **2**.[1–3]

FIRST EPISODE PSYCHOSIS—WORKUP OF SECONDARY CAUSES
Data Behind Current Practices

Background
Evidence examining the usefulness of a particular workup test in FEP is generally limited to studies of imaging procedures and does not exist for most of the laboratory tests routinely ordered. As such, most recommendations reviewing laboratory workup for FEP remain extrapolations of studies linking psychosis with the medical disorders in question. The studies investigating the strength of this link are often limited to case series and retrospective cohorts, with reviews and meta-analyses available only for a few commonly used tests. In **Table 1**, the investigators sought to summarize some of the data that were found linking psychosis with the medical condition being tested. The authors then assigned recommendations per the Strength of Recommendation Taxonomy[4] guidelines based on the strength and quantity of studies available, also preferentially selecting for patient-oriented outcomes.

Findings
Stronger cohort and review data were identified supporting testing for folate,[5,6] and vitamin D,[7,8] followed by thyroid-stimulating hormone,[9] antinuclear antibody,[10,11]

Box 1
Possible medical illnesses with secondary or co-occurring psychosis

- Central Nervous System

  o Head trauma
  o Congenital/anoxic brain injury
  o Epilepsy
  o Delirium
  o Dementias
  o Prion disease
  o Stroke (ischemic, hemorrhagic)
  o Hydrocephalus
  o Agenesis of corpus callosum
  o Parkinson disease
  o Huntington disease
  o Migraine (familial hemiplegic migraine)
  o Masses (brain tumor, AVM, abscess, cyst, tuberous sclerosis, sarcoidosis)
- Demyelinating Disease

  o Multiple sclerosis
  o Metachromatic leukodystrophy
  o Schilder disease
  o Marchiafava-Bignami disease
- Autoimmune Disorders

  o Systemic lupus erythematosus
  o Rheumatic fever
  o Myasthenia gravis
  o Paraneoplastic syndrome
  o Anti-NMDA encephalitis
  o Acute disseminated encephalomyelitis
- Infections

  o Human immunodeficiency virus
  o Viral encephalitis (HSV, CMV, EBV, measles, rubella, varicella, rabies)
  o Bacterial encephalitis (tuberculosis, Mycoplasma pneumoniae, Brucella)
  o Neurosyphilis
  o Neuroborreliosis (Lyme disease)
  o CNS parasitic infections (toxoplasmosis, malaria, cysticercosis, cryptococcus)

- Endocrinopathies

  o Hypoglycemia
  o Addison disease
  o Pheochromocytoma
  o Cushing disease
  o Hyper- and hypothyroid
  o Hypo- and hyperparathyroid
- Sleep Disorders

  o Narcolepsy
  o Hypnagogic and hypnopompic hallucinations
- Nutritional Deficiencies

  o Mg, Vit A, D, B1, B3, B12
- Substance Use–Related Problems

  o Recreational (hallucinogens, stimulants, cannabis, synthetics, kratom, benzodiazepines, alcohol)
  o Iatrogenic (steroids, antimalarials, isoniazid, anticholinergics)
- Metabolic Disorders

  o Amino acid aberrations (Hartnup, homocystinuria, phenylketonuria)
  o Porphyria
  o Wilson disease
  o GM2 gangliosidosis
  o Fabry disease
  o Niemann-Pick type C disease
  o Gaucher disease (adult type)
- Chromosomal Abnormalities

  o Sex chromosome abnormalities (Kleinfelter syndrome XXY, Turner syndrome XO)
  o Fragile X syndrome
  o Friedreich ataxia
  o VCFS chromosome 22.11q
  o Prader-Willi syndrome
  o Fahr syndrome

Abbreviations: AVM, arteriovenous malformation; CMV, cytomegalovirus; CNS, central nervous system; EBV, Epstein-Barr virus; HSV, herpes simplex virus; NMDA, N-methyl-d-aspartate.

Adapted from Freudenreich O, Brown HE, Holt DJ. Psychosis and Schizophrenia. In: Stern TA, Fava M, Wilens TE, et al, editors. Massachusetts General Hospital Comprehensive Clinical Psychiatry, 2nd edition. London: Elsevier; 2016; with permission.

---

and ceruloplasmin.[12,13] Data were compelling for the testing of HIV due to higher all-cause mortality,[14,15] as well as urinary tract infections due to their role in premature mortality[16] and the etiopathology of relapse.[17] The highest-quality evidence exists from systematic reviews linking drugs of abuse with psychosis onset,[18–23] yielding the strongest recommendation for toxicology screens in FEP workup. Imaging studies also had some of the strongest evidence via systematic reviews,[24,25] with findings and cost implications arguing against routine screening in psychosis alone and supporting

---

Box 2
Possible diagnostic tests to rule-out[a] medical illnesses with cooccurring psychosis

- Clinical/History

  ○ Parkinson, dementias (Lewy-body, frontotemporal, Alzheimer)

- Laboratory:

  ○ Wilson—ceruloplasmin
  ○ SLE – Antitreponemal Ab
  ○ Drug intoxication/withdrawal—UDS
  ○ Pheochromocytoma—metanephrines
  ○ Rheumatic fever—ASO titers
  ○ Myasthenia gravis—anti-AChR Ab
  ○ Paraneoplastic—panel, anti-NMDA Ab
  ○ Neurosyphilis—antitreponemal IgG
  ○ Neuroborreliosis (Lyme) —serum titer
  ○ HIV—HIV ELISA/PCR
  ○ Sarcoidosis—amyloid, ACE, chest X ray
  ○ Endocrinopathies (hypoglycemia, Addison, Cushing, hyper- and hypothyroid, hypo-/hyperparathyroidism, hypopituitarism)—TFTs, Glu, BMP, PTH, Na, K, Ca, AM cortisol
  ○ Homocystinuria—homocysteine, methionine
  ○ Porphyrias—porphyrins
  ○ Nutritional deficiencies—Mg, Vit A, D, B1, B3, B12

- Lumbar Puncture:

  ○ Prion disease, MS, viral encephalitis (HSV, measles, CMV, rubella, EBV, varicella)—CSF CBC, gluc, cultures, 14-3-3 proteins, oligoclonal bands

- EEG

  ○ Epilepsy/seizures

- MRI

  ○ Head trauma, dementias, prion disease, stroke, hydrocephalus, demyelinating diseases (multiple sclerosis, metachromatic leukodystrophy, Schilder disease, Marchiafava-Bignami disease,) masses (tumor, AVM, abscess, tuberous sclerosis, sarcoidosis,) CNS parasitic infections (malaria, toxoplasma, cysticercosis, cryptococcus, tuberculosis)

- Genetic test

  ○ Huntington, Friedrich ataxia, chromosomal aberrations (XXY, XO, fragile X syndrome, VCFS 22.11q) Prader-Willi, GM2 gangliosidosis, Fabry disease, Niemann-Pick type C disease, Gaucher disease, Hartnup, phenylketonuria

- Other:

  ○ Sleep disorders (narcolepsy, hypnagogic & hypnapompic hallucinations)—polysomnography
  ○ Tuberculosis—skin test

Some tests are screens and would require additional testing to confirm diagnosis.
Abbreviations: Ab, antibody; ACE, angiotensin-converting enzyme; AChR, acetylcholine receptor; ASO, antistreptolysin O; CBC, complete blood count; CMV, cytomegalovirus; CNS, central nervous system; CSF, cerebrospinal fluid; EBV, Epstein-Barr virus; EEG, electrocardiogram; ELISA, enzyme-linked immunosorbent assay; Gluc, glucose; HSV, herpes simplex virus; IgG, immunoglobulin G; Mg, magnesium; MS, multiple sclerosis; NMDA, N-Methyl-d-aspartate; PCR, polymerase chain reaction; PTH, parathyroid hormone; SLE, systemic lupus erythematosus; UDS, urine drug screen.
[a] Tests listed earlier are suggested diagnostic tests that, if negative, would make named condition less likely but do not exclude the possibility of a diagnosis. Furthermore, additional testing may be necessary, particularly if there is high clinical suspicion for such condition.

---

instead a clinically guided approach. Despite this being commonly done in clinical practice, studies of structural imaging in the workup of patients with pediatric FEP as young as 12 years also did not yield support for routine screening without additional neurologic or atypical symptoms.[48,49] Because of the lack of existing studies evaluating the usefulness of structural neuroimaging in children younger than 12 years, a recommendation could not be made for this younger age group and clinical judgment with a survey of accompanying symptoms remains key. Evidence is stronger, however, in support of the earlier screening for genetic conditions in children and early

Table 1
Commonly ordered tests and supporting data

CBC W/Diff	UA	HIV	Antitreponemal IgG

• R/o medical causes: delirium, infection, anemia
• Baseline: if starting med
• ANC
• 2010 retrospective study: monocytosis in 54/66 patients correlating with worse psychotic symptoms[26]
• 2013 cohort: immune symptom dysregulation in FEP (postpartum).[27]
• Difficult to accurately assess the value of this test, given it is an indirect marker of several illnesses, yet studies are limited
  ○ Level 3 Consensus (1 or 2 if consider delirium)
  ○ Recommendation B/C
	• R/o medical causes: delirium, infection
	• Prognosis: etiopathology of relapse and mortality
	• 2013 cross-sectional study: ↑ risk of relapse of psychotic symptoms[17]
	• 2014 chart review: associated with increased premature mortality risk[16]
	• UTI prevalence in psychosis[16].
	  ○ 21% primary psychoses
	  ○ 18% affective psychoses
	  ■ Level 2 (mortality and prevention)
	  ■ Recommendation B
		• R/o medical causes: HIV
		• Prognosis: morbidity and mortality
		• 1991 study: 12/31 patients with psychosis as presenting symptom. Up to 15% of all patients with HIV develop psychosis[28]
		• 1996, 2015 studies: all cause mortality higher when HIV and psychosis were co-morbid[14,15]
		• Acute psychosis risk higher in first year of HIV. Risk diminishes with ART[15]
		  ○ Level 2 (mortality and prevention)
		  ○ Recommendation B
			• R/o medical causes: neurosyphilis
			• 2004 study: 30 cases. In patients with syphilis and psychiatric symptoms, psychosis was the presenting symptom for 4/17 patients[29]
			  ○ Level 3 consensus
			  ○ Recommendation B/C

(continued on next page)

CMP	TSH	ANA	Ceruloplasmin

• R/o medical causes: delirium, Addison, hyper PTH, hyper-/hypoglycemia
• Baseline: Na, LFTs
• 2014 case series: (6 cases) psychosis/catatonia due to hypoNa[30] Another reported in 2009[31]
• Electrolyte abnormalities may be a clue to workup Addison disease[32] and VCFS where appropriate[33]
• Difficult to accurately assess the value of this test, given it is an indirect marker of several illnesses, yet studies are limited
  ○ Level 3 (1 or 2 if include delirium data)
  ○ Relevant for baseline
  ○ Recommendation B
	• R/o medical causes: hyper-/hypothyroidism, subacute thyroiditis Hashimoto disease
	• 2011 case series: 10 people with psychosis secondary to thyroid disease (1980–2009)[34]
	• 2000 retrospective cohort study: (18 cases older than 20 y) Affective psychoses were most common[9]
	  ○ Level 2
	  ○ Recommendation B
		• R/o medical causes: systemic lupus erythematosus (SLE) P = 1/415
		• 2008 cohort study: acute psychosis in 89/520 (17.1%) SLE patients. Psychosis primary to other CNS symptoms in 59 of these patients[10]
		• 2015 study: neuropsychiatric symptoms were presenting SLE symptoms in 28%–40% of patients and developed within 1 y of onset in 63% of all patients[11]
		  ○ Level 2
		  ○ Recommendation B
			• R/o medical causes: Wilson disease (WD) P = 1/30,000
			• 2018 study: 40%–50% of patients present with CNS symptoms first. Of these 10%–25% are psychiatric. With time 100% of patients experience psychiatric symptoms[12]
			• 2014 review: psychiatric symptoms can precede other WD symptoms by 2.5 y[13]
			• 20% of patients saw psychiatrist before WD diagnosis[13]
			• Suspect particularly with sensitivity to neuroleptics
			  ○ Level 2
			  ○ Recommendation B

Toxicology	25-OH Vit D	Folate	Methylmalonic Acid/B12

• R/o medical causes: drug intoxication, drug withdrawal, substance-induced psychosis
• Multiple reviews and meta-analyses:
  ○ Cannabis[18,19]
  ○ Stimulants[20,21]
  ○ Alcohol[22]
  ○ Benzodiazepines[23]
• Hallucinogens; cause psychosis via primary drug mechanism; may not be in routine toxicology screen.
  ○ Level 1
  ○ Recommendation A
	• R/o medical causes: vitamin D deficiency
	• 2018 meta-analysis: vitamin D levels are reduced in FEP. 3/7 studies found correlation between low vitamin D and worse psychiatric symptoms[7]
	• 2012 cross-sectional study: teens with psychiatric disorders and low vitamin D levels were 3.5 times more likely to have psychotic symptoms[8]
	  ○ Level 1,2—prevention, morbidity
	  ○ Recommendation A
		• R/o medical cause: folate deficiency
		• 2003 review: low levels of folate were found to be an independent risk factor for psychosis[5]
		• Levels <10% of normal carry 4- to 7-fold increased risk of schizophrenia. A dose-response benefit was found with supplementation[5]
		• 2017 meta-analysis: also found that low folate levels may be risk factor for schizophrenia[6]
		  ○ Level 1—prevention
		  ○ Level 1,2—dx
		  ○ Recommendation A
			• R/o medical causes: B12 deficiency, pernicious anemia
			• 1983, 2013, 2017 case series: can present as psychosis without anemia. Supplementation helpful even when levels in low- normal range[35–37]
			• B12 levels in low-normal range underestimate tissue levels by 50%; test not sensitive or specific[38]
			• Homocysteine or MMA are better predictors of tissue levels than serum B12[39]
			  ○ Level 2,3 (stronger for at risk population with low dietary intake)
			  ○ Recommendation B/C

EEG	CT[a]	MRI[a]	OTHERS[a]

• R/o medical causes: seizures, temporal lobe epilepsy, interictal psychosis of epilepsy
• Prognosis: worse with EEG abnormalities[40]
• Systematic review: 27 studies linking psychosis with epilepsy.[41]
• 2012 study: 240 patients with acute psychosis. Study did not find support for routine use of EEG.[42]
• >10 case reports of epilepsy presenting as psychosis. Only a few are cited.[43–47]
• Mixed findings regarding usefulness as screen.
  ○ Level 2
  ○ Recommendation B/C
	• R/o medical causes: masses, hemorrhage
	• 2009 systematic review findings in 1.7% (n = 384)
	• In FEP routine CT or MRI is of little benefit and should be clinically guided with co-occurring neurologic symptoms[24]
	• Less helpful than MRI
	  ○ Level 1
	  ○ Recommendation A AGAINST screening unless clinically indicated[a]
		• R/o medical causes: masses, hemorrhage, demyelinating conditions, other neurologic conditions
		• 2008 systematic review: 4 MRI studies; none causative. Less than 5% with results that would influence management. Not cost-effective[25]
		• Retrospective studies in young patients with FEP (12–30 y). Diagnostic utility of imaging "minimal."[48] Another study concluded "no diagnostic utility" of routine screening.[49] In FEP routine CT or MRI is of little benefit and should be clinically guided with co-occurring neurologic symptoms[24]
		  ○ Level 1
		  ○ Recommendation B AGAINST screening unless clinically indicated[a]
			• Not enough evidence to clinically recommend
			• Functional MRI
			• PET
			• SPECT (single-photon emission computerized tomography)

Abbreviations: ANC, absolute neutrophil counts; ART, assisted reproductive technologies; CNS, central nervous system; CT, computed tomography; HIV, human immunodeficiency virus; LFTs, liver function tests; MMA, methylmelonic acid; PTH, parathyroid hormone; UTI, urinary tract infection; VCFS, velocardiofacial syndrome; WD, Wilson disease.

[a] In FEP, routine/indiscriminate CT & MRI screening of young, otherwise medically healthy individuals is of little diagnostic benefit. Recommend clinically guided screening for people with neurologic signs, and those with FEP aged 50 y and older. For children with FEP younger than twelve, data is lacking, and clinician judgment is advised.

adolescents with FEP.[50] It is worthwhile mentioning that the usefulness of complete blood count and comprehensive metabolic panel testing was particularly difficult to assess, as these laboratory tests are both direct and indirect markers of a vast number of illnesses, which could not be wholly captured by the search parameters. Therefore the "Level" evaluation of the quality of available data and ensuing "Recommendation" are likely underestimates of the true value of these tests in FEP. Data are summarized in **Table 1**.

Recommendation rating for each test (denoted by a letter above) was based on strength of supporting data (denoted by "level" above) and relevance for patient centered measures and outcomes per the Strength of Recommendation Taxonomy (SORT).[4] The letter A represents the strongest "recommendation" for a test and C the weakest based on available data and outcomes. The "level" of data score assigns a 1 to the strongest supporting data (meta-analyses and systematic reviews), whereas 3 represents the weakest (generally case reports and consensus data).

RECOMMENDED TESTING—TIERED APPROACH

Recommended workup of secondary causes of psychosis for all patients with FEP is shown in **Table 2**.

Table 2
First tier

Infectious	Metabolic/ Immune	Toxicity/Deficiency	Neurologic/Other
• CBC with differential • Urinalysis • HIV • Antitreponemal IgG	• CMP • TSH • ANA • Ceruloplasmin	• Toxicology screen • Vitamin D (25-OH) • Folate (Vit B9) • Methylmalonic acid (B12)	• EEG • Physical/neurologic examination[a] (as discussed later) • Survey of history and review of symptoms[a] (as discussed later)

Baseline/Monitoring

• Hemoglobin A1C
• Fasting lipids
• Pregnancy test
• Electrocardiogram

Abbreviations: ANA, antinuclear antibody; CBC, complete blood count; CMP, comprehensive metabolic panel; EEG, electrocardiogram; HIV, human immunodeficiency virus; IgG, immunoglobulin G; TSH, thyroid-stimulating hormone.
[a] Findings will dictate need for additional (second-tier) clinically guided testing.

Additional clinically guided workup for secondary causes of psychosis is shown in **Table 3**.

A Note About Treatment Response

A lack of response to conventional treatment with neuroleptics and other psychiatric agents over time, as well as persisting altered mental status, should lower the threshold for additional, second-tier tests.

Additional Comments

Erythrocyte sedimentation rate and C-reactive protein (CRP) were not included in the initial recommendation, given they are nonspecific markers of inflammation. The

Table 3
Second tier—clinically guided

History-Guided	If Affirmative Then Consider
Biographic	
Is the patient <13 year old (very early onset)?	Genetic testing MRI (if additional atypical symptoms)
Is the patient >45 year old at the time of FEP onset?	MRI (neurologic disorders and tumors more likely)
Does the patient have neurodegenerative symptoms or developmental delay? Especially if of Ashkenazi Jewish ancestry	MRI, genetic testing • GM2 gangliosidosis • Fabry Dz • Niemann-Pick type C Dz • Gaucher Dz • 22q11.2 deletion
Home	
Was the patient's current home/residence built before 1978?	Lead level
Occupation	
Plumbing, auto mechanics, construction work, glass manufacturing, production of metal, batteries, ammunition explosives, jet engines, ceramic glaze, surgical equipment	Lead level
Waste disposal, gold and coal miner, production of metal, batteries, cement, explosives, fluorescent light bulbs, human cremation, amalgam dental restoration	Mercury level
Work around zinc or copper ores, farming work in Asia (arsenic in pesticides) ingesting well water	Arsenic level
Diet	
Is the patient homeless or malnourished?	Mg, Vit A, B1, B3, B12
Is the patient vegan or vegetarian?	Mg, Vit A, B1, B3, B12
Does the patient eat a raw-food diet that includes undercooked meat?	Toxoplasma antibodies
Is the diet fish predominated?	Mercury level
Pets	
Is the patient exposed to cats/cat litter?	Toxoplasma antibodies
Review of Symptoms-Guided	**If Affirmative Then Consider**
Neurologic	
Staring spells, episodic loss of consciousness, myoclonic movements/rigidity?	Longer EEG/EMU (seizures)
Recent onset seizures?	MRI, paraneoplastic panel
AVH are associated with sleep onset/waking?	Sleep study
Waxing and waning neurologic symptoms?	MRI (multiple sclerosis)

(continued on next page)

Table 3
(continued)

Review of Symptoms-Guided	If Affirmative Then Consider
Impairment in gait, memory, aphasia nystagmus/ocular palsy (with heavy alcohol use)?	MRI and B1 (Marchiafava-Bignami, Korsakoff psychosis)
Altered mental status/confusion (+/− weight changes, hair loss, cold/heat intolerance)?	T4, antithyroperoxidase Ab, antithyroglobulin Ab, paraneoplastic panel
Confusion, headache, nausea/vomiting (+/− fever, myalgias)	MRI, EEG (acute disseminated encephalomyelitis, elevated ICP)
Confusion, memory changes, unsteady gait, incontinence	MRI (hydrocephalus)
Other	
Headache, palpitations, sweating/flushing, (with ↑BP)	Metanephrines (pheochromocytoma)
Sore throat/recent throat or ear infection?	Antistreptolysin Ab (PANDAS)
GI symptoms, fatigue, muscle weakness, orthostasis, low BP/HR, skin hyperpigmentation, weight loss	↑K, ↓Na, AM Cortisol (Addison)
Abdominal pain, GI symptoms, renal stones, bone and joint pain, fatigue	PTH, phosphorus (hyperparathyroid)
Fatigue, dizziness, tingling/paresthesias, weakness, paleness	Homocysteine
Fatigue, weight loss, night sweats, cough, (with ↑calcium)?	MRI, IM consultation (sarcoidosis, malignancy)
Skin lesions, abdominal pain, dark urine?	Porphyrins; urine or serum
Skin lesions and joint pains?	ANA/Lupus Abs, antistreptolysin Ab
Recent or multiple prior blood clots?	Antiphospholipid Ab

Exam-Guided	
General	• Tall, thin (Marfanoid)—homocystinuria (homocystine—serum/urine) • Flu-like symptoms (myalgias, fatigue) in immunocompromised (toxoplasma Ab)
HEENT	• Abnormal facies/cleft palate (small, low-set ears, wide-set eyes, hooded eyes, short flattened groove in upper lip)—DiGeorge 22q11.2 deletion (genetic testing) • Kayser-Fleischer Rings—Wilson disease (ceruloplasmin, urine copper) • Oral/mouth sores—Behcet disease (pathergy test)
Cardiovascular	• Profound elevations in BP & HR—pheochromocytoma (urine VMA)
Musculoskeletal/Skin	• Joint pain/swelling (+skin lesions)—SLE, porphyria (ANA, ESR, porphyrins) • Mees' lines (transverse white lines on nail)—arsenic (urine metalloproteins)
Skin	• Cutaneous lesions—porphyria, SLE—eczematous/psoriatic/malar (ANA, porphyrins) • Skin discoloration, desquamation (Mercury) • Erythema nodosum, sores, disfiguring nodules—Sarcoid—W > M (MRI)

(continued on next page)

Table 3 (continued)		
Exam-Guided		
Neurologic Cranial nerves, strength & sensory testing, reflexes, finger-nose-finger, and gait	Unilateral mydriasis	Temporal lobe seizures (*EEG*), migraines
	Pupils accommodate but do not react to light	Neurosyphilis (*antitreponemal IgG*)
	Supranuclear gaze palsy, ataxia	Neimann-Pick (*genetic testing*)
	Myoclonus, ataxia, aphasia, hyperreflexia/clonus, seizures, stupor/coma	Hashimoto (*anti-TPO, anti-TG Ab, TFTs*)
		Encephalitis (viral, paraneoplastic) (*LP, serum anti-NMDA Ab, paraneoplastic panel*)
		Marchiafava-Bignami, leukodystophy, gangliosidoses, prion disease (*LP, MRI*)
	Asymmetric focal findings	Multiple sclerosis, tumor, abscess, stroke, sarcoid (facial palsy) (*MRI/CT*)
	Sensory changes (vision, hearing, smell)	Neurosarcoid (*MRI/CT*)
		Neuroborreliosis/ Lyme (*Ab*)
	Choreiform movements, progressive behavioral and cognitive impairment	Huntington disease (*genetic testing*)

Studies/tests are not diagnostic; however, they may increase pretest probability when co-occurring with psychosis.

Abbreviations: Ab, antibody; ANA, antinuclear antibody; AVH, auditory verbal hallucinations; BP, blood pressure; Dz, disease; EEG, electrocardiogram; EMU, epilepsy monitoring unit; ESR, erythrocyte sedimentation rate; HR, heart rate; IM, internal medicine; LP, lumbar puncture; NMDA, N-methyl-d-aspartate; PTH, parathyroid hormone; SLE, systemic lupus erythematosus; TFT, thyroid function tests; TG, thyroglobulin; TPO, thyroperoxidase; VMA, vanillylmandelic acid.

authors recommend that these tests are ordered if the pretest probability of an underlying, causative autoimmune condition is high. In addition, CRP elevation is also found in FEP secondary to schizophrenia,[51] rendering it a less helpful test in differentiating between primary and secondary psychoses.

ACKNOWLEDGMENTS

Johnathan Daniel Smith, Assistant Professor, Department of Psychiatry, Consult-Liaison Psychiatry, Vanderbilt University Medical Center, Nashville, TN, United States of America. Margarita Abi Zeid Daou, Assistant Professor, Department of Psychiatry, University of Massachusetts Medical School, Worcester, MA, United States of America.

REFERENCES

1. Freudenreich O, Brown HE, Holt DJ. Psychosis and schizophrenia. In: Stern TA, Fava M, Wilens TE, et al, editors. Massachusetts general Hospital comprehensive clinical Psychiatry. 2nd edition. London: Elsevier; 2016. p. 307–23.e7. Print. 28.

2. Freudenreich O, Schulz SC, Goff DC. Initial medical work-up of first-episode psychosis: a conceptual review. Early Interv Psychiatry 2009;3(1):10–8.

3. Keshavan MS, Kaneko Y. Secondary psychoses: an update. World Psychiatry 2013;12(1):4–15.

4. Ebell MH, Siwek J, Weiss BD, et al. Strength of recommendation taxonomy (SORT): a patient-centered approach to grading evidence in the medical literature. Am Fam Physician 2004;69(3):548–56.

5. Muntjewerff JW, van der Put NMJ, Eskes TKAB, et al. Homocysteine metabolism and B-vitamins in schizophrenic patients: low plasma folate as a possible independent risk factor for schizophrenia. Psychiatry Res 2003;121:1–9 (4-7 fold; independ risk factor).

6. Ding Y, Ju M, He L, et al. Association of folate level in blood with the risk of schizophrenia. Comb Chem High Throughput Screen 2017;20(2):116–22. Decr folate risk factor for schiz.

7. Firth J, Carney R, Stubbs B, et al. Nutritional deficiencies and clinical correlates in first-episode psychosis: a systematic review and meta-analysis. Schizophr Bull 2018;44(6):1275–92.

8. Gracious BL, Finucane TL, Freidman-Campbell M, et al. Vitamin D deficiency and psychotic features in mentally ill adolescents: a cross-sectional study. BMC Psychiatry 2012;12(1):38.

9. Brownlie BE, Rae AM, Walshe JW, et al. Psychoses associated with thyrotoxicosis: 'thyrotoxic psychosis'. A report of 18 cases, with statistical analysis of incidence. Eur J Endocrinol 2000;142:438–44.

10. Appenzeller S, Cendes F, Costallat LTL. Acute psychosis in systemic lupus erythematosus. Rheumatol Int 2008;28:3 p237–p243.

11. Chandra SR, Issac TG, Ayyappan K. New onset psychosis as the first manifestation of neuro-psychiatric lupus. A situation causing diagnostic dilemma. Indian J Psychol Med 2015;37(3):333–8.

12. Litwin T, Dusek P, Szafrański T, et al. Psychiatric manifestations in Wilson's disease: possibilities and difficulties for treatment. Ther Adv Psychopharmacol 2018;8(7):199–211.

13. Zimbrean PC, Schilsky ML. Psychiatric aspects of Wilson disease: a review. Gen Hosp Psychiatry 2014;36(1):53–62.

14. Sewell DD. Schizophrenia and HIV. Schizophr Bull 1996;22:465–73, all cause mortality and morbidity higher.

15. Helleberg M, Pedersen MG, Pedersen CB, et al. Associations between HIV and schizophrenia and their effect on HIV treatment outcomes: a nationwide population-based cohort study in Denmark. Lancet HIV 2015;2(8):e344–50.

16. Graham KL, Carson CM, Ezeoke A, et al. Urinary tract infections in acute psychosis. J Clin Psychiatry 2014;75(4):379–85 (21%, 18%).

17. Miller BJ, Graham KL, Bodenheimer CM, et al. A prevalence study of urinary tract infections in acute relapse of schizophrenia. J Clin Psychiatry 2013;74(3):271–7.

18. Wilkinson ST, Radhakrishnan R, D'Souza DC. Impact of cannabis use on the development of psychotic disorders. Curr Addict Rep 2014;1(2):115–28.

19. Kraan T, Velthorst E, Koenders L, et al. Cannabis use and transition to psychosis in individuals at ultra-high risk: review and meta-analysis. Psychol Med 2016;46(4):673–81.

20. Grant KM, LeVan TD, Wells SM, et al. Methamphetamine-associated psychosis. J Neuroimmune Pharmacol 2012;7(1):113–39.

21. Roncero C, Daigre C, Grau-López L, et al. An international perspective and review of cocaine-induced psychosis: a call to action. Subst Abus 2014;35(3): 321–7.
22. Masood B, Lepping P, Romanov D, et al. Treatment of alcohol-induced psychotic disorder (alcoholic hallucinosis)-A systematic review. Alcohol Alcohol 2018;53(3): 259–67.
23. Pétursson H. The benzodiazepine withdrawal syndrome. Addiction 1994;89(11): 1455–9.
24. Goulet K, Deschamps B, Evoy F, et al. Use of brain imaging (computed tomography and magnetic resonance imaging) in first-episode psychosis: review and retrospective study. Can J Psychiatry 2009;54(7):493–501.
25. Albon E, Tsourapas A, Frew E, et al. Structural neuroimaging in psychosis: a systematic review and economic evaluation. Health Technol Assess 2008;12(18): iii–iv, ix-163.
26. Dimitrov DH. Correlation or coincidence between monocytosis and worsening of psychotic symptoms in veterans with schizophrenia? Schizophr Res 2011;126: 306–7.
27. Bergink V, Burgerhout KM, Weigelt K, et al. Immune system dysregulation in first-onset postpartum psychosis. Biol Psychiatry 2013;73(10):p1000–7.
28. Harris MJ, Jeste DV, Gleghorn A, et al. New-onset psychosis in HIV-infected patients. J Clin Psychiatry 1991;52(9):369–76.
29. Lair L, Naidech AM. Modern neuropsychiatric presentation of neurosyphilis. Neurology 2004;63(7):1331–3.
30. Novac AA, Bota D, Witkowski J, et al. Special medical conditions associated with catatonia in the internal medicine setting: hyponatremia-inducing psychosis and subsequent catatonia. Perm J 2014;18(3):78–81.
31. Singh RK, Chaudhury S. Hyponatremia-induced psychosis in an industrial setting. Ind Psychiatry J 2009;18(2):137–8.
32. Anglin RE, Rosebush PI, Mazurek MF. The neuropsychiatric profile of addison's disease: revisiting a forgotten phenomenon. J Neuropsychiatry Clin Neurosci 2006;18(4):450–9.
33. Thomas ZS. Psychosis, electrolyte imbalance, and velocardiofacial syndrome. Psychosomatics 2003;44(4):348–50.
34. Khemka D, Ali JA, Koch C. Primary hypothyroidism associated with acute mania: case series and literature review. Exp Clin Endocrinol Diabetes 2011;119:513–7.
35. Evans DL, Edelsohn GA, Golden RN. Organic psychosis without anemia or spinal cord symptoms in patients with vitamin B12 deficiency. Am J Psychiatry 1983; 140(2):218–21.
36. Jayaram N, Rao MG, Narasimha A, et al. Vitamin B12 levels and psychiatric symptomatology: a case series. J Neuropsychiatry Clin Neurosci 2013;25(2): 150–2.
37. Carvalho AR, Vacas S, Klut C. Vitamin B12 deficiency induced psychosis – a case report. Eur Psychiatry 2017;41. S805 0924-9338.
38. Lachner C, Steinle NI, Regenold WT. The neuropsychiatry of vitamin B12 deficiency in elderly patients. J Neuropsychiatry Clin Neurosci 2012;24(1):5–15, understimates by 50%.
39. Vashi P, Edwin P, Popiel B, et al. Methylmalonic acid and homocysteine as indicators of vitamin B-12 deficiency in cancer. PLoS One 2016;11(1):e0147843.
40. Manchanda R, Norman R, Malla A, et al. EEG abnormalities and 3-year outcome in first episode psychosis. Acta Psychiatr Scand 2008;117:277–82.

41. Irwin LG, Fortune DG. Risk factors for psychosis secondary to temporal lobe epilepsy: a systematic review. J Neuropsychiatry Clin Neurosci 2014;26(1):5–23.

42. Raybould JE, Alfers C, Cho Y, et al. EEG screening for temporal lobe epilepsy in patients with acute psychosis. J Neuropsychiatry Clin Neurosci 2012;24(4):452–7.

43. Ramsey BJ. Frontal lobe epilepsy presenting as a psychotic disorder with delusions and hallucinations: a case study. CNS Spectr 1999;4(9):64–82.

44. Bowe A. New-onset psychosis: consider epilepsy. Curr Psychiatr 2011;10(4):104.

45. Needham E, Hamelijnck J. Temporal lobe epilepsy masquerading as psychosis – a case report and literature review. Neurocase 2012;18(5):400–4.

46. Naha S, Naha K, Hande HM, et al. A young woman with seizures and psychosis. BMJ Case Rep 2014;2014. bcr2014203635.

47. Sultan S, Fallata EO. A case of complex partial seizures presenting as acute and transient psychotic disorder. Case Rep Psychiatry 2019;2019:1901254.

48. Williams SR, Koyanagi CY, Hishinuma ES. On the usefulness of structural brain imaging for young first episode inpatients with psychosis. Psychiatry Res Neuroimaging 2014;224(2):104–6.

49. Adams M, Kutcher S, Antoniw E, et al. Diagnostic utility of endocrine and neuroimaging screening tests in first-onset adolescent psychosis. J Am Acad Child Adolesc Psychiatry 1996;35(1):67–73.

50. Giannitelli M, Consoli A, Raffin M, et al. An overview of medical risk factors for childhood psychosis: implications for research and treatment. Schizophr Res 2018;192:39–49.

51. Johnsen E, Fathian F, Kroken RA, et al. The serum level of C-reactive protein (CRP) is associated with cognitive performance in acute phase psychosis. BMC Psychiatry 2016;16:60.

Medical Etiologies of Secondary Psychosis in Children and Adolescents

Jessica Merritt, MD[a], Yasas Tanguturi, MBBS, MPH[b],
Catherine Fuchs, MD, DFAACAP[a], Allyson Witters Cundiff, MD[a],*

KEYWORDS

- Secondary psychosis • Pediatric • Child • Adolescent • Medical etiologies
- Somatic • Physically ill child

KEY POINTS

- Psychosis in children and adolescents as a primary disorder is not common and careful exploration of other etiologies must occur.
- Etiologies of psychosis in child and adolescence could include neurologic, infectious, genetic, inborn errors of metabolism, autoimmune, rheumatologic, endocrine, nutritional, metabolic, and iatrogenic categories.
- Child and adolescent psychiatrists should consider medical explanations for symptoms of psychosis.
- Somatic psychoses in children and adolescents range from typical to atypical presentations.
- Treatment of the somatic disorder may lead to resolution of psychosis.

INTRODUCTION

Classification of psychosis into primary psychiatric versus secondary to an underlying somatic disorder requires careful attention to patterns of psychosis or physical symptom onset and course, family history, and collateral history.[1] The *Diagnostic and Statistical Manual of Mental Disorders* (Fifth Edition) (*DSM-5*) classifies those conditions where the pathophysiology of psychosis is due to a known neurologic or medical condition, as "psychotic disorder due to another medical condition".[2] The child and adolescent psychiatrist must acknowledge the variability of somatic diseases

Disclosure Statement: The authors have nothing to disclose.
[a] Department of Child and Adolescent Psychiatry, Vanderbilt University Medical Center, 1500 21st Avenue South, Suite 2200, Nashville, TN 37212, USA; [b] Department of Psychiatry, Child and Adolescent Psychiatry, Vanderbilt University Medical Center, 1601 23rd Avenue South, Nashville, TN 37212, USA
* Corresponding author.
E-mail address: allyson.e.witters@vumc.org

Child Adolesc Psychiatric Clin N Am 29 (2020) 29–42
https://doi.org/10.1016/j.chc.2019.08.005
1056-4993/20/© 2019 Elsevier Inc. All rights reserved.

childpsych.theclinics.com

contributing to mental status changes when developing a systematic plan for clinical/laboratory investigation.[3] Child and adolescent psychiatrists should consider both common and rare medical contributors to psychosis presenting in childhood.

The authors provide an updated review of pediatric somatic disorders associated with psychosis. When possible, the symptom patterns and underlying neurobiology described in these diverse conditions are identified. The authors have organized the somatic disorders associated with psychosis into neurologic, infectious, genetic, inborn errors of metabolism (IEMs), autoimmune, rheumatologic, endocrine, nutritional/metabolic, and iatrogenic categories. In some categories there is limited information in the pediatric literature.

NEUROLOGIC DISORDERS

Various neurologic diseases are associated with psychosis. Epilepsy, head trauma, and neoplastic disease are associated more frequently with psychosis in early life to midlife.[4] Clinical symptomatology includes atypical patterns, such as multimodal hallucinations (predominantly visual), significant confusion, disorientation, delusions of mistaken identity, and catatonic features.[5] Risk of psychosis with stroke in infants, children, and adolescents is not addressed due to overlaps in the literature with epilepsy.

Alice in Wonderland syndrome, more commonly seen in children and adolescents, includes altered perception of either body or objects, which affects all sensory modalities. These hallucinations or illusions may occur with migraines, epilepsy, delirium, brain lesions (including tumors), infections, and substance use. Patients may express paranoia and children may struggle with descriptions of their perceptions.[6]

The prevalence of psychiatric symptoms in children with epilepsy is 26% to 44% compared with 7% in the general population. In 1 cross-sectional study of 59 children with frontal lobe epilepsy, 69.4% had psychiatric disorders; of those, 20% had either bipolar disorder or psychosis. There was also a high association with intellectual disability.[7] In population-based studies, psychosis of epilepsy (POE), especially focal temporal and frontal lobe epilepsy, seems bidirectional, with psychosis and epilepsy each a risk factor for the other.[8] Primary schizophreniform disorders in the general population have a prevalence of 0.4% to 1%; in comparison, POE has a prevalence of 7% to 10% in the general population. Clinical symptoms of psychosis vary with stage of epilepsy (**Table 1**). The neuropathogenesis of POE, although not well understood, may include abnormalities in dopamine[9] or abnormal serotonin affecting γ-aminobutyric acid (GABA) and glutamate transmission, genetic, neuroendocrine, or inflammatory mediators[7] or focal lesions in the limbic brain structures.[8] A review of cross-sectional studies identified a range of 2.5 times to 10.9 times increased risk of first episode psychosis after onset of epilepsy.[10]

Migraine headaches may present with psychosis. Familial hemiplegic migraine is a rare, autosomal dominant form of migraine that includes a motor aura. The diagnosis requires reversible motor weakness and at least 1 other temporary neurologic symptom. One case report describes a father and son with episodes of auditory and visual hallucinations temporally associated with familial hemiplegic migraine; the episodes include confusion, affective instability, and sleep cycle disruption. Psychosis is hypothesized to be a manifestation of a prolonged aura or delirium.[11]

A review of childhood survivors of central nervous system (CNS) tumors identified psychotic symptoms in 2.8% of patients over a 9-year period.[12] The investigators reviewed the risk related to both the primary lesion and the effects of treatment,

Table 1
Psychosis of epilepsy subtypes

Epilepsy Stage	Psychosis of Epilepsy: Primarily Associated with Temporal Lobe and Frontal Lobe Epilepsy
Ictal	• Psychotic symptoms are clinical expression of the seizure itself
Postictal	• Increase in secondary generalized tonic-clonic seizures prior to onset of POE • Often bilateral independent ictal foci • Psychotic symptoms occur up to 120 h after the seizure • May be psychotic episode or isolated psychotic symptoms • Short duration • Affective psychosis with grandiose and religious delusions • Feelings of impending death • Onset typically 10 y postdiagnosis of epilepsy • Insomnia as presenting symptom • Family history of psychiatric disorders • Accounts for 25% of POE
Interictal	• Psychotic episodes are independent of the seizure • Resemble schizophreniform disorders but with better premorbid function • Intact personality • Absence of negative symptoms • Later onset • May occur within days or months to years after seizure • 0.3%–0.4% adults with epilepsy
Alternative psychosis or forced normalization	• Psychotic episodes occur after relative or complete normalization of EEG/after remission of seizures • Reported in temporal lobe epilepsy and generalized epilepsies • Paranoid psychosis without clouding of consciousness • Affective symptoms • Rare: 3 out of 2267 children with epilepsy in 1 report

Data from Kanner AM, Rivas-Grajales AM. Psychosis of epilepsy: a multifaceted neuropsychiatric disorder. CNS Spectr 2016;21(3):247-57; and Kawakami Y, Itoh Y. Forced Normalization: Antagonism Between Epilepsy and Psychosis. Pediatr Neurol 2017;70:16-19.

especially radiation, on the developing brain. Identified factors include location of the tumor, premorbid neurologic state, and surgical morbidity. Dose of radiation and age at time of treatment were identified as factors linked to psychosis.

Narcolepsy is defined as excessive daytime sleepiness, cataplexy, sleep paralysis, hypnagogic/hypnopompic hallucinations, and disrupted nocturnal sleep. Onset is bimodal (ages 15 years or 35 years). In pediatric populations, presentation may include behavioral, metabolic, endocrine, and mood changes. Hallucinations occur in 39% to 50% of children, typically at sleep onset (hypnagogic) and offset (hypnopompic). The hallucinations are multimodal, associated with sleep, and usually without delusions. One retrospective study of narcolepsy identified 1.8% comorbidity with psychosis, clinically similar to schizophrenia, often within 3 years after onset of narcolepsy. Another study identified 9.8% of children with narcolepsy who developed schizophrenia.[13]

Delirium is a syndrome of brain dysfunction seen in critically ill, including infants and children, defined in the *DSM-5* by 6 domains (**Fig. 1**), including psychotic symptoms, such as abnormalities of perception and thought.[4] Mental status assessment requires a developmental approach. Malas and colleagues[14] reviewed the inflammatory, metabolic, and neurochemical processes that contribute to risk of delirium and identified patterns of abnormal thought.

Traumatic brain injury (TBI) is associated with delirium[15] and psychosis.[16] In studies of patients 16 years and older, the early period after TBI is described as a posttraumatic confusional state, a form of delirium, with neurobehavioral deficits, including psychotic-like symptoms. The presence of psychotic symptoms is a predictor of outcome 1 year after injury, indicating a poorer prognosis even when the symptoms resolve prior to discharge. Other risk factors include sleep disturbance and greater cognitive impairment, male gender, and age.[17] Psychotic disorders due to TBI include delusional disorders and schizophrenia-like psychoses.[16] Delusional patterns are predominantly Capgras syndrome (32%), reduplicative paramnesia (32%), delusional jealousy (16%), Cotard syndrome (16%), and others. Negative symptoms are uncommon (25%). Presentations are notable for an absence of psychotic symptoms or prodrome before the TBI. The onset of psychotic symptoms may be sudden, with mean latency of presentation up to 3.3 years after TBI. Psychotic symptoms may be preceded by affective instability, social withdrawal, and decline in performance. Neurologic studies post-TBI with psychosis show abnormal magnetic resonance imaging (MRI)/computed tomography lesions in 94%, predominantly frontal and temporal regions, and abnormal electroencephalogram (EEG) in 71%, affecting both temporal and frontal regions with slowing and spiking patterns. Psychosis may occur with a range of severity of TBI. Risk factors include positive family history of psychotic illness and history of neurodevelopmental or neurologic disorder. Posttraumatic stress disorder may occur in TBI with trauma-related delusions and hallucinations. Proposed pathogenic models include frontal and temporal circuit injury, combined with genetic and environmental risk factors, having an impact on the brain circuits.[16]

INFECTIOUS DISORDERS

Psychiatric symptoms may be the primary or secondary presentation in infectious diseases. Symptoms may occur in the active phase or chronic phase of the infection.[18] Numerous infectious agents have been known to cause psychotic symptoms,

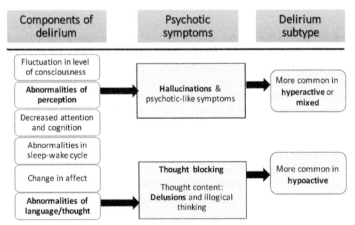

Fig. 1. Psychosis in delirium. (*Data from* American Psychiatric Association. Diagnostic and Statistical Manual of Mental Disorders. 5th ed. Washington D.C.: 2013; and Malas N, Brahmbhatt K, McDermott C, et al. Pediatric Delirium: Evaluation, Management, and Special Considerations. Curr Psychiatry Rep 2017;19(9):65.)

including viruses, bacteria, and protozoa (**Table 2**).[3,18,19] Occult infections can present with psychiatric symptoms including irritability, depression, delirium, cognitive dysfunction, or psychosis.[18]

Mycoplasma pneumonia with progression to encephalitis may present with psychotic symptoms.[20] Lyme disease is caused by a tick-borne spirochete (*Borrelia burgdorferi*); psychiatric symptoms typically are depressive episodes but may include psychosis, especially with chronic infection.[21] Brucellosis may present with acute psychosis in adolescents and young adults.[22]

The clinical presentation of multiple, acute viral infections (herpes simplex virus, Epstein-Barr virus, cytomegalovirus, influenza, measles, rubella, and mumps) may present with psychosis,[19] usually associated with acute encephalitis. Psychiatric presentation of rabies infection may include anxiety, agitation, bizarre behavior and hallucinations, approximately 10 days after infection.[18] Human immunodeficiency virus (HIV) infection is a chronic disease that may be associated with neuropsychiatric complications. Psychosis is an uncommon manifestation of HIV/AIDS, more frequent in elderly patients with AIDS-related neurocognitive impairments or those with HIV-associated dementia.[23] Opportunistic infections in those with AIDS can cause psychosis (eg, cryptococcal meningitis and neurosyphilis). Acute parasitic infections (toxoplasmosis or cerebral malaria) also may exhibit psychotic symptoms.[18]

Multiple pathogenic mechanisms for neuropsychiatric symptoms have been proposed. Viruses are thought to directly invade the CNS through hematogenous spread or through infected leukocytes, leading to infection of the vascular endothelial cells, subarachnoid space, or neural tissues. Similar mechanisms may happen in cell wall–deficient bacteria (*Mycoplasma*, *Chlamydia*, *Borrelia*, and *Brucella*), which are implicated in neurodegenerative and neurobehavioral diseases. Other mechanisms include immune-mediated damage resulting in vasculopathy (*Mycoplasma*) or through direct alterations in dopamine synthesis (*Toxoplasma*).[18]

GENETIC DISORDERS

Several genetic conditions predispose to development of primary psychotic disorders (such as schizophrenia). Examples include common (DiGeorge syndrome) or rare

Table 2
Infectious agents known to be associated with psychotic symptoms

Viruses	Bacteria	Protozoa
Herpes simplex virus	*Treponema pallidum*	*Toxoplasma gondii*
Epstein-Barr virus	*Borrelia burgdorferi*	*Neurocysticercosis*
Cytomegalovirus	*Mycoplasma pneumonia*	*Plasmodium falciparum*
Influenza	*Brucella*	
Measles		
Rubella		
Mumps		
Polio		
Vaccinia		
Coxsackie B4 virus		
Eastern equine encephalitis		
HIV		
Rabies (endogenous retrovirus)		
Borna (human retrovirus)		

Data from Refs.[3,18,19]

(copy number variant) conditions.[3] Additional childhood disorders caused by chromosomal abnormalities associated with secondary psychotic symptoms include juvenile-onset Huntington disease, Prader-Willi syndrome, Turner syndrome, and Klinefelter ayndrome.[3] Congenital disorders are often associated with psychiatric symptoms and are well described by Benjamin and colleagues.[24] Psychotic symptoms co-occurring in congenital disorders with clinical symptoms (as listed in **Box 1**) warrant further diagnostic assessment.

INBORN ERRORS OF METABOLISM

IEMs are specific forms of genetic disorders resulting from full or a partial loss of a gene function due to mutation. The pathology of IEMs may involve accumulation of harmful enzymatic substrates or absence of a necessary neural product.[25] Typical pathophysiology for IEMs includes disrupted neuronal function or neuronal cell death.[5] Presentation of psychiatric symptoms, especially psychosis, may occur years prior to onset of neurologic symptoms.[25] Sedel and colleagues[26] reviewed the psychiatric manifestations in both adolescents and adults and proposed 2 categories of IEMs associated with psychosis (**Fig. 2**). A subset of patients with intellectual disability, behavioral, or personality changes was not associated with psychiatric syndromes.

Reported psychotic symptoms include visual hallucinations (in urea cycle disorders, homocysteine metabolism disorders, and Niemann-Pick disease) and delusions with catatonia (porphyrias).[25] Specific symptoms may be associated with each condition; for example, abdominal pain, peripheral neuropathy (porphyria), liver dysfunction, jaundice, splenomegaly (Wilson disease or Niemann-Pick disease), ataxia, supranuclear gaze palsy (Niemann-Pick), juvenile cataracts, seizures (cerebrotendinous

---

Box 1
Clinical symptoms comorbid with psychosis indicative of need for further assessment of possible congenital disorders

Atypical body size

Ataxia

Cardiovascular abnormalities

Cognitive impairment/intellectual disability

Dermatologic abnormalities (skin conditions in tuberous sclerosis and neurofibromatosis)

Dysmorphia

Endocrine abnormalities

Hearing and/or vision abnormalities

Hematologic abnormalities (hemolytic anemia in G6PD deficiency)

Movement disorders

Peripheral neuropathy

Renal abnormalities

Seizures

Hepatic abnormalities

Adapted from Benjamin S, Lauterbach MD, Stanislawski AL. Congenital and acquired disorders presenting as psychosis in children and young adults. Child Adolesc Psychiatr Clin N Am 2013;22(4):581-608; with permission.

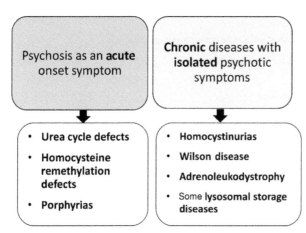

Fig. 2. Psychotic symptoms associated with IEMs. (*From* Sedel F, Baumann N, Turpin JC, et al. Psychiatric manifestations revealing inborn errors of metabolism in adolescents and adults. J Inherit Metab Dis 2007;30(5):631-41; with permission.)

xanthomatosis), eye disorders (disorders of homocysteine metabolism), or skeletal abnormalities (cystathionine β-synthase deficiency).[25] Clinical signs to consider include atypical or delayed development (hypotonia, dysmorphia, microcephaly, and intellectual disability/cognitive decline), growth delays, gastrointestinal signs, or catatonia.[26] Recognition of IEMs may inform treatment of psychosis, because patients with IEMs may show sensitivity to antipsychotics,[3] treatment resistance, and development of metabolic adverse effects.[25] In some cases, symptoms may be corrected with simple dietary modifications or replacements.

AUTOIMMUNE ENCEPHALOPATHIES

Studies have linked autoimmune disease and psychosis. Inflammation may be the common pathway through increased permeability of the blood-brain barrier (BBB), production of proinflammatory cytokines, and priming of microglia.[27] Psychosis can occur with autoimmune encephalitis.[28] Correlations have been reported between proxy inflammatory markers, such as elevated neutrophil:lymphocyte ratios,[29] and inflammatory biomarkers, such as interleukin 6 and C-reactive protein,[30] in those with psychosis.

Autoimmune encephalitis typically presents with subacute onset of psychiatric symptoms (delusions, hallucinations, paranoia, insomnia, and agitation) and neurologic symptoms (seizures, speech impairment, ataxia, dyskinesias, choreoathetosis, tremor, dystonia, and autonomic instability). Prodromal symptoms of fever, malaise, headache, gastrointestinal, and upper respiratory symptoms were noted in 50% of cases.[31] Many antibodies have been identified in case reports of autoimmune encephalitis (**Box 2**).

Anti–N-methyl-D-aspartate (NMDA) receptor (anti-NMDAR) antibodies are a more commonly identified cause of autoimmune-mediated encephalitis, with more than 40% of cases occurring below the age of 18%, and 80% of pediatric cases occurring in girls.[32] Symptoms are thought to result from anti-NMDA antibodies binding to GluN1 subunit of NMDAR, leading to internalization and decreased NMDAR expression, which may align with glutamate hypothesis of schizophrenia.[31,32] Paraneoplastic processes have been associated with anti-NMDAR encephalitis with 30% of girls

---

Box 2
Antibodies associated with autoimmune encephalitis

Antibodies to cell surface components

NMDAR

Voltage-gated K channel complex

Glycine receptor

GABA-A and GABA-B receptor

Dopamine D_2 receptor

Glutamate receptor

Contactin-associated protein-like 2

Leucine-rich glioma-inactivated 1

Other antibodies

Glutamic acid decarboxylase

Ma2 (also referred to as Ta)

Antineuronal nuclear antibody type 1, also known as anti-Hu

Data from Refs.[28,31,32]

---

younger than 18 years and 10% of girls younger than 14 years having ovarian teratoma. Up to 80% have abnormal EEG patterns, typically extreme delta brush; nonspecific MRI findings are identified in fewer than half of pediatric patients.[32] In 1 review of anti-NMDAR encephalitis, 54% had psychotic symptoms. Of those with psychosis, 32.9% had delusions (73% described as persecutory), and 77% had perceptual disturbances (64% visual, 59% auditory, and 3% olfactory/tactile). Thought blocking and disorganized thinking were present at combined rate of 13%, with disorganized behaviors in 87% of children.[31] Presentation in children differs from that in adolescents and adults, with higher rates of neurologic symptoms and increased rates of developmental regression, temper tantrums, and inattention in children.[32]

Pediatric acute-onset neuropsychiatric syndrome (PANS)/pediatric autoimmune neuropsychiatric disorder associated with streptococcal infection is described as precipitous onset of obsessive-compulsive symptoms or food refusal and concurrent mood/anxiety, cognitive and sleep disturbances, and motor abnormalities.[33] Psychotic symptoms have been documented in 14% to 37% of PANS patients, with hallucinations (36%) most common, equally likely to be auditory or visual (70%) and described as complex, nonderogatory, and nonthreatening. Delusions were less common (6.3%) with reported increased severity in those with psychotic symptoms compared with those without. The pathogenesis of psychotic symptoms is hypothesized to be molecular mimicry involving the basal ganglia and striatum.[33]

RHEUMATOLOGIC/OTHER AUTOIMMUNE DISORDERS

Psychosis has been associated with rheumatologic disorders, including sarcoidosis, antiphospholipid syndrome (APS), and systemic lupus erythematosus (SLE).[28] Acute disseminated encephalomyelitis (ADEM) is characterized by abrupt and diffuse demyelination within the CNS due to T cell–mediated targeting of myelin. Typically, symptoms occur after an infection (measles) or vaccination (small pox or rabies).[34] Estimated occurrence of ADEM is approximately 0.4 per 100,000 of those under

20 years old with a mortality rate of 2%.[35] Headache, fever, nausea, vomiting, and changes in mentation occur 1 week to 3 weeks after prodromal illness of fever, malaise, and myalgias. Isolated, acute psychosis characterized by paranoia, delusions of persecution, agitation/aggression, and hallucinations have been described as primary presenting symptoms. EEG often is abnormal, with moderate to severe diffuse, high-voltage theta-delta activity and nonspecific CSF findings. MRI findings of multiple areas of increased signal intensity typically involving white matter are common.[34]

Multiple sclerosis, an autoimmune demyelinating condition of CNS, is rare in the pediatric population (3%–5% of cases). One study found that in the 1 year to 5 years after the first demyelinating episode, a significantly increased risk for development of psychotic disorders among this population exists. Presence of temporal lobe lesions or the common pathway of inflammation as a cause of psychosis associated with multiple sclerosis has been postulated.[36]

Sarcoidosis, a multisystem, noncaseating granulomatous inflammatory disease, occurs in 3/100,000 to 10/100,000 adults with unknown prevalence in children. Isolated neurosarcoidosis has been reported in 10 pediatric cases, with at least 1 patient described as experiencing auditory hallucinations.[37]

SLE commonly presents as headache (72%), mood disorders (57%), cognitive disorders (55%), and psychosis (12%). Children exhibit psychotic symptoms more often than adults.[38] Neuropsychiatric SLE may feature neurologic symptoms, such as mononeuritis multiplex, myelitis, and neuropathy, in addition to psychiatric symptoms. Neuropsychiatric SLE–associated psychosis is thought to be secondary to autoantibodies causing direct damage to brain parenchyma with risk of generalized brain dysfunction. An alternative hypothesis is that psychosis may be related to blood vessel damage and vasculitis.[39]

Antiphospholipid antibody syndrome (APS), an autoimmune condition characterized by thrombosis in the presence of positive circulating antiphospholipid antibodies, can be primary or secondary to other rheumatologic condition, such as SLE. Psychosis is a rare symptom of APS with case reports in patients as young as 9 years. Symptoms include delusions, paranoia, and hallucinations (auditory more common than visual).[40]

Neuropathophysiologic changes contributing to psychosis in autoimmune diseases may include inflammation associated with permeability of the BBB and presence of proinflammatory cytokines. Rheumatologic and other autoimmune disorders may have similar presentations of psychoses due to different underlying processes, including inflammatory white matter demyelination (MS),[41] APS,[40] or antibodies directly damaging brain parenchyma (SLE).[39]

IATROGENIC CAUSES

Psychosis secondary to autoimmune conditions must be carefully distinguished from iatrogenic causes, because many treatments can precipitate psychosis. Steroid-induced psychosis occurs rarely in pediatric populations compared with adults, although case reports have been described. Pathogenesis of steroid-induced psychosis is thought to be due to neuronal cell death within the amygdala, alterations in the cortical dendritic spines, and changes in the level of nerve growth factor expression in septal nuclei.[38] Agents, such as isoniazid, antimalarial, antibiotics, antiretrovirals, and stimulants, also have been associated with psychosis.[23,41–45]

ENDOCRINE DISORDERS

Secondary psychoses have been associated with several endocrine disorders. In Cushing disease, a pituitary gland tumor secretes excess cortisol, causing insulin resistance, moon face, central obesity, hirsutism. Patients may present with psychiatric symptoms, including depression, mania and psychosis, thought to be secondary to excess glucocorticoids.[46]

Hypothyroidism is a common disorder with inadequate synthesis and release of thyroid hormone. Iodine deficiency is the most common cause worldwide; Hashimoto thyroiditis is most prevalent in developed countries. Myxedema psychosis, an uncommon manifestation of hypothyroidism, was described in a case report of a 12-year-old patient with acute confusional state and psychotic features, including bizarre statements, paranoia, auditory and visual hallucinations, and inability to recognize family members, resolving rapidly with thyroxine.[47]

Hyperthyroid patients may present with a myriad of clinical findings, including cardiac, structural, ophthalmologic, constitutional, and neuropsychiatric symptoms, such as decreased attention, concentration, executive planning, and memory. Psychosis associated with hyperthyroidism is less prevalent.[48] Patients with hyperthyroidism-associated psychosis, however, also have been identified.[49] Delusional symptoms typically occur in combination with other psychiatric symptoms (depression, mania, and hallucinations). It remains undetermined if the etiology of the thyrotoxic state (Graves disease, Hashimoto thyroiditis, toxic goiter, or exogenous thyroid hormone poisoning) influences either the onset or type of psychiatric symptomatology.[50]

Psychosis in the context of diabetes mellitus occurs most commonly with hypoglycemia but may occur with hyperglycemia (usually in diabetic ketoacidosis or hyperglycemic hyperosmolar states in patients with type 1 diabetes mellitus).[51]

Hypothalamic pituitary adrenal (HPA) axis dysregulation has been associated with primary psychotic disorders, including schizophrenia. Basal cortisol levels may be elevated in people at risk for psychosis.[52] Catamenial (menstrual) psychosis highlights the role of hormones and HPA axis involvement in psychosis. Menstrual psychosis (divided into premenstrual, catamenial, para menstrual, midcycle, and epochal types) is better understood to have a cyclical presentation with return of baseline behavior between episodes.[53]

Pheochromocytomas and paragangliomas are associated with anxiety and depression, but perhaps less well known is associated psychosis. Earliest reports of pheochromocytomas with psychosis were described in the 1960s; Pratt[54] described psychosis associated with cases of familial carotid body tumors (a specific type of paraganglioma). Pheochromocytomas and paragangliomas are types of neural crest cell tumors that secrete catecholamines. They should be considered when patients present with autonomic instability plus psychosis. Psychosis may be the initial symptom. Case reports of resections of such tumors describe remission of psychotic symptoms.[55] The mechanism of how elevated peripheral catecholamines may lead to psychosis is unclear. It is generally recognized that primary psychosis is associated with elevated dopamine in the striatum, although it is less clear how peripherally elevated dopamine could cross the BBB. Johansson hypothesizes[56] that the BBB may be damaged by extreme hypertension resulting from pheochromocytomas and paragangliomas.

NUTRITIONAL DISORDERS

Psychosis can be a result of malnutrition and malnutrition can result from psychosis.[57] Early-life nutrition affects neurodevelopment. Critical nutrients include long-chain polyunsaturated fatty acids, micronutrients (including zinc, iodine, and iron), folate, vitamin D, vitamin A, and vitamin-like nutrients, such as choline.[58] The relationship between nutrition and epigenetics (DNA methylation, post-translational histone modifications, and micro-RNAs) has been linked to immune function and inflammation, further contributing to the potential development of neuropathic disease.[58]

A case of psychotic symptoms due to vitamin B_{12} and folate deficiency in a 12 year old has been reported.[59] In addition to secondary psychosis, there is evidence to suggest that there are significant reductions in folate, vitamin D, and vitamin C with first-episode psychosis, with suggestion that severity of psychiatric symptoms is related to level of vitamin D.[60]

Eating disorders also may present with psychotic symptoms. Transient psychosis is estimated to occur in 10% to 15% of patients with anorexia nervosa,[61] most likely related to electrolyte disturbances.

DISCUSSION

Somatic disorders associated with psychosis in children and adolescents are numerous. The authors provide a reference to facilitate recognition of potential medical etiologies for psychotic symptoms in children and adolescents. When assessing a patient with psychosis, clinicians should always evaluate for possible comorbid somatic disorders by carefully obtaining a history of events and symptoms leading to psychotic symptom presentation. A recent review by Staal and colleagues[1] found that the symptoms of both primary and secondary psychoses resemble each other, indicating the need for a standard and thorough history and physical examination. This should include a thorough history of medication exposure, prior medical conditions, family members' medical and psychiatric conditions, psychosocial factors, and substance use histories. Detailed history should be followed by physical, including neurologic and mental status, examinations as well as appropriate laboratory analysis. The recommended standard psychosis work-up (as described in adults) is further described in detail by Maja Skikic and Jose Alberto Arriola's article, "First Episode Psychosis Medical Workup: Evidence-Informed Recommendations and Introduction to a Clinically-Guided Approach," in this issue.

Factors increasing suspicion for an underlying organic cause include acute or subacute onset of psychotic symptoms, accompanied by regression (behavioral or cognitive), or associated with apparent triggers (infection, medication, and so forth). Additionally, the presence of unique physical symptoms (ie, seizures, dysmorphic facies, and malar rash) or psychiatric symptoms (ie, confusion and catatonia) raises suspicion for a psychosis associated with a somatic disorder.[3,24] Identification of medical conditions or iatrogenic causes that contribute to psychosis is imperative, because it determines treatment and disease course.[3] Psychosis secondary to a neurodevelopmental or genetic disorder has implications regarding genetic counseling.[24]

Clinicians should assess psychiatric and medical clinical symptom patterns; unique presenting features should increase suspicions for secondary causes and guide further evaluation, keeping in mind the implications for disease course and development. A nuanced and balanced clinical approach is vital.[1]

REFERENCES

1. Staal M, Panis B, Schieveld JNM. Early warning signs in misrecognized secondary pediatric psychotic disorders: a systematic review. Eur Child Adolesc Psychiatry 2018. [Epub ahead of print].
2. Arciniegas DB. Psychosis. Continuum (Minneap Minn) 2015;21(3 Behavioral Neurology and Neuropsychiatry):715–36.

3. Giannitelli M, Consoli A, Raffin M, et al. An overview of medical risk factors for childhood psychosis: implications for research and treatment. Schizophr Res 2018;192:39–49.

4. American Psychiatric Association (APA). Diagnostic and statistical manual of mental disorders (DSM-5®). Washington, DC: APA; 2013.

5. Keshavan MS, Kaneko Y. Secondary psychoses: an update. World Psychiatry 2013;12(1):4–15.

6. Farooq O, Fine EJ. Alice in Wonderland syndrome: a historical and medical review. Pediatr Neurol 2017;77:5–11.

7. Ticci C, Luongo T, Valvo G, et al. Clinical and electroencephalographic correlates of psychiatric features in children with frontal lobe epilepsy. Epilepsy Behav 2019; 92:283–9.

8. Kanner AM, Rivas-Grajales AM. Psychosis of epilepsy: a multifaceted neuropsychiatric disorder. CNS Spectr 2016;21(3):247–57.

9. Kawakami Y, Itoh Y. Forced normalization: antagonism between epilepsy and psychosis. Pediatr Neurol 2017;70:16–9.

10. Hesdorffer DC. Comorbidity between neurological illness and psychiatric disorders. CNS Spectr 2016;21(3):230–8.

11. LaBianca S, Jensen R, van den Maagdenberg AM, et al. Familial hemiplegic migraine and recurrent episodes of psychosis: a case report. Headache 2015; 55(7):1004–7.

12. Turkel SB, Tishler D, Tavare CJ. Late onset psychosis in survivors of pediatric central nervous system malignancies. J Neuropsychiatry Clin Neurosci 2007; 19(3):293–7.

13. Postiglione E, Antelmi E, Pizza F, et al. The clinical spectrum of childhood narcolepsy. Sleep Med Rev 2018;38:70–85.

14. Malas N, Brahmbhatt K, McDermott C, et al. Pediatric delirium: evaluation, management, and special considerations. Curr Psychiatry Rep 2017;19(9):65.

15. Leentjens AF, Schieveld JN, Leonard M, et al. A comparison of the phenomenology of pediatric, adult, and geriatric delirium. J Psychosom Res 2008;64(2): 219–23.

16. Fujii DE, Ahmed I. Psychotic disorder caused by traumatic brain injury. Psychiatr Clin North Am 2014;37(1):113–24.

17. Sherer M, Yablon SA, Nick TG. Psychotic symptoms as manifestations of the posttraumatic confusional state: prevalence, risk factors, and association with outcome. J Head Trauma Rehabil 2014;29(2):E11–8.

18. Mufaddel A, Omer AA, Salem MO. Psychiatric aspects of infectious diseases. Open J Psychiatr 2014;4(03):202.

19. Yolken RH, Torrey EF. Are some cases of psychosis caused by microbial agents? A review of the evidence. Mol Psychiatry 2008;13(5):470–9.

20. Waites KB, Talkington DF. Mycoplasma pneumoniae and its role as a human pathogen. Clin Microbiol Rev 2004;17(4):697–728.

21. Nicolson GL, Haier J. Role of chronic bacterial and viral infections in neurodegenerative, neurobehavioural, psychiatric, autoimmune and fatiguing illnesses: part 2. Br J Med Pract 2010;3(1):24–33.

22. Karsen H, Akdeniz H, Karahocagil MK, et al. Toxic-febrile neurobrucellosis, clinical findings and outcome of treatment of four cases based on our experience. Scand J Infect Dis 2007;39(11–12):990–5.

23. Dube B, Benton T, Cruess DG, et al. Neuropsychiatric manifestations of HIV infection and AIDS. J Psychiatry Neurosci 2005;30(4):237–46.

24. Benjamin S, Lauterbach MD, Stanislawski AL. Congenital and acquired disorders presenting as psychosis in children and young adults. Child Adolesc Psychiatr Clin N Am 2013;22(4):581–608.

25. Bonnot O, Herrera PM, Tordjman S, et al. Secondary psychosis induced by metabolic disorders. Front Neurosci 2015;9:177.

26. Sedel F, Baumann N, Turpin JC, et al. Psychiatric manifestations revealing inborn errors of metabolism in adolescents and adults. J Inherit Metab Dis 2007;30(5):631–41.

27. Benros ME, Eaton WW, Mortensen PB. The epidemiologic evidence linking autoimmune diseases and psychosis. Biol Psychiatry 2014;75(4):300–6.

28. AlHakeem AS, Mekki MS, AlShahwan SM, et al. Acute psychosis in children: do not miss immune-mediated causes. Neurosciences 2016;21(3):252–5.

29. Bustan Y, Drapisz A, Ben Dor DH, et al. Elevated neutrophil to lymphocyte ratio in non-affective psychotic adolescent inpatients: evidence for early association between inflammation and psychosis. Psychiatry Res 2018;262:149–53.

30. Enderami A, Fouladi R, Hosseini SH. First-episode psychosis as the initial presentation of multiple sclerosis: a case report. Int Med Case Rep J 2018;11:73–6.

31. Sarkis RA, Coffey MJ, Cooper JJ, et al. Anti-N-Methyl-D-Aspartate receptor encephalitis: a review of psychiatric phenotypes and management considerations: a report of the American Neuropsychiatric Association Committee on Research. J Neuropsychiatry Clin Neurosci 2018;31(2):137–42.

32. Brenton JN, Goodkin HP. Antibody-mediated autoimmune encephalitis in childhood. Pediatr Neurol 2016;60:13–23.

33. Silverman M, Frankovich J, Nguyen E, et al. Psychotic symptoms in youth with Pediatric Acute-onset Neuropsychiatric Syndrome (PANS) may reflect syndrome severity and heterogeneity. J Psychiatr Res 2019;110:93–102.

34. Nasr JT, Andriola MR, Coyle PK. ADEM: literature review and case report of acute psychosis presentation. Pediatr Neurol 2000;22(1):8–18.

35. Neeki MM, Au C, Richard A, et al. Acute disseminated encephalomyelitis in an incarcerated adolescent presents as acute psychosis case report and literature review. Pediatr Emerg Care 2019;35(2):E22–5.

36. Pakpoor J, Goldacre R, Schmierer K, et al. Psychiatric disorders in children with demyelinating diseases of the central nervous system. Mult Scler 2018;24(9):1243–50.

37. Rao R, Dimitriades VR, Weimer M, et al. Neurosarcoidosis in pediatric patients: a case report and review of isolated and systemic neurosarcoidosis. Pediatr Neurol 2016;63:45–52.

38. Alpert O, Marwaha R, Huang H. Psychosis in children with systemic lupus erythematosus: the role of steroids as both treatment and cause. Gen Hosp Psychiatry 2014;36(5):2.

39. Boeke A, Pullen B, Coppes L, et al. Catatonia associated with systemic lupus erythematosus (SLE): a report of two cases and a review of the literature. Psychosomatics 2018;59(6):523–30.

40. Hallab A, Naveed S, Altibi A, et al. Association of psychosis with antiphospholipid antibody syndrome: a systematic review of clinical studies. Gen Hosp Psychiatry 2018;50:137–47.

41. Camara-Lemarroy CR, Ibarra-Yruegas BE, Rodriguez-Gutierrez R, et al. The varieties of psychosis in multiple sclerosis: a systematic review of cases. Mult Scler Relat Disord 2017;12:9–14.

42. Baytunca MB, Erermis S, Bildik T, et al. Isoniazid-induced psychosis with obsessive-compulsive symptoms (Schizo-Obsessive disorder) in a female child. J Child Adolesc Psychopharmacol 2015;25(10):819–20.

43. Przybylo HJ, Przybylo JH, Davis AT, et al. Acute psychosis after anesthesia: the case for antibiomania. Paediatr Anaesth 2005;15(8):703–5.

44. Biswas PS, Sen D, Majumdar R. Psychosis following chloroquine ingestion: a 10-year comparative study from a malaria-hyperendemic district of India. Gen Hosp Psychiatry 2014;36(2):181–6.

45. Martinez-Aguayo JC, Arancibia M, Meza-Concha N, et al. Brief psychosis induced by methylphenidate in a child with attention deficit disorder: a case report and literature review. Medwave 2017;17(5):6.

46. Sharma A, Sawant N, Shah N. A study on psychiatric disorders, body image disturbances, and self-esteem in patients of Cushing's disease. Indian J Endocrinol Metab 2018;22(4):445–50.

47. Mavroson MM, Patel N, Akker E. Myxedema psychosis in a patient with undiagnosed hashimoto thyroiditis. J Am Osteopath Assoc 2017;117(1):50–4.

48. Lo Y, Tsai SJ, Chang CH, et al. Organic delusional disorder in psychiatric inpatients: comparison with delusional disorder. Acta Psychiatr Scand 1997;95(2):161–3.

49. Brownlie BE, Rae AM, Walshe JW, et al. Psychoses associated with thyrotoxicosis - 'thyrotoxic psychosis.' A report of 18 cases, with statistical analysis of incidence. Eur J Endocrinol 2000;142(5):438–44.

50. Adediran KI, Alapati D, Rasimas JJ. Delusional psychosis in Graves' disease. Prim Care Companion CNS Disord 2018;20(1) [pii:17l02145].

51. Lopes R, Pereira BD. Delirium and psychotic symptoms associated with hyperglycemia in a patient with poorly controlled type 2 diabetes mellitus. Innov Clin Neurosci 2018;15(5–6):30–3.

52. Chaumette B, Kebir O, Mam-Lam-Fook C, et al. Salivary cortisol in early psychosis: new findings and meta-analysis. Psychoneuroendocrinology 2016;63:262–70.

53. Fernando MD, Grizzaffi J, Crapanzano KA, et al. Catamenial psychosis in an adolescent girl. BMJ Case Rep 2014;2014 [pii:bcr2014206589].

54. Pratt L. Familial carotid body tumors. Arch Otolaryngol 1973;97(4):334–6.

55. Brown JS Jr. Cases of remission of psychosis following resection of pheochromocytoma or paraganglioma. Schizophr Res 2016;176(2–3):304–6.

56. Johansson BB. Neurogenic modification of the vulnerability of the blood-brain barrier during acute hypertension in conscious rats. Acta Physiol Scand 1983;117(4):507–11.

57. Seeman MV. Eating disorders and psychosis: seven hypotheses. World J Psychiatry 2014;4(4):112–9.

58. Yan X, Zhao X, Li J, et al. Effects of early-life malnutrition on neurodevelopment and neuropsychiatric disorders and the potential mechanisms. Prog Neuropsychopharmacol Biol Psychiatry 2018;83:64–75.

59. Dogan M, Ozdemir O, Sal EA, et al. Psychotic disorder and extrapyramidal symptoms associated with vitamin B12 and folate deficiency. J Trop Pediatr 2009;55(3):205–7.

60. Firth J, Carney R, Stubbs B, et al. Nutritional deficiencies and clinical correlates in first-episode psychosis: a systematic review and meta-analysis. Schizophr Bull 2018;44(6):1275–92.

61. Sarro S. Transient psychosis in anorexia nervosa: review and case report. Eat Weight Disord 2009;14(2–3):e139–43.

Violence and Suicide Risk Assessment in Youth with Psychotic Disorders

Practical Considerations for Community Clinicians

Charles L. Scott, MD*, Anne B. McBride, MD

KEYWORDS

• Violence • Suicide • Risk • Psychosis • Early psychosis • Adolescent • Teenager

KEY POINTS

• Although most youth with psychosis do not exhibit violence, psychosis is a significant independent risk factor for violent and suicidal behaviors and warrants special consideration.

• Specific psychotic symptoms (eg, command hallucinations, delusions, paranoia) can be identified and should be considered when assessing violence and suicide risk.

• Youth with psychotic disorders exhibit higher levels of suicidal behaviors than nonpsychotic peers, and earlier onset of psychosis is associated with increased suicidal thinking and behavior.

INTRODUCTION

Although the majority of youth with psychotic symptoms do not experience an increased risk of violence, psychosis is a significant risk factor for violence and suicidal behavior in children and adolescents. Mental health providers play an important role in the identification of psychotic symptoms in youth because early treatment improves long-term outcome and can lower the risk of harm to self or others. This article provides a practical overview for clinicians and forensic evaluators on risk factors for future violence and suicidal behavior uniquely associated with psychotic symptoms.

Disclosure Statement: The authors have nothing to disclose.
Department of Psychiatry and Behavioral Sciences, University of California, Davis Medical Center, 2230 Stockton Boulevard, Sacramento, CA 95817, USA
* Corresponding author.
E-mail address: clscott@ucdavis.edu

Child Adolesc Psychiatric Clin N Am 29 (2020) 43–55
https://doi.org/10.1016/j.chc.2019.08.015   childpsych.theclinics.com
1056-4993/20/© 2019 Elsevier Inc. All rights reserved.

Abbreviations	
FEP	first episode psychosis
SAVRY	structured assessment of violence risk in youth
TCO	threat/control override

PSYCHOSIS AND VIOLENCE RISK ASSESSMENT
Case Vignette

Jason is a 16-year-old boy referred to your outpatient clinic by his school counselor. He was suspended from school because he brought a hunting knife on campus, which was discovered when it accidently fell out of his backpack during gym class. In seventh grade, Jason associated with peers who were involved in using alcohol and drugs. He was later caught by his science teacher using marijuana in the school bathroom. Although Jason was adjudicated delinquent for vandalism and shoplifting when he was in the eighth grade, he successfully completed his supervisory aftercare requirements. He has no other prior mental health or treatment history.

Jason's mother, a single parent owing to his father's incarceration, reports she is concerned that Jason may have relapsed on marijuana despite his denials and started to "act strange." She describes that he no longer socializes with anyone, isolates in his room after school, spends "hours" on the computer, and rarely showers.

During your evaluation, Jason seems to be extremely guarded. When asked, he tells you that he hears "his coach's voice" calling him "a fag" and saying that "other students hate you and want to kill you." He describes that this "voice" makes him angry and he feels sad that his peers wish him harm. He reports that the coach's voice is "strong" and "may be telling me I have to kill or be killed." When asked, he states that he brought the hunting knife to school to "protect myself." His urine drug screen is negative for all tested substances, including marijuana. Jason refuses all treatment and wants to go home so he can "be safe in my room." His mother relates that after he shuts his bedroom door, he barricades himself in his room. She adds that she found more than 20 knives hidden underneath his bed.

You are concerned that Jason may be developing a psychotic illness. How would you assess the relationship of a possible psychotic illness to his risk of future violence or aggression?

Psychosis and Future Violence Risk Overview

Although most individuals with a psychotic disorder are not violent, psychotic symptoms are important to explore when assessing a youth's future violence risk.[1]

Large and Nielssen[2] conducted a systematic review of violence occurring in first episode psychosis (FEP). Serious violence was defined as an assault that caused an injury, any use of a weapon, or any sexual assault. Severe violence was defined as violence that resulted in physical harm to the victim or required hospital treatment. These authors found that 34.5% of patients experiencing their first-episode of psychosis exhibited some form of violent behavior before treatment and 16.6% had exhibited serious violence. **Box 1** summarizes those risk factors that were associated with violence of any severity in this population.

The primary risk factors associated with serious violence were a history of prior violence or convictions, the duration of untreated psychosis, and total symptom scores.

Risk factors for future violence have also been identified in those individuals at risk to develop psychosis or who have some symptoms of psychosis, but do not yet meet diagnostic criteria for a psychotic disorder. For example, Hutton and colleagues[3]

Box 1
Risk factors associated with any form of violence in individuals with FEP

- Involuntary treatment
- History of prior violence or any criminal convictions
- Hostile affect
- Symptoms of mania
- Illicit substance use
- Lower levels of education
- Younger age
- Male sex
- Duration of untreated psychosis

Data from Large MM, Nielssen O. Violence in first-episode psychosis: a systematic review and meta-analysis. Schizophr Res 2011;125(2–3):209–220.

---

looked specifically at violence risk factors present in 34 people at ultra-high risk of developing psychosis and found the following risk factors present: convictions for violence, current thoughts or plans, violent past, concerns expressed by others regarding violence, jealousy, suspiciousness, impulsiveness, persecutory beliefs, anger, and irritability.

Specific Psychotic Symptoms and Violence

Because most individuals diagnosed with a psychotic disorder are not violent, are there particular psychotic symptoms that are noted to increase a person's risk to act aggressively? Most of the research evaluating the relationship of specific psychotic symptoms to violence derives from the adult literature[1] and should be considered when evaluating children and adolescents. Paranoia, delusions, and auditory hallucinations are 3 of the most common psychotic symptoms that have shown a unique relationship to future violence risk.

Paranoia and future violence

In the MacArthur Study of Mental Disorder and Violence, adults experiencing nondelusional suspiciousness, such as misperceiving others' behavior as indicating hostile intent, were at an increased risk of violence when followed prospectively after psychiatric hospital release.[4] In their meta-analysis from 7 UK general population surveys (including >23,000 adults), Coid[5] found that paranoid ideation was associated with violence, severity, and frequency independent of other psychotic-like symptoms. Paranoid individuals also described more incidents involving the police. These associations were independent of comorbid substance abuse or other psychiatric comorbidity.

Delusions and violence

Threat/control override (TCO) type delusions are characterized by the presence of beliefs that one is being threatened (eg, being followed or poisoned) or that one is losing control to an external source (eg, one's mind is dominated by forces beyond the person's control).[6] Swanson and colleagues,[7] using data from the Epidemiologic Catchment Area surveys, found that people who reported TCO symptoms were about twice as likely to engage in assaultive behavior as those with other psychotic symptoms. In contrast, results from the MacArthur Study of Mental Disorder and Violence[5] showed that the presence of delusions did not predict higher rates of violence among recently discharged psychiatric patients. In particular, a relationship between the presence of TCO delusions and violent behavior was not found. Similarly, in their study of 224 detained male adolescents (ages 12–17), Colins and colleagues[8] found detained youth with paranoid delusions or TCO delusions did not have a higher rate of violent future crimes when compared with detained youth without TCO delusions.

Nederlof and associates[9] conducted a cross-sectional multicenter study to further examine whether the experience of TCO symptoms is related to aggressive behavior. The investigators determined that TCO symptoms were a significant correlate of aggression in their study sample. When the 2 domains of TCO symptoms were evaluated separately, only threat symptoms made a significant contribution to aggressive behavior. In their attempt to reconcile conflicting findings from earlier research regarding the relationship of TCO symptoms to aggressive behavior, the authors suggested that various methods of measuring TCO symptoms may underlie the seemingly contradictory findings among various studies.[10] These authors findings, however, suggest that inquiring as to specific threat delusions remain an important aspect of evaluating psychotic symptoms and future dangerousness.

In addition to research examining the potential relationship of delusional content to aggression, Appelbaum and coworkers[10] used the MacArthur-Maudsley Delusions Assessment Schedule to examine the contribution of non–content-related delusional material to violence. The 7 dimensions covered by the MacArthur-Maudsley Delusions Assessment Schedule (with brief definitions) are:

1. *Conviction*: The degree of certainty about the delusional belief.
2. *Negative affect*: Whether the delusional belief makes the individual unhappy, frightened, anxious, or angry.
3. *Action*: The extent to which the individual's actions are motivated by the delusional belief.
4. *Inaction*: Whether the individual has refrained from any action as a result of the delusional belief.
5. *Preoccupation*: The extent to which the individual indicates that their thoughts focus exclusively on the delusion.
6. *Pervasiveness*: The degree to which the delusional belief penetrates all aspects of the individual's experiences.
7. *Fluidity*: The degree to which the delusional belief changed frequently during the interview.

These authors found that individuals with persecutory delusions had significantly higher scores on the dimensions of "action" and "negative affect," indicating that persons with persecutory delusions may be more likely to react in response to the dysphoric aspects of their symptoms.[11] Other research has demonstrated that individuals suffering from persecutory delusions and negative affect are more likely to act on their delusions[11] and to act violently.[12] When evaluating a patient with persecutory delusions, the clinician should also inquire if the patient has used safety actions. Safety actions are specific behaviors (such as avoidance of a perceived persecutor or an escape from a fearful situation) that the individual has used with the intention of minimizing a misperceived threat. In a study of 100 patients with current persecutory delusions, more than 95% reported using safety behaviors in the past month.[13] **Box 2** provides sample questions to further investigate potential delusions and risk of further violence based on the research summarized elsewhere in this article.

Box 2
Sample questions to evaluate possible delusions associated with violence

- Do you worry that any one wishes you harm?
- What ways do you believe that others are attempting to harm you?
- Do you ever worry you are being spied on? Is it possible that you are being followed?
- Do you believe others are plotting against you?
- Have you had the experience that others can insert thought in your head?
- Have you had any concerns that you are under the external control of another power?
- How certain are you that this is happening?
- Is there anything that could convince you that this was not true?
- How does this belief make you feel (eg, unhappy, frightened, anxious, or angry)?
- Have you thought about any actions to take as a result of these beliefs? If so, what?
- Have you taken any actions as a result of your beliefs? If so, what specific actions?
- Have you stopped doing something you would normally have done based on these beliefs?
- How much time do you spend thinking about this?
- In what ways have these beliefs impacted your life?

Command hallucinations and violence

Auditory hallucinations that command the patient to do something are experienced by approximately one-half of psychiatric patients who experience auditory hallucinations.[14] The majority of command hallucinations are nonviolent in nature and patients are more likely to obey nonviolent instructions than violent commands.[15] However, between 30% and 65% of individuals comply with the command to harm others.[14,16]

Research establishing specific factors associated with a person acting on harm-other command hallucinations has been mixed. In a review of 7 controlled studies examining the relationship between command hallucinations and violence, no study demonstrated a positive relationship between command hallucinations and violence, and one found an inverse relationship.[17] In contrast, McNiel and associates[18] found in their study of 103 civil psychiatric inpatients that 33% of patients reported having had command hallucinations to harm others during the prior year and 22% of the patients reported that they complied with such commands. The authors concluded that patients in their study who experienced command hallucinations to harm others were more than twice as likely to be violent than those without such commands.

Four factors have been described as increasing a person's willingness to comply with harm-other command hallucinations. First, persons are more likely to act on auditory hallucinations to harm others when they perceive the voice they hear as powerful.[14,16] Birchwood and Chadwick[19] noted that persons who perceive a voice as powerful experience a subjective loss of control over the voice with associated feelings of powerlessness and helplessness. Evaluators should ask the individual what he or she believes would be the consequence for failing to obey the voice with more dire perceived outcomes increasing compliance.[20] Second, if the person believes that following the directive of the command hallucination will benefit them, they are more likely to comply.[14] Third, persons are more likely to follow harmful command hallucinations when they are associated with a congruent delusion.[15] As an example, an adolescent who hears a voice to kill his mother is more likely to act on this command if he has the delusional belief that his mother has been invaded by an evil alien who is preparing to kill him. Finally, Cheung and colleagues[12] noted in their study of patients with schizophrenia that those whose hallucinations generated negative emotions (eg, anger, anxiety, and sadness) were more likely to act violently than those individuals with voices that generated a positive emotion. **Box 3** provides sample questions to further investigate auditory hallucinations and their potential risk of further violence based on the research summarized elsewhere in this article.

General Violence Risk Assessment in Youth with Psychosis or Psychotic-Like Symptoms

Clinical risk factors
In addition to understanding risk factors uniquely associated with psychotic symptoms and aggression, the clinician should also evaluate nonpsychotic risk factors for future violence. Bushman and colleagues[21] outline personal and environmental risk factors for youth violence and these are summarized in **Box 4**.

Structured instruments in assessing youth's violence risk
In addition to a clinical assessment of violence risk, a variety of structured assessments to evaluate a youth's risk of future violence have also been developed. Most of these instruments, however, do not include risk factors specific to psychotic symptoms and their relationship to aggression. One of the most well-studied and empirically supported structured assessments for youth violence is the Structured Assessment of Violence Risk in Youth (SAVRY).[22] The SAVRY is based on the structured professional judgment model and can be used in youth between ages 12 and 18. The SAVRY has been found to have strong predictive validity for violent recidivism in juvenile offenders specifically, across gender and ethnicity.[23,24] However, because the SAVRY does not include a rating specific to psychosis, the evaluator should be aware that use of this instrument may augment their evaluation but cannot substitute for evaluation of those risks uniquely associated with youth with psychotic symptoms.

Case vignette review
As an evaluator, you note that Jason has numerous risk factors for future violence specific to his psychotic symptoms. These include general paranoia, a threat delusion that other students wish to kill him, fear and sadness related to this belief, powerful auditory command hallucinations that he has acted on by obtaining knives for his protection, safety behaviors to protect himself (eg, barricading himself in the room and collecting knives), treatment refusal, and social isolation. He also has numerous

---

Box 3
Sample questions to evaluate auditory hallucinations associated with risk of future violence

- What are the voices saying?
- Is the voice of someone you know or are familiar with?
- How confident are you that the voices are real?
- Do you believe that the voices are well-meaning?
- What coping strategies do you have to deal with the voices?
- Do you feel you can resist doing what the voices are telling you to do?
- Do you feel the voice is powerful?
- Do you benefit in any way from acting on the voices?
- How do these voices make you feel?

general risk factors, independent of psychosis, for potential violence that include a prior history of juvenile delinquency, marijuana use, antisocial peer group, and family disruption because his father is incarcerated. Although he has numerous readily identified risk factors for future violence, the evaluator should attempt to review other known risk factors as outlined to better estimate the level of his future risk. Jason should have treatment initiated as soon as possible because early treatment can make a meaningful impact on lowering his violence risk. For example, in a 10-year prospective follow-up study of individuals with FEP, Langeveld and colleagues[25] found that once treatment was initiated, the prevalence of violence in psychotic individuals declined gradually to approach base rates of violence in the general population. However, persistent substance use remained a risk factor for violence even after treatment initiation, indicating the need for Jason to have ongoing substance use monitoring and treatment independent of treatment for his psychotic symptoms.

PSYCHOSIS AND SUICIDE RISK ASSESSMENT
Case Vignette

Terry is a 13-year-old girl who has been diagnosed with depression and is being treated in your outpatient clinic. She was initially brought to you when her mother found her cutting on her wrists and thighs in her bedroom when she was 12 years old. She has become increasingly isolated and completely alienated from her friends owing to her odd appearance. A former honor student, she is now failing all her classes. Her teachers describe that she stares ahead without moving for the entire hour of every class and, when questioned, her answers seem unrelated to the classroom material presented. She is admitted to the inpatient psychiatric unit to evaluate for a potential psychotic depressive disorder.

During her hospitalization, she confides to her therapist that she started having a visual hallucination at age 8 of her grandmother after she died from a heart attack. She reports a belief that her grandmother died because she did not complete the meal that she had cooked for her granddaughter on the night before her death. She describes extreme guilt and believes that she must be punished for "killing Nana."

She states that she hears her voice telling her to "join Nana in heaven" so that they both can be "at peace." She acknowledges that during the week after her grandmother's death, she attempted to hang herself in the room with her belt, but the closet rod holding the belt noose broke. When asked, she states that she first heard her grandmother's voice at age 9 and she began hearing her voice again about 3 months before her hospital admission.

You are concerned about Terry's risk for suicide based on her apparently psychotic presentation and wonder if antipsychotic medications should be initiated. What specific factors should you consider regarding her psychotic symptoms that may increase her risk of suicide?

Suicide in Youth with Psychotic Symptoms

Psychosis represents a significant risk factor for suicidal behaviors (ie, ideation, attempts, or completed suicide) in children and adolescents. Youth with psychotic disorders exhibit significantly higher levels of suicidal behaviors than their typically developing peers.[26] In addition, research indicates that individuals with onset of psychosis before entering adulthood report suicidal ideation and attempts at increased rates compared with individuals whose psychosis begins in adulthood.[27] In their prospective cohort study of 1112 adolescents (aged 13–16 years), Kelleher and colleagues[28] found that those youth who reported psychotic symptoms at baseline had a nearly 70-fold increased odds of acute suicide attempts compared with youth without psychotic symptoms.

In their study of clinical high-risk and psychotic disorder children ages 7 to 13 years, Sinclair-McBride and colleagues[29] likewise found an elevated risk of suicidal thoughts and behaviors, although many of these young children had never expressed their suicidal plant or intent. In addition, the severity of the suicidal thoughts and behaviors was significantly correlated with reported social anhedonia (a lack of close friends, preferring to spend time alone) and odd behavior or appearance in this young subpopulation.

Various researchers have attempted to examine additional factors that may pose a particular risk for suicidal behaviors in youth with psychotic symptoms. In their review of 110 youth (ages 9–17 years) with positive psychotic symptoms of less than 6 months duration, Sanchez-Gistau and colleagues[30] noted that participants were more likely to be classified as a high suicide risk if they had attempted suicide before the current psychotic episode, had severe depressive symptoms, and were taking antidepressants. Neither the subtype of psychosis (ie, affective or nonaffective psychosis) or positive versus negative Positive and Negative Syndrome Scale scores differentiated attempters from nonattempters in this sample. Bjorkenstam and colleagues[31] reviewed cases of more than 2800 individuals (ages 15–30 years) diagnosed with their FEP and discharged from a psychiatric facility. The 2 strongest risk factors in this sample for a suicide after a FEP hospital discharge were a history of self-harm or a conviction for a violent crime.

In their systematic review and meta-analysis of controlled studies, Challis and colleagues[32] examined factors associated with suicide attempts or deliberate self-injury (referred to as deliberate self-harm), in individuals before and after treatment for FEP. These researchers noted that substance abuse and depressed mood were associated with deliberate self-harm, but positive psychotic symptoms were not. In addition, individuals with a longer duration of untreated psychosis before FEP treatment had higher rates of deliberate self-harm before and after treatment. Coentre and colleagues[33] noted that, in those with FEP, suicidal behavior was particularly high in the first years after FEP. In this study, suicidal behavior was associated with a previous suicide attempt, sexual abuse, comorbid polysubstance use, lower baseline functioning, a longer time in treatment, recent negative events, older patients, a longer duration of untreated psychosis, higher positive and negative psychotic symptoms, family history of severe mental disorder, substance use, depressive symptoms, and cannabis use.

Specific Psychotic Symptoms and Suicidality in Youth

Hallucinations and suicide risk

As with research studying the relationship of specific psychotic symptoms to violence, most research examining the relationship of specific psychotic symptoms to suicide and/or suicidal behavior derives from the adult literature. In their study of 148 adult inpatients with a psychotic spectrum disorder, Wong and colleagues[34] noted that the presence of command auditory hallucinations was significantly associated with active suicidal ideation and a greater percentage of patients with command auditory hallucinations endorsed a recent suicide attempt. Individuals in this study who experienced noncommand auditory hallucinations did not demonstrate an increase in suicide ideation. In contrast, Harkavy-Friedman and colleagues[35] found that, in 100 individuals diagnosed with schizophrenia or schizoaffective disorder and experiencing command hallucinations, only those who had a past suicide attempt were at an increased risk for a future suicide attempt.

In one of the few studies examining the presence of auditory hallucinations in youth, Connell and colleagues[36] noted that most adolescents who experience hallucinations do not have an increased rate of mental disorder as an adult. However, those youth who experience hallucinations at more than 1 point in time (between ages 14 and 21 in this study) had an increased risk of developing a psychotic illness and an increased risk of suicidal behavior. Therefore, evaluators assessing hallucinations should evaluate whether the youth has experienced hallucinations at a prior point in time to help assess suicide risk.

Younger children's risk of suicide related to hallucinations may be unique when compared with adolescents. For example, Livingston and Bracha[37] found that psychotic children did not have an increased risk owing to auditory hallucinations; instead, their risk of suicide was elevated if they experienced visual hallucinations of dead relatives.

Delusions and suicide risk

Various studies have substantiated that delusions represent an independent risk factor for suicidal behaviors in certain populations. For example, individuals with psychotic (delusional) depression have a 2-fold higher risk of committing a suicidal attempt than patient with nonpsychotic depression.[38] Guilt delusions in youth may increase the risk of suicidal ideation. For example, in their study of children and adolescents diagnosed with bipolar 1 disorder (aged 6–15 years), Duffy and colleagues[39] noted that the delusions of guilt were uniquely associated with increased odds of suicidal ideation.

Delusional-like experiences in the general population are common. Saha and colleagues[40] evaluated the relationship of delusional-like experiences to suicidal ideation, suicide plan, and suicide attempts in 8841 Australian adults drawn from a national survey of mental health. In this study, 3 questions (with subsequent probes for affirmative responses) were asked to screen for delusional-like experiences:

1. Have you ever felt that your thoughts were being directly interfered with or controlled by another person?
2. Have you ever had a feeling that people were too interested in you?
3. Do you ever have any special powers that most people lack?

> **Box 5**
> **Risk factors for suicide in youth with psychosis**
>
> - Severe depression
> - Prior suicide attempts
> - History of self-harm
> - Violent crime convictions
> - Substance abuse (particularly cannabis)
> - Longer duration of untreated psychosis
> - Command auditory hallucinations to kill combined with past suicide attempt
> - Hallucinations at more than 1 point in time
> - Visual hallucinations of dead relatives (in younger children)
> - Delusions of guilt (particularly in bipolar 1 disorder)

These researchers found that participants endorsing one or more delusional-like experiences were approximately 2 to four times as likely to report suicidal ideation, plans, or attempts.

Box 5 summarizes key factors that evaluators should investigate when assessing a youth with psychotic symptoms and their risk for future violence.

General Factors Associated with Suicide Risk

In addition to evaluating for psychotic symptoms that may specifically increase a youth's risk for suicidal behavior, the clinical should also be familiar with general

> **Box 6**
> **Key risk factors for suicide in youth**
>
> - Mental disorders with the most common being
>   - Affective disorder
>   - Substance abuse
>   - Personality disorder
> - Previous suicide attempts
> - Specific personality characteristics
>   - Impulsivity
>   - Poorer problem-solving skills
> - Family structure and process risk factors
>   - History of mental disorder in a first-degree relative (particularly depression and substance abuse)
>   - Family history of suicide
>   - Violence in the home
> - Specific life events traits
>   - Interpersonal losses
>   - School problems and academic stress
>   - Acute conflicts with parental figures
> - Exposure to inspiring models who have committed suicide
> - Availability of means to commit suicide
>
> *Data from* Bilsen J. Suicide and youth: risk factors. Front Psychiatry 2018;9:540.

risk factors for suicide in children and adolescents, independent of psychosis. Bilsen[41] reviewed the most important risk factors for suicide in late school age-children and adolescents based on his review of the scientific literature. **Box 6** summarizes these key factors that are important in assessing general suicide risk factors in this population.

Case Vignette Review

Terry has numerous specific factors related to her psychotic symptoms that increase her suicide risk. These include her comorbid depression, history of self-harm, auditory hallucinations at separate points in her life, visual hallucinations of her dead grandmother, delusions of guilt, social anhedonia, odd appearance, long period of untreated psychosis, and command hallucinations combined with a prior suicide attempt. Terry is at high risk to attempt suicide and a thorough review of other general risk factors described in **Box 6** is warranted. In addition, the treatment providers should carefully consider the initiation of appropriate pharmacotherapy to manage her psychotic depression as soon as possible.

SUMMARY

Although most youth with psychosis are not a danger to self or others, the presence of psychotic symptoms carries unique risk for aggression and suicidal behaviors. Key points regarding this relationship are as follows:

- Although most youth with psychosis do not exhibit violence, psychosis is a significant independent risk factor for violent and suicidal behaviors and warrants special consideration.
- Specific psychotic symptoms (eg, command hallucinations, delusions, paranoia) can be identified and should be considered when assessing violence and suicide risk.
- Youth with psychotic disorders exhibit higher levels of suicidal behaviors than nonpsychotic peers, and earlier onset of psychosis is associated with increased suicidal thinking and behavior.

REFERENCES

1. Scott CL, Resnick PJ. Clinical assessment of psychotic and mood disorder symptoms for risk of future violence. CNS Spectr 2014;19:468–73.
2. Large MM, Nielssen O. Violence in first-episode psychosis: a systematic review and meta-analysis. Schizophr Res 2011;125(2–3):209–20.
3. Hutton P, Parker S, Bowe S, et al. Prevalence of violence risk factors in people at ultra-high risk of developing psychosis: a service audit. Early Interv Psychiatry 2012;1:91–6.
4. Monahan J, Steadman HJ, Silver E, et al. Rethinking risk assessment: the MacArthur study of mental disorder and violence. New York: Oxford University Press; 2001.
5. Coid J. The epidemiology of abnormal homicide and murder followed by suicide. Psychol Med 1983;13:855–60.
6. Link BG, Stueve A. Evidence bearing on mental illness as a possible cause of violent behavior. Epidemiol Rev 1995;17:172–81.
7. Swanson JW, Borum R, Swartz M. Psychotic symptoms and disorders and risk of violent behavior in the community. Crim Behav Ment Health 1996;6:317–38.

8. Colins OF, Vermeiren RR, Noom M, et al. Psychotic-like symptoms as a risk factor of violent recidivism in detained male adolescents. J Nerv Ment Dis 2013;6: 478–83.

9. Nederlof A, Peter M, Hovens J. Threat/control-override symptoms and emotional reactions to positive symptoms as correlates of aggressive behavior in psychotic patients. J Nerv Ment Dis 2011;199:342–7.

10. Appelbaum PS, Robbins PC, Roth LH. Dimensional approach to delusions: comparison across types and diagnoses. Am J Psychiatry 1999;156:1938–43.

11. Buchanan A, Alison RM, Wessely S, et al. Acting on delusions, II: the phenomenological correlates of acting on delusions. Br J Psychiatry 1993;163:77–81.

12. Cheung P, Schweitzer I, Crowley K, et al. Violence in schizophrenia: role of hallucinations and delusions. Schizophr Res 1997;26:181–90.

13. Freeman D, Garety PA, Kuipers E, et al. Acting on persecutory delusions: the importance of safety seeking. Behav Res Ther 2007;45(1):89–99.

14. Shawyer F, Mackinnon A, Farhall J, et al. Command hallucinations and violence: implications for detention and treatment. Psychiat Psychol Law 2003;10:97–107.

15. Chadwick P, Birchwood M. The omnipotence of voices: a cognitive approach to hallucinations. Br J Psychiatry 1994;164:190–201.

16. Fox J, Gray N, Lewis H. Factors determining compliance with command hallucinations with violent content: the role of social rank, perceived power of the voice and voice malevolence. Journal Foren Psychi Psych 2004;15:511–31.

17. Rudnick A. Relation between command hallucinations and dangerous behavior. J Am Acad Psychiatry Law 1999;27:253–7.

18. McNiel DE, Eisner JP, Binder RL. The relationship between command hallucinations and violence. Psychiatr Serv 2000;51:1288–92.

19. Birchwood M, Chadwick P. The omnipotence of voices: testing the validity of a cognitive model. Psychol Med 1997;27:1345–53.

20. Barrowcliff A, Haddock G. Factors affecting compliance and resistance to auditory command hallucinations: perceptions of a clinical population. J Ment Health 2010;19:542–52.

21. Bushman BJ, Coyne SM, Anderson CA, et al. Risk factors for youth violence: youth violence commission, International Society for Research on Aggression (ISRA). Aggress Behav 2018;44:331–6.

22. Borum R, Bartel P, Forth A. Structured assessment of violence risk in youth professional manual. Lutz (FL): Psychological Assessment Resources; 2006.

23. Catchpole REH, Gretton HM. The predictive validity of risk assessment with violent young offenders: a 1-year examination of criminal outcome. Crim Justice Behav 2003;30(No. 6):688–708.

24. Meyers JR, Schmidt F. Predictive validity of the structured assessment for violence risk in youth (SAVRY) with juvenile offenders. Crim Justice Behav 2008;35(No. 3):344–55.

25. Langeveld J, Bjørkly S, Auestad B, et al. Treatment and violent behavior in persons with first episode psychosis during a 10-year prospective follow-up study. Schizophr Res 2014;156(2–3):272–6.

26. Lincoln SH, Norkett E, Graber K, et al. Suicidal behaviors in children and adolescents with psychotic disorders. Schizophr Res 2017;179:13–6.

27. Joa I, Johannessen JO, Friis S, et al. Baseline profiles of adolescent vs. adult-onset first-episode psychosis in an early detection program. Acta Psychiatr Scand 2009;119:99–500.

28. Kelleher I, Corcoran P, Keeley H, et al. Psychotic symptoms and population risk for suicide attempt: a prospective cohort study. JAMA Psychiatry 2013;70:940–8.

29. Sinclair-McBride K, Morelli N, Tembulka S, et al. Young children with psychotic symptoms and risk for suicidal thoughts and behaviors: a research note. BMC Res Notes 2019;11:568.
30. Sanchez-Gistau V, Baeza I, Arango C, et al. Predictors of suicide attempt in early-onset, first-episode psychosis: a longitudinal 24-month follow-up study. J Clin Psychiatry 2013;74:59–66.
31. Bjorkenstam C, Bjorkenstam E, Hjern A, et al. Suicide in first episode psychosis; a nationwide cohort study. Schizophr Res 2014;195:58–66.
32. Challis S, Nielssen O, Harris A, et al. Systematic meta-analysis of the risk factors for deliberate self-harm before and after treatment for first-episode psychosis. Acta Psychiatr Scand 2013;127:442–54.
33. Coentre R, Talina MC, Góis C, et al. Depressive symptoms and suicidal behavior after first-episode psychosis: a comprehensive systematic review. Psychiatry Res 2017;253:240–8.
34. Wong Z, Ongur D, Cohen B, et al. Command hallucinations and clinical characteristics of suicidality in patient with psychotic disorders. Compr Psychiatry 2013;54:511–617.
35. Harkavy-Friedman JM, Kimy D, Nelson EA, et al. Suicide attempts in schizophrenia: the role of command auditory hallucinations for suicide. J Clin Psychiatry 2003;64:871–4.
36. Connell M, Betts K, McGrath JJ, et al. Hallucinations in adolescents and risk for mental disorders and suicidal behavior in adulthood: prospective evidence from the MUSP birth cohort study. Schizophr Res 2016;176:546–51.
37. Livingston R, Bracha H. Psychotic symptoms and suicidal behavior in hospitalized children. Am J Psychiatry 1992;149:1585–6.
38. Gournellis R, Tournikioti K, Touloumi G, et al. Psychotic (delusional) depression and suicidal attempts: a systematic review and meta-analysis. Acta Psychiatr Scand 2018;137:18–29.
39. Duffy ME, Gai AR, Rogers ML, et al. Psychotic symptoms and suicidal ideation in child and adolescent bipolar 1 disorder. Bipolar Disord 2019;00:1–8.
40. Saha S, Sott JG, Johnston AK, et al. The association between delusional-like experiences and suicidal thoughts and behavior. Schizophr Res 2011;132:197–202.
41. Bilsen J. Suicide and youth: risk factors. Front Psychiatry 2018;9:1–5.

The Prodrome of Psychotic Disorders

Identification, Prediction, and Preventive Treatment

Barnaby Nelson, PhD[a,b],*, Patrick McGorry, PhD, MD[a,b]

KEYWORDS

- Psychosis • Prodrome • High risk • Prediction • Transdiagnostic
- Preventive treatment

KEY POINTS

- The last 25 years have seen a substantial focus on the prodromal period of psychotic disorders, triggered by the introduction of "at risk" criteria.
- Prediction studies have identified a range of risk factors involved in the transition from "at risk" status to first episode psychotic illness, with the field now moving in the direction of dynamic and multimodal prediction approaches.
- Treatment studies indicate that risk of transition to psychotic disorder can at least be delayed in this clinical population, with the strongest evidence to date being for cognitive behavioral therapy.
- The optimal type and sequence of treatment in this clinical population remains an active area of research.
- Psychosis risk criteria have been broadened to transdiagnostic pluripotent risk criteria that are currently being trialed in prospective follow-up studies.

INTRODUCTION

Over the last 25 years the early recognition of schizophrenia and other psychotic disorders has become a principal focus of psychiatric research and clinical services.[1,2] The early phase of psychotic disorders refers to both the first episode of psychosis and the preonset or "prodromal" phase. In this article, the authors provide a general overview of attempts to identify the prodromal phase of psychotic disorders, predictors of outcome in this clinical population, and preventive treatment trials. They

Disclosure Statement: The authors have nothing to disclose.
[a] Orygen, The National Centre of Excellence in Youth Mental Health, The University of Melbourne, Parkville, Victoria 3052, Australia; [b] Centre for Youth Mental Health, The University of Melbourne, 35 Poplar Road (Locked Bag 10), Parkville, Victoria 3052, Australia
* Corresponding author.
E-mail address: Barnaby.Nelson@orygen.org.au

Child Adolesc Psychiatric Clin N Am 29 (2020) 57–69
https://doi.org/10.1016/j.chc.2019.08.001   **childpsych.theclinics.com**
1056-4993/20/© 2019 Elsevier Inc. All rights reserved.

conclude by summarizing recent work that takes a broader, transdiagnostic approach to identifying risk for serious mental disorder.

IDENTIFICATION OF THE PRODROMAL PHASE OF PSYCHOTIC DISORDERS

The early psychosis movement, starting in Melbourne in the early 1990s, initially focused on timely recognition and phase-specific treatment of first episode psychosis. Strong evidence has now accumulated for the benefit of providing comprehensive specialized treatment of the first episode of psychosis.[3] However, it was also recognized that for most patients a prolonged period of nonspecific psychiatric symptoms, attenuated psychotic symptoms, and impaired functioning precedes the first psychotic episode.[4–6] This prodromal phase of psychotic illness (from the Greek "prodromos," meaning "running before") is akin to prodromal phases of other illnesses marked by precursor symptoms—for example, fever, headache, lack of energy, and appetite frequently occur in the prodrome of many infective disorders.[7,8] Much of the disability associated with psychotic disorders, particularly schizophrenia, develops long before the onset of frank psychosis and is difficult to reverse even if the first psychotic episode is successfully treated.[9] Within the context of the early intervention paradigm, it was suspected that pushing the point of intervention even further back from the first episode of psychosis to the prodromal phase may result in even better outcomes.[10–13] The rationale was that intervening during this phase may ameliorate, delay, or even prevent onset of fully fledged disorder,[7] thereby reducing the burden of disability, prevalence, and possibly even the incidence of psychotic disorders.

One of the challenges in this field is that the nonspecific nature of the most common prodromal features means that prodromal intervention may be provided for a substantial proportion of "false-positive" cases, that is, people who were falsely identified as being at risk of progressing to a psychotic disorder. This does not necessarily mean that intervention is not required however, as there is typically a genuine need for care given the presence of distress, impairment, and help-seeking[14] and because of the fact that the great majority ($\sim 75\%$) of this patient group suffer from nonpsychotic disorders at clinic entry, mainly mood and anxiety disorders.[15] Meta analytical evidence indicates that approximately two-thirds of cases do not go on to develop psychosis (see later discussion).[16] Indeed, the term "prodrome" should strictly only be used once the full-blown syndrome has developed.[4] The original thinking by the authors' group was that before diagnosis with a psychotic disorder, the prodrome should be thought of as a *risk state for psychosis*, not as a specific disease entity (ie, the presence of the syndrome implies that the affected person is at that time more likely to develop psychosis in the near future than someone without the syndrome). However, if the symptoms resolve then this degree of increased risk may remit as well. The terms and criteria that were introduced in the mid 1990s—the "ultra-high risk" (UHR) criteria and "at risk mental state" (ARMS)[13,17,18]—reflected these concepts. The term "ultra" (and more recently "clinical") was used in order to differentiate this approach from the traditional "high risk" approach based purely on familial risk. The UHR criteria were an attempt to identify people with a high likelihood of developing a psychotic disorder within the near future (eg, within 12 months). However, in more recent years, particularly driven by the issue of whether to include attenuated psychosis syndrome (APS) in the Diagnostic and Statistical Manual of Mental Disorders-5 (DSM-5), arguments have been made that the ARMS concept should be thought of as a disease entity in its own right,[14,19,20] particularly given that it is associated with reduction in quality of life and functioning commensurate with other disorders listed in the DSM[14,a]. Rather than being seen as a "disease entity," a more flexible perspective is that this is a heterogenous phenotype with diffuse comorbidity, which justifies a "need for care" and as such qualifies for being seen as a "disorder."

In the formulation of the UHR criteria it was recognized that the nonspecific nature of prodromal symptoms make it problematic to use these features alone to identify people at imminent risk of psychotic disorder. Psychotic-like experiences have been found to occur commonly in the general population, especially among adolescents and young adults.[24–27] Therefore, symptoms alone would result in a high false-positive rate and poor sensitivity. A "close-in" strategy[28] was used to maximize the possibility of identifying people who may truly be in the prodromal phase of a psychotic disorder. This strategy included the risk factor of age, as the age of highest incidence of psychotic disorder is adolescence and young adulthood.[5] Clinical need for care was another factor. The criteria required that a young person must be seeking help, or be identified by someone, such as a parent or teacher, as needing help. Although the UHR criteria have undergone minor changes over the years (**Table 1**), they are based around 3 groups:

- *APS group:* patients who have experienced subthreshold positive psychotic symptoms (eg, overvalued ideas, perceptual disturbances) during the past year.
- *Brief limited intermittent psychotic symptoms group:* patients who have experienced an episode of frank psychotic symptoms that have lasted less than a week and resolved without treatment.
- *Trait and state risk factor group:* patients with a schizotypal personality disorder or who have a first-degree relative with a psychotic disorder and have experienced chronic poor functioning or a significant decrease in functioning during the previous year.

The main instruments used to operationalize these criteria consist of the Comprehensive Assessment of At-Risk Mental States[29] and the Structured Interview for Prodromal Symptoms.[30] The UHR criteria, sometimes with minor modifications, have been adopted extensively across European, Asian, and US early intervention services.[31]

Another approach that has been used to identify psychosis risk has been the basic symptoms approach that emerges out of European psychopathologic research.[32] Basic symptoms refer to subjective disturbances in thought, affect, motor functioning, bodily sensation, perception, and tolerance of stress.[33] There is some evidence that basic symptoms may identify people earlier in the prodromal phase than the UHR criteria, with the attenuated psychotic symptoms that form part of the UHR criteria appearing later during the prodromal phase, closer to the onset of frank psychosis.[34] The main instruments used to identify basic symptoms consist of the Bonn Scale for the Assessment of Basic Symptoms and the shorter Schizophrenia Prodromal Instrument-Adult Version.[35]

CLINICAL OUTCOMES OF ULTRA-HIGH RISK FOR PSYCHOSIS PATIENTS

A substantial body of research has accumulated indicating that the UHR criteria have strong predictive validity for psychotic disorder when applied to a help-seeking population, with 22% progressing to psychotic disorder over a 1-year period and 36%

---

[a] The proposal to include attenuated psychosis syndrome in DSM 5 was vigorously debated. A decision was ultimately made to include the diagnosis in the section "Conditions requiring further research" rather than in the coded disorders section based primarily on concerns regarding reliability of assessment.[21–23]

Table 1
Melbourne ultra high risk for psychosis criteria

Criteria	Attenuated Psychotic Symptoms (APS)	Brief Limited Intermittent Psychotic Symptoms (BLIPS)	Trait and State Risk Factors (Trait)
Symptom/trait requirement	Presence of attenuated (subthreshold) positive psychotic symptoms within past 12 mo	Presence of frank psychotic symptoms for <1 wk that spontaneously resolve (ie, without treatment) within the past 12 mo	Presumed genetic vulnerability based on presence of schizotypal personality disorder or a first-degree relative with a psychotic disorder
Drop in functioning/ sustained low functioning requirement	*1994–2006:* N/A *2006–2016:* 30% drop in SOFAS score for a month within the past year or SOFAS score of 50 or less for the past 12 mo or longer. *2016 onwards:* N/A	*1994–2006:* N/A *2006–2016:* 30% drop in SOFAS score for a month within the past year or SOFAS score of 50 or less for the past 12 mo or longer. *2016 onwards:* N/A	*1994–2006:* 30% drop in GAF score within the past 12 mo *or* GAF score of 50 or less for the past 12 mo or longer. *2006 onwards:* 30% drop in SOFAS score for a month within the past year *or* SOFAS score of 50 or less for the past 12 mo or longer.
Age range	*1994–2006:* 14–30 y *2006 onwards:* 15–25 y		

Operationalized using the Comprehensive Assessment of At-Risk Mental States (CAARMS).

over a 3-year period,[36] which is several thousand-fold greater than the expected incidence rate for first episode psychosis in the general population.[37] A long-term follow-up study of UHR patients indicated risk for psychosis onset occurring up to 10 years after service entry.[38] A trend in the data has been a reducing rate of transition to psychosis in more recently ascertained UHR cohorts (10%–20% over 12 months), which seems to be due to a combination of factors including earlier intervention, treatment changes, minor changes in clinical characteristics of cohorts, and lead time bias (length of follow-up period in relation to symptom duration).[39–41]

The long-term follow-up study of UHR patients referred to earlier revealed that 70% of UHR patients who did not develop psychosis ("nontransitioned" cases) had nonpsychotic disorders over a 2- to 14-year follow-up period, mainly mood disorders (49%) and anxiety disorders (35%).[42] Similar figures have been reported in US and European samples.[43] A recent systematic review of nonpsychotic outcomes in this clinical population found that most nontransitioned UHR cases (22%–82%) had at least one nonpsychotic clinical diagnosis at 2 to 7.5 years after clinic entry.

The persistence of attenuated psychotic symptoms (both positive and negative symptoms) has also been a focus of interest. In their systematic review, Beck and colleagues[43] found that 28% to 71% of nontransitioned UHR patients had not remitted from UHR status (ie, still presented with attenuated positive psychotic symptoms) over the long term. The authors' group recently found that UHR patients who had persistent attenuated psychotic symptoms displayed poorer functioning and more severe general psychopathology and negative and depressive symptoms at follow-up compared with those without persistent attenuated psychotic symptoms and that persistent attenuated psychotic symptoms were associated with reduced gray matter volume at baseline.[44] Persistent negative symptoms have also been observed in 6.1% of UHR patients at long-term follow-up and are associated with poor psychosocial functioning and deficits in processing speed.[45]

At long-term follow-up, UHR patients have been reported to have mild-moderate psychosocial functioning on the group level (a social and occupational functioning assessment scale score of ~68).[46,47] However, there are important subgroup differences, with about 25% of patients categorized as having poor functional outcome and 75% with good outcome.[47] Although transition to psychosis is related to poor functional outcome, other variables, most notably childhood maltreatment, also have a predictive role.[47] Half of UHR patients who do not transition to psychosis present with poor psychosocial outcomes at 2-year and 6-year follow-up[43] (**Fig. 1** for summary).

PREDICTORS OF TRANSITION TO PSYCHOSIS

A range of variables have been identified that predict those who transition to psychosis among the group who have already been identified as being at risk (for comprehensive reviews see[48] and[49]). In terms of clinical variables, negative symptoms, thought disorder, poor baseline social functioning, as well as decline in social functioning, and longer duration of symptoms before clinic entry have been identified as the more reliable predictors of transition to psychosis. Of environmental risk factors, a history of childhood trauma and cannabis abuse have been identified most consistently as related to transition (however, caution should be used when interpreting these findings given contradictory findings and the limited range of variables assessed to date[48]). Other potential factors such as migration, urbanicity, and perceived discrimination have not been sufficiently studied to date. Mizrahi has suggested that a common feature underlying environmental risk factors associated with psychosis may be exposure to social stress.[50] There is some evidence for neurocognitive deficits as predictive of transition but limited evidence to support specific cognitive domains. Social cognition has not been widely studied to date in this population. Changes in brain structure, particularly increased rate of gray matter loss, and changes in thalamic connectivity have also been identified as related to transition. Although the literature to date has been limited, there is evidence for elevated plasma levels of certain inflammatory markers, oxidative stress and that dysregulation of the hypothalamic-pituitary-adrenal axis might be associated with transition. The research on neurophysiology has been limited, with the most promising predictive variable being mismatch negativity.

Models that include several different variables (ie, multimodal prediction models[51–53]) as well as dynamic risk models (ie, models that account of changes over time[54–57]) seem to offer improved prediction than models limited to one type of assessment modality or static variable assessment. Methodological limitations in the research to date have included modest sample sizes, lack of external validation, variations in sample ascertainment, as well as the challenge of the lower rate of transition to psychosis (the main outcome of interest) in recently recruited samples.[58]

TREATMENTS FOR ULTRA-HIGH-RISK PATIENTS

There have been 20 randomized controlled trials (RCTs) published in the UHR population, with the primary outcome of interest generally being reduction in rate of transition to psychotic disorder. The RCTs have varied in quality and size and have consisted of a range of psychosocial, pharmacologic, and nutritional supplement

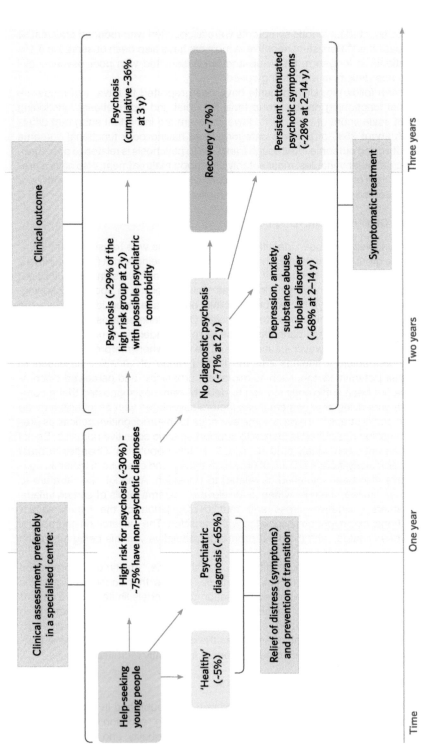

Fig. 1. Clinical outcomes of ultra-high risk for psychosis patients. (*Adapted from* Millan MJ, Andrieux A, Bartzokis G, et al. Altering the course of schizophrenia: progress and perspectives. Nat Rev Drug Discov 2016;15(7):485–515; with permission.)

interventions including cognitive behavioral therapy (CBT), family therapy, cognitive remediation, integrated psychological therapy, risperidone plus CBT, omega-3 fatty acids, N-methyl-D-aspartate-receptor modulators, and antipsychotic medications. Overall, these specific treatments are associated with a lower rate of transition to psychosis over 12 months compared with treatment as usual or monitoring. However, the medium- to longer-term findings have been mixed (see[46] for summary). It remains unclear what the most effective type of specific intervention is.[59,60] The most effective duration and sequence of interventions is also not established. In order to inform these issues, the authors are currently conducting a large-scale sequential multiple assignment randomized trial with a UHR sample (n = 342), trialing a sequence of psychosocial and pharmacologic interventions.[61] Given the heterogeneity of the UHR population, future intervention trials may benefit from stratifying UHR patients to treatment type (ie, matching treatment to patient profile), as well as including multiple treatment steps in the intervention design.

Several clinical guidelines for the treatment of UHR patients have been published.[62–65] The main recommendations that emerge from these guidelines include the following:

- Assessment of a suspected at-risk mental state by a trained mental health specialist.
- Individual CBT with or without family intervention.
- Treatment for presenting problems, such as mood or anxiety disorders.
- Treatments to prevent development or persistence of social, educational, or vocational problems.
- A psychological treatment approach should be trialed to being with. If psychological treatments are ineffective and there are severe and progressive attenuated psychotic symptoms, or the attenuated psychotic symptoms are associated with risk to self or others, then a low-dose second-generation antipsychotic could be trialed.
- After treatment, if symptoms, poor functioning, or distress continue, monitor regularly for changes for up to 3 years using structured and validated assessment tools.

CASE EXAMPLE OF TREATMENT OF AN ULTRA-HIGH-RISK PATIENT

Below, the investigators present a brief case example of a UHR young person who was assessed and treated at the authors' UHR clinic, the PACE clinic, at Orygen in Melbourne (please see[66] for further examples). Simon is a 17-year-old young man who was referred to Orygen by his General Practitioner (GP, ie, primary care doctor). Simon's mother had made an appointment for Simon to see his GP because she was concerned that he seemed depressed, anxious, and "not quite himself." Simon's family is from an Anglo-Saxon background. His father works as a plumber and his mother as a sales assistant. The GP referral noted a 1-year deterioration in social and educational functioning with worsening anxiety and attenuated psychotic symptoms over the past 6 months. Simon was brought to the initial appointment at the PACE clinic by his mother. He presented with a range of anxiety symptoms, sleep disturbance, increased avoidance of friends, poor school attendance and increased time spent playing online computer games, and occasional thoughts of harming himself, which he had not yet acted on. Simon's teachers had expressed concern to his mother that they had noticed him being more distractible and anxious in class. Simon disclosed during the assessment that he believed that people were watching him or secretly talking or laughing about him at school and on the street. Although he recognized that it was unlikely that this was actually happening, he found these thoughts confusing and distressing. Simon also reported occasional perceptual disturbances over the past 6 months, such as hearing his name or his brother's name being called and seeing fleeting movements in the corner of his visual field. Simon reported a history of significant bullying over his late primary and early high school years. This included being called derogatory names and physical taunts by school peers, as well as being excluded from social groups. Simon reported no drug or alcohol abuse.

A shared formulation of Simon's presenting complaints was developed. Given the severity of the bullying that Simon had experienced, this formulation postulated that he had developed a sense that he must be guarded and aware of others around him at all times, and this possibly contributed to his long-standing anxiety symptoms and beliefs that he is vulnerable and that others should not be trusted and a general hypervigilance, which may also have contributed to his mild perceptual disturbances. There were no clear biological predisposing factors reported and no reported family history of mental illness. Simon's ongoing avoidant behavior meant that he had lost contact with some of his friends, exacerbating his fears about what they might think of him. His hypervigilant behavior when he left the house led him to misinterpret the responses of others, leading to him feeling safest when he remains in his room at home. His poor school attendance led to increased attention from teachers when Jack did go to class, which would compound his anxiety. In the absence of alternative means of coping with distress and confusion about his beliefs and perceptual disturbances, Simon's avoidance had worsened, maintaining both his symptoms and the situational triggers. A diagram was developed with Simon to summarize these ideas. Protectively, Simon's parents, particularly his mother, were very supportive of him and had been actively involved in helping him to access treatment. He previously performed well at school academically and has a small group of close friends who have continued to try and keep in touch with him, particularly online.

Simon received weekly-fortnightly sessions with a clinical psychologist at PACE as well as a review by a psychiatrist every 3 weeks. Simon was brought to the sessions by his mother and engaged well with the therapist. Most sessions were individual sessions with Simon, but occasionally, with Simon's permission, his parents joined the sessions. The sessions included psychoeducation regarding anxiety, attenuated psychotic symptoms, and the concept of psychosis risk. This included discussion of the fact that approximately one-third of young people who meet the "risk" criteria experience a worsening of symptoms to the point where an episode of psychosis is diagnosed and medication may be required. Although being careful not to alarm Simon and his family, the importance of monitoring symptoms closely and engaging with treatment was conveyed. Psychoeducation regarding anxiety symptoms and the contributing role of cognitive and behavioral avoidance was discussed.

The sessions adopted a cognitive behavioral approach, including the identification of underlying beliefs (eg, "I am vulnerable", "Others can't be trusted"), rules and assumptions (eg, "If I avoid others then I will be safe"), and negative automatic thoughts (eg, "They are watching me"), as well as the interaction between his thoughts, emotions, physical sensations, and behaviors (eg, between thoughts of being watched, sense of fear, physiologic arousal, and hypervigilant behavior). Thought monitoring records and cognitive and behavioral techniques were used to address Simon's cognitive biases (eg, Socratic dialogue, cognitive challenging, examining the evidence, testing others' reactions, etc.). Physical exercise and anxiety management strategies such as active relaxation strategies were also used. Medication was not prescribed.

Over 6 months of treatment Simon's anxiety and attenuated psychotic symptoms reduced substantially and he no longer experienced perceptual disturbances. His symptoms no longer met UHR criteria and his school attendance and social functioning improved. He was discharged from the PACE clinic with the arrangement of regular mental state monitoring by his GP.

PLURIPOTENT RISK: BROADENING THE "AT RISK" APPROACH

Over recent years, the pattern of clinical pathways to first episode psychosis and the outcomes of UHR patients described earlier (ie, heterotypic and pluripotent symptom evolution) have prompted the authors to consider a broader approach to identifying young people at risk of psychosis and other serious mental disorders, informed by the transdiagnostic clinical staging model in psychiatry.[67–69] The concept of pluripotent risk is central to this thinking. "Pluripotent risk," observed in many areas of general medicine, refers to clinical signs and symptoms that are *not fixed* as to their potential development—that is, they may evolve into a range of different syndromes. Although both uni- and pluripotent approaches may be worth pursuing,[70] the latter approach is consistent with the growing body of research indicating shared risk architecture across the range of mental disorders[71] and may be more efficient with regard to power to conduct studies in disorders with relatively low incidence rates such as schizophrenia or bipolar disorder.[72] Recently, the authors' group developed a set of criteria, the "Clinical High At Risk Mental State" (CHARMS) criteria, based on available evidence and expert clinical opinion and experience to capture a composite definition of risk for multiple syndromes, extending the ARMS for psychosis approach.[73] The criteria are currently being validated in a prospective follow-up study being conducted across *headspace* and OYH services, with a similar approach also being trialed in Canada.[74] The CHARMS approach provides an operational definition of a broad-spectrum UHR or pluripotent state, identifying young people at risk of a range of serious mental disorders whose symptoms might evolve through either homotypic or heterotypic routes. This approach might identify from within a general cohort of distressed and help-seeking young people the enriched subset at greatly enhanced risk of serious mental illness, paving the way for a range of prediction, aetiological, and preventive treatment studies.

SUMMARY

The last 25 years have seen substantial focus on the prodromal period of psychotic disorders, triggered by the introduction of "at risk" criteria. Prediction studies have identified a range of risk factors involved in the transition from at risk status to first episode psychotic illness, with the field now moving in the direction of dynamic and multimodal prediction approaches. Larger samples and external validation are also key requirements for this field in order to generate prediction tools that can reliability be used in clinical practice. Treatment studies have indicated that risk of transition to psychotic disorder can at least be delayed in this clinical population. Although the strongest evidence to date is for CBT, the optimal type and sequence of treatment remains an active area of research. Over the last 10 years, the early intervention for psychosis approach has widened to include the full spectrum of youth mental health and new specially designed youth clinical service structures have been established. A transdiagnostic pluripotent risk state has been identified through the authors' work in psychosis risk, conceptually supported by the clinical staging model, leading to the development of broader "at risk" criteria, which are currently being validated in prospective follow-up studies.

REFERENCES

1. McGorry PD, Killackey E, Yung A. Early intervention in psychosis: concepts, evidence and future directions. World Psychiatry 2008;7(3):148–56.
2. McGorry PD, Ratheesh A, O'Donoghue B. Early intervention-an implementation challenge for 21st century mental health care. JAMA Psychiatry 2018;75(6): 545–6.
3. Correll CU, Galling B, Pawar A, et al. Comparison of early intervention services vs treatment as usual for early-phase psychosis: a systematic review, meta-analysis, and meta-regression. JAMA Psychiatry 2018;75(6):555–65.
4. Yung AR, McGorry PD, McFarlane CA, et al. Monitoring and care of young people at incipient risk of psychosis. Schizophr Bull 1996;22(2):283–303.
5. Häfner H, Maurer K, Loffler W, et al. The influence of age and sex on the onset and early course of schizophrenia. Br J Psychiatry 1993;162(80):80–6.
6. Yung AR, McGorry PD. The prodromal phase of first-episode psychosis: past and current conceptualizations. Schizophr Bull 1996;22(2):353–70.
7. Yung AR. The schizophrenia prodrome: a high-risk concept. Schizophr Bull 2003; 29(4):859–65.
8. Huber G, Gross G, Schuttler R. Schizophrenie. Verlaufs- und sozialpsychiatrische Langzeituntersuchungen an den 1945-1959 in Bonn hospitalisierten schizophrenen Kranken. Bonn (Germany): Springer; 1979.
9. Häfner H, Maurer K, Loffler W, et al. Modeling the early course of schizophrenia. Schizophr Bull 2003;29(2):325–40.
10. Yung AR, Phillips LJ, McGorry PD, et al. The prediction of psychosis: a step towards indicated prevention of schizophrenia? Br J Psychiatry 1998;(Supplement 33):14–20.
11. McGorry PD, Phillips LJ, Yung AR. Recognition and treatment of the pre-psychotic phase of psychotic disorders: frontier or fantasy?. In: Miller T, Mednick SA, McGlashan TH, et al, editors. Early intervention in psychiatric disorders. Amsterdam: Kluwer; 2001. p. 101–22.
12. McGorry PD, Yung A, Phillips L. Ethics and early intervention in psychosis: keeping up the pace and staying in step. Schizophr Res 2001;51:17–29.
13. McGorry PD, Singh BS. Schizophrenia: risk and possibility. In: Raphael B, Burrows GD, editors. Handbook of preventive psychiatry. Amsterdam: Elsevier; 1995. p. 492–514.
14. Fusar-Poli P, Rocchetti M, Sardella A, et al. Disorder, not just state of risk: meta-analysis of functioning and quality of life in people at high risk of psychosis. Br J Psychiatry 2015;207(3):198–206.
15. Fusar-Poli P, Nelson B, Valmaggia L, et al. Comorbid depressive and anxiety disorders in 509 individuals with an at-risk mental state: impact on psychopathology and transition to psychosis. Schizophr Bull 2014;40(1):120–31.
16. Fusar-Poli P, Borgwardt S, Bechdolf A, et al. The psychosis high-risk state: a comprehensive state-of-the-art review. JAMA Psychiatry 2013;70(1):107–20.
17. Yung AR, Phillips LJ, Yuen HP, et al. Psychosis prediction: 12-month follow up of a high-risk ("prodromal") group. Schizophr Res 2003;60(1):21–32.
18. Yung AR, Phillips LJ, Yuen HP, et al. Risk factors for psychosis in an ultra high-risk group: psychopathology and clinical features. Schizophr Res 2004;67(2–3): 131–42.
19. Fusar-Poli P, Carpenter WT, Woods SW, et al. Attenuated psychosis syndrome: ready for DSM-5.1? Annu Rev Clin Psychol 2014;10:155–92.

20. Carpenter WT, Regier D, Tandon R. Misunderstandings about attenuated psychosis syndrome in the DSM-5. Schizophr Res 2014;152(1):303.
21. Woods SW, Walsh BC, Saksa JR, et al. The case for including attentuated psychotic symptoms syndrome in DSM-5 as a psychosis risk syndrome. Schizophr Res 2010;123(2–3):199–207.
22. Carpenter WT. Attenuated psychosis syndrome: need for debate on a new disorder. Psychopathology 2014;47(5):287–91.
23. Nelson B. Attenuated psychosis syndrome: don't jump the gun. Psychopathology 2014;47(5):292–6.
24. van Os J, Hanssen M, Bijl RV, et al. Prevalence of psychotic disorder and community level of psychotic symptoms: an urban-rural comparison. Arch Gen Psychiatry 2001;58(7):663–8.
25. Tien AY. Distributions of hallucinations in the population. Soc Psychiatry Psychiatr Epidemiol 1991;26(6):287–92.
26. Verdoux H, van Os J. Psychotic symptoms in non-clinical populations and the continuum of psychosis. Schizophr Res 2002;54:59–65.
27. Johns LC, Cannon M, Singleton N, et al. Prevalence and correlates of self-reported psychotic symptoms in the British population. Br J Psychiatry 2004; 185:298–305.
28. McGorry PD, Yung AR, Phillips LJ. The "close-in" or ultra high-risk model: a safe and effective strategy for research and clinical intervention in prepsychotic mental disorder. Schizophr Bull 2003;29(4):771–90.
29. Yung AR, Yuen HP, McGorry PD, et al. Mapping the onset of psychosis: the comprehensive assessment of at-risk mental states. Aust N Z J Psychiatry 2005;39(11–12):964–71.
30. Miller TJ, McGlashan TH, Rosen JL, et al. Prodromal assessment with the structured interview for prodromal syndromes and the scale of prodromal symptoms: predictive validity, interrater reliability, and training to reliability. Schizophr Bull 2003;29(4):703–15.
31. Olsen KA, Rosenbaum B. Prospective investigations of the prodromal state of schizophrenia: assessment instruments. Acta Psychiatr Scand 2006;113(4): 273–82.
32. Huber G, Gross G. The concept of basic symptoms in schizophrenic and schizoaffective psychoses. Recenti Prog Med 1989;80(12):646–52.
33. Schultze-Lutter F. Subjective symptoms of schizophrenia in research and the clinic: the basic symptoms concept. Schizophr Bull 2009;35(1):5–8.
34. Schultze-Lutter F, Ruhrmann S, Berning J, et al. Basic symptoms and ultrahigh risk criteria: symptom development in the initial prodromal state. Schizophr Bull 2010;36(1):182–91.
35. Schultze-Lutter F, Addington J, Ruhrmann S, et al. Schizophrenia proneness instrument, adult version (SPI-A). Rome (Italy): Giovanni Fioriti Editore s.r.l.; 2007.
36. Fusar-Poli P, Bonoldi I, Yung AR, et al. Predicting psychosis: meta-analysis of transition outcomes in individuals at high clinical risk. Arch Gen Psychiatry 2012;69(3):220–9.
37. McGrath J, Saha S, Welham J, et al. A systematic review of the incidence of schizophrenia: the distribution of rates and the influence of sex, urbanicity, migrant status and methodology. BMC Med 2004;2:13.
38. Nelson B, Yuen HP, Wood SJ, et al. Long-term follow-up of a group at ultra high risk ("Prodromal") for psychosis: the PACE 400 study. JAMA Psychiatry 2013; 70(8):793–802.

39. Nelson B, Yuen HP, Lin A, et al. Further examination of the reducing transition rate in ultra high risk for psychosis samples: the possible role of earlier intervention. Schizophr Res 2016;174(1–3):43–9.

40. Hartmann JA, Yuen HP, McGorry PD, et al. Declining transition rates to psychotic disorder in "ultra-high risk" clients: investigation of a dilution effect. Schizophr Res 2016;170(1):130–6.

41. Yung AR, Yuen HP, Berger G, et al. Declining transition rate in ultra high risk (prodromal) services: dilution or reduction of risk? Schizophr Bull 2007;33(3):673–81.

42. Lin A, Wood SJ, Nelson B, et al. Outcomes of nontransitioned cases in a sample at ultra-high risk for psychosis. Am J Psychiatry 2015;172(3):249–58.

43. Beck K, Andreou C, Studerus E, et al. Clinical and functional long-term outcome of patients at clinical high risk (CHR) for psychosis without transition to psychosis: a systematic review. Schizophr Res 2019;210:39–47.

44. Cropley VL, Lin A, Nelson B, et al. Baseline grey matter volume of nontransitioned "ultra high risk" for psychosis individuals with and without attenuated psychotic symptoms at long-term follow-up. Schizophr Res 2015;173(3):152–8.

45. Yung AR, Nelson B, McGorry PD, et al. Persistent negative symptoms in individuals at Ultra High Risk for psychosis. Schizophr Res 2019;206:355–61.

46. Nelson B, Amminger GP, Yuen HP, et al. NEURAPRO: a multi-centre RCT of omega-3 polyunsaturated fatty acids versus placebo in young people at ultra-high risk of psychotic disorders—medium-term follow-up and clinical course. NPJ Schizophr 2018;4(1):11.

47. Yung AR, Cotter J, Wood SJ, et al. Childhood maltreatment and transition to psychotic disorder independently predict long-term functioning in young people at ultra-high risk for psychosis. Psychol Med 2015;45(16):3453–65.

48. Addington J, Farris M, Stowkowy J, et al. Predictors of transition to psychosis in individuals at clinical high risk. Curr Psychiatry Rep 2019;21(6):39.

49. Riecher-Rossler A, Studerus E. Prediction of conversion to psychosis in individuals with an at-risk mental state: a brief update on recent developments. Curr Opin Psychiatry 2017;30(3):209–19.

50. Mizrahi R. Social stress and psychosis risk: common neurochemical substrates? Neuropsychopharmacology 2016;41(3):666–74.

51. Clark SR, Schubert KO, Baune BT. Towards personalized secondary prevention of psychosis: using probabilistic assessments of transition risk in psychosis prodrome. J Neural Transm 2015;122:155–69.

52. Clark SR, Baune BT, Schubert KO, et al. Prediction of transition from ultra-high risk to first-episode psychosis using a probabilistic model combining history, clinical assessment and fatty-acid biomarkers. Transl Psychiatry 2016;6(9):e897.

53. Koutsouleris N, Kambeitz-Ilankovic L, Ruhrmann S, et al. Prediction models of functional outcomes for individuals in the clinical high-risk state for psychosis or with recent-onset depression: a multimodal, multisite machine learning analysis. JAMA Psychiatry 2018;75(11):1156–72.

54. Nelson B, McGorry PD, Wichers M, et al. Moving from static to dynamic models of the onset of mental disorder: a review. JAMA Psychiatry 2017;74(5):528–34.

55. Yuen HP, Mackinnon A. Performance of joint modelling of time-to-event data with time-dependent predictors: an assessment based on transition to psychosis data. PeerJ 2016;4:e2582.

56. Yuen HP, Mackinnon A, Hartmann J, et al. Dynamic prediction of transition to psychosis using joint modelling. Schizophr Res 2018;202:333–40.

57. Yuen HP, Mackinnon A, Nelson B. A new method for analysing transition to psychosis: joint modelling of time-to-event outcome with time-dependent predictors. Int J Methods Psychiatr Res 2018;27(1):1–12.
58. Studerus E, Ramyead A, Riecher-Rossler A. Prediction of transition to psychosis in patients with a clinical high risk for psychosis: a systematic review of methodology and reporting. Psychol Med 2017;47(7):1163–78.
59. Davies C, Cipriani A, Ioannidis JPA, et al. Lack of evidence to favor specific preventive interventions in psychosis: a network meta-analysis. World Psychiatry 2018;17(2):196–209.
60. Davies C, Radua J, Cipriani A, et al. Efficacy and acceptability of interventions for attenuated positive psychotic symptoms in individuals at clinical high risk of psychosis: a network meta-analysis. Front Psychiatry 2018;9:187.
61. Nelson B, Amminger GP, Yuen HP, et al. Staged Treatment in Early Psychosis: a sequential multiple assignment randomised trial of interventions for ultra high risk of psychosis patients. Early Interv Psychiatry 2018;12(3):292–306.
62. Galletly C, Castle D, Dark F, et al. Royal Australian and New Zealand College of Psychiatrists clinical practice guidelines for the management of schizophrenia and related disorders. Aust N Z J Psychiatry 2016;50(5):410–72.
63. International Early Psychosis Association Writing Group. International clinical practice guidelines for early psychosis. Br J Psychiatry 2005;187(suuplement 48):s120–4.
64. Schmidt SJ, Schultze-Lutter F, Schimmelmann BG, et al. EPA guidance on the early intervention in clinical high risk states of psychoses. Eur Psychiatry 2015; 30(3):388–404.
65. Addington J, Addington D, Abidi S, et al. Canadian treatment guidelines for individuals at clinical high risk of psychosis. Can J Psychiatry 2017;62(9):656–61.
66. Nelson B, Hughes A, Leicester S, et al. A stitch in time: interventions for young people at ultra high risk of psychosis. Melbourne, Australia: Orygen, The National Centre of Excellence in Youth Mental Health; 2014.
67. McGorry P, Keshavan M, Goldstone S, et al. Biomarkers and clinical staging in psychiatry. World Psychiatry 2014;13(3):211–23.
68. McGorry PD. Issues for DSM-V: clinical staging: a heuristic pathway to valid nosology and safer, more effective treatment in psychiatry. Am J Psychiatry 2007;164(6):859–60.
69. McGorry PD, Hickie IB, Yung AR, et al. Clinical staging of psychiatric disorders: a heuristic framework for choosing earlier, safer and more effective interventions. Aust N Z J Psychiatry 2006;40(8):616–22.
70. McGorry PD, Hartmann JA, Spooner R, et al. Beyond the "at risk mental state" concept: transitioning to transdiagnostic psychiatry. World Psychiatry 2018; 17(2):133–42.
71. Hyman SE. New evidence for shared risk architecture of mental disorders. JAMA Psychiatry 2019;76(3):235–6.
72. Cuijpers P. Examining the effects of prevention programs on the incidence of new cases of mental disorders: the lack of statistical power. Am J Psychiatry 2003; 160:1385–91.
73. Hartmann JA, Nelson B, Spooner R, et al. Broad clinical high-risk mental state (CHARMS): methodology of a cohort study validating criteria for pluripotent risk. Early Interv Psychiatry 2019;13(3):379–86.
74. Addington J, Goldstein BI, Wang JL, et al. Youth at-risk for serious mental illness: methods of the PROCAN study. BMC Psychiatry 2018;18(1):219.

Childhood-Onset Schizophrenia and Early-onset Schizophrenia Spectrum Disorders: An Update

David I. Driver, MD[a],*, Shari Thomas, MD[b], Nitin Gogtay, MD[c], Judith L. Rapoport, MD[d]

KEYWORDS

- Schizophrenia • Childhood-onset schizophrenia • Childhood psychosis

KEY POINTS

- Childhood-onset schizophrenia (COS) is an extraordinarily rare illness, with an incidence less than 0.04%. In both healthy children and children with a variety of other psychiatric illnesses, hallucinations are not uncommon; diagnosis should not be based on these alone.
- The evaluation of a child with suspected COS includes collecting extensive collateral information, observing patients/families over several visits, excluding underlying medical illnesses, and evaluating, with a high index of suspicion, for speech/language/educational deficits and comorbid mood or anxiety disorders.
- Once a diagnosis is established and other comorbidities are addressed, treatment planning should encompass aggressive psychopharmacologic, psychotherapeutic, and psychosocial interventions.
- Clozapine is an excellent third-line medication for use in COS. Epidemiologic studies demonstrate that its use often occurs much later than recommended by the clinical guidelines, despite having superior efficacy in the treatment refractory population.

The authors declare no conflicts of interest.

This is an update of an article that first appeared in the *Child and Adolescent Psychiatric Clinics of North America*, Volume 22, Issue 4, October 2013.

[a] Child Psychiatry Branch, National Institutes of Mental Health (NIMH), National Institutes Health (NIH), Building 10, Room 4N313C, 10 Center Drive, Bethesda, MD 20814, USA; [b] Healthy Foundations Group, 4350 East West Highway, Suite 200, Bethesda, Maryland 20814, USA; [c] National Institutes Health (NIH), NSC Building, Room 6104, 6001 Executive Boulevard, Rockville, MD 20852, USA; [d] National Institutes Health (NIH), Building 10-CRC, Room 6-5332, 10 Center Drive, Bethesda, MD 20814, USA

* Corresponding author.

E-mail address: david.driver@nih.gov

INTRODUCTION

The clinical severity, impact on development, and poor prognosis of childhood-onset schizophrenia (COS) may represent more homogeneous forms of the disorder.[1,2] In addition, the deleterious effects of incorrectly diagnosing COS are equally important to recognize. Despite the relatively high (up to 5%) prevalence of psychotic symptoms in otherwise healthy children,[3,4] COS is rare, so epidemiologic incidence data with diagnoses based on standardized clinical assessments are lacking. It is generally accepted that the incidence of COS is less than 0.04% based on the observations from the National Institute of Mental Health (NIMH) cohort. Approximately 30% to 50% of patients with affective or other atypical psychotic symptoms are misdiagnosed as COS,[5–9] and greater than 90% of the initial referrals to the NIMH study of COS received alternate diagnoses. Because the goal of NIMH study of COS was to study schizophrenia in its most homogeneous form, children with a diagnosis of schizoaffective disorder were excluded. In general, few schizoaffective children were seen by the authors during the study period, precluding any meaningful data analyses.

Although neurobiologically and phenomenologically continuous with its adult counterpart, COS represents a more severe form of the disorder,[10,11] with more prominent prepsychotic developmental disorders, brain abnormalities, and genetic risk factors.[2,9] The use of various screening and diagnostic tools has not proved as valuable as the longitudinal assessment by a judicious clinician. A unique benefit of the NIMH COS study was the washout period, whereby patients are observed as inpatients, medication-free, for up to 3 weeks. If a provisional diagnosis of COS was appropriate based on the screening process (clinical interview, records review, and structured interview), the patient was admitted to the unit and began the rigorous process of tapering all medications (up to 4 weeks). During this period, and the subsequent medication-free phase (up to 3 weeks), patients were observed by staff, received weekly ratings and had the support of up to 2 individually assigned staff members (ie, 2:1 staffing). This process ruled out COS in approximately 40% of the children provisionally diagnosed as COS.

Realizing the framework and limitations of the environment in which psychiatric providers operate, the authors' model is not feasible outside of the NIMH. The keys to attaining accurate diagnoses and optimizing treatment planning, however, lie in evaluating children suspected of having COS for speech/language/educational deficits, obtaining extensive collateral information, and observing patients and their families over several visits. Furthermore, COS carries with it a commitment to use a class of medications with a significant side-effect profile and significant long-term health risks.[12] Given the implications of the diagnosis, it is important for clinicians to exercise a considerable amount of caution and care when evaluating children with COS, being careful not to focus solely on addressing the psychotic symptoms and subsequently overlooking common comorbidities, such as receptive and expressive language disorders.

Research on the effects of a delayed diagnosis in COS is sparse, and this study design excluded children whose diagnosis may have been delayed, occurring after the age of 13. Even the adult literature is limited by the lack of a standardized measurement.[13,14] In adults and in early-onset schizophrenia (EOS), it has been shown that a delay in diagnosis results in a longer duration of untreated psychosis (DUP) and a subsequent robust, but moderate, effect on clinical outcome.[14,15] Furthermore, a 2016 review found that the mean DUP for EOS was 3.5-times longer than the mean DUP for adult-onset patients,[16] This may be due to the prevalence of comorbidities that complicate the presentation for EOS patients.

Although a measured, thoughtful approach to diagnosis is essential, making a timely diagnosis is also important.

PREMORBID PHENOTYPE

Of children with COS, 67% show premorbid disturbances in social, motor, and language domains as well as demonstrating learning disabilities and having what seem to be comorbid mood or anxiety disorders.

In addition, although not reported in studies of the premorbid history of adult-onset schizophrenia (AOS),[16,17] 27% have met criteria for autism/autism spectrum disorders (ASD) before the onset of their psychotic symptoms.[18] Outcome and prognosis have been positively correlated with the presence and severity of these developmental abnormalities,[16,19–21] with some studies suggesting the severity of these deficits may actually represent a premorbid phenotype for COS.[22–27]

The data on the premorbid functioning and symptomatology of the NIMH patients confirm and extend these findings. A review of the authors' cohort (n = 47) in 2000 showed that 55% had language abnormalities, 57% had motor abnormalities, and 55% had social abnormalities several years before the onset of psychotic symptoms. There was also a high rate of failed grades and special education placement.[24,28] Gender, familial psychopathology, and familial eye-tracking dysfunction have shown significant relationships with at least some aspect of the probands' premorbid development (**Table 1**).[24]

These results have been strengthened by a 2012 review of the authors' cohort (n = 118). Of the 118 children in the cohort, 65 (55.08%) had premorbid academic impairments, 85 (72.03%) had premorbid social/behavioral impairments, 60 (50.85%) had

Table 1 Relation of premorbid impairments to schizophrenia risk factors for 49 patients with childhood-onset schizophrenia			
Premorbid Impairment and Risk Factor	**Present (N)**	**Absent (N)**	**P Value**
Speech and language impairment			
Sex	27	22	.57
Score for family loading for schizophrenia spectrum disorders	27	21	.04
Mean family score for eye tracking	22	17	.04
Motor impairment			
Sex	28	21	.009
Score for family loading for schizophrenia spectrum disorders	28	20	.50
Mean family score for eye tracking	22	17	.25
Social impairment			
Sex	27	22	.56
Score for family loading for schizophrenia spectrum disorders	27	21	.15
Mean family score for eye tracking	19	20	.37

Table 2	
Realms of premorbid developmental problems based on 2012 chart review	
	N (%)
Social/behavioral	85 (72.03)
Academic	65 (55.08)
Language	60 (50.85)
Motor	52 (44.07)
Pervasive developmental disorder	24 (20.34)

premorbid language impairments, 52 (44.07%) had premorbid motor impairments, and 24 (20.34%) screened positive for pervasive developmental disorder (**Table 2**). The average number of abnormalities (15 domains) in each child was 3.89, and 103 (87.29%) children had premorbid impairment in at least one domain. In addition, 47% of children who did not have a pervasive developmental disorder (eg, autism, Asperger, or pervasive developmental disorder not otherwise specified) received pre-psychotic mental health treatment and/or a psychiatric or psychological evaluation.

DEFINITION/SYMPTOM CRITERIA

Since Kolvin's classic studies,[29] it is generally agreed on that COS can be diagnosed with the unmodified *Diagnostic and Statistical Manual of Mental Disorders* (Fourth Edition, Text Revision) *(DSM-IV-TR)* criteria for schizophrenia.[30] In addition, the NIMH study has defined COS, whereby the onset of psychotic symptoms is before the 13th birthday, combined with a premorbid intelligence quotient of 70 or above and absence of any significant neurologic problem. The *Diagnostic and Statistical Manual of Mental Disorders* (Fifth Edition) amends the criteria to reflect a gradient of psychopathology, from least to most severe, and provided updated severity dimensions.[31]

CLINICAL FINDINGS
Physical Examination

A diagnosis of COS requires exclusion of an underlying medical or psychiatric illness. It is only after all other identifiable causes of organic psychosis have been excluded that a diagnosis of COS can appropriately be considered. Details regarding the components of the physical examination of individuals suspected of having a primary psychiatric illness are discussed by Maja Skikic and Jose Alberto Arriola's article, "First Episode Psychosis Medical Workup: Evidence-Informed Recommendations and Introduction to a Clinically-Guided Approach," in this issue. A physical examination, including a thorough neurological examination is essential to the diagnostic process and clinicians should be vigilant to any abnormal physical and/or neurologic findings because COS is a diagnosis of exclusion. It is also important to bear in mind the rare medical causes and frequently missed diagnoses during the evaluation. Although discussed elsewhere in this issue, a select summary list is provided in **Table 3**.

Rating Scales and Diagnostic Modalities

For the NIMH COS study, the Social Communication Questionnaire, previously known as the Autism Screening Questionnaire, and the Kiddie Schedule for Affective Disorders and Schizophrenia–Present and Lifetime Version (K-SADS-PL) were used, with the supplemental ratings as indicated by the results of the K-SADS-PL, for all probands. The Schedule for Affective Disorders and Schizophrenia and the Structured

Table 3 Differential diagnoses of childhood-onset schizophrenia	
Medical etiologies	• Seizure disorder • Anti–N-methyl-ᴅ-aspartate receptor encephalitis • Herpes simplex encephalitis • Lysosomal storage diseases • Neurodegenerative disorders • Central nervous system tumors • Progressive organic central nervous system disorder (eg, sclerosing panencephalitis) • Metabolic disorders • Chromosomal disorders: 22q11 deletion syndrome[a]
Misdiagnosed psychiatric illnesses	• Psychotic depression • Bipolar disorder • ASDs; pervasive developmental disorders • Obsessive-compulsive disorder • Generalized anxiety disorder • Posttraumatic stress disorder • Multidimensionally impaired (not a formal *Diagnostic and Statistical Manual of Mental Disorders* diagnosis, but discussed later in the article): individuals with multiple language or learning disorders, mood lability, and transient psychotic symptoms

[a] Rates significantly higher than expected.[29,32,33]

Interview for DSM-III Personality Disorders were used to evaluate all family members for axis I and axis II disorders, respectively. During follow-up visits, the probands were evaluated using the Scale for the Assessment of Positive Symptoms, Scale for the Assessment of Negative Symptoms, Brief Psychiatric Rating Scale for Children, Clinical Global Impressions Scale, Children's Global Impressions Scale, Bunny-Hamburg Global Ratings, Simpson-Angus Scale, and Abnormal Involuntary Movement Scale.[34]

As discussed previously, it is simply not feasible to apply what was done at NIMH in the community. In clinical practice, it is routinely recommended to outpatient providers that they use the Scale for the Assessment of Positive Symptoms and Scale for the Assessment of Negative Symptoms to monitor clinical progress and the Abnormal Involuntary Movement Scale to monitor for potential side effects of the medication regimen (**Table 4**).

The NIMH COS branch developed a 2-item screen that identified children with COS and distinguished them from peers with nontrivial levels of psychosis with sensitivity and specificity of 79% and 78%, respectively.[35–53] The 2 items are the NIMH global scale depression and psychosis ratings, which are single items scored on a scale of 1 to 15, with higher numbers reflecting greater severity. This screen was validated on the sample of patients who presented to the NIMH COS branch and thus does not represent the heterogeneity of patients in the community.

Genetics

As discussed by Jennifer K. Forsyth and Robert F. Asarnow's article, "Genetics of Childhood-Onset Schizophrenia: 2019 Update," in this issue, genetic studies of COS and EOS demonstrate several variants, as opposed to a few highly penetrant mutations, contribute to the genetic risk of schizophrenia[54–58] and may even have an impact on response to antipsychotics.[59] Identification of common risk alleles in schizophrenia has allowed for composite polygenic risk scores to be calculated.

Table 4
Tools used by the National Institute of Mental Health child branch in the evaluation of childhood-onset schizophrenia

Tool	Description
Initial evaluation	
Social Communication Questionnaire, previously known as the Autism Screening Questionnaire	Brief instrument helps evaluate communication skills and social functioning in children who may have autism or ASDs. Completed by a parent or other primary caregiver in less than 10 min
K-SADS-PL	A semistructured diagnostic interview designed to assess current and past episodes of psychopathology in children and adolescents according to *Diagnostic and Statistical Manual of Mental Disorders* (Third Edition Revised) and *DSM-IV* criteria
Psychotic disorders supplement[a] Affective disorders supplement[a] Anxiety disorders supplement[a] Behavioral disorders supplement[a] Substance abuse and other disorders supplement[a]	Supplements to the K-SADS-PL used for diagnostic exploration and clarification; administered in the order in which symptoms appeared
Follow-up	
Scale for the Assessment of Positive Symptoms[b]	Assessment of positive symptoms of psychosis devised primarily to focus on schizophrenia
Scale for the Assessment of Negative Symptoms[b]	Assessment of negative symptoms of psychosis devised primarily to focus on schizophrenia
Brief Psychiatric Rating Scale for Children	A 21-item, clinician-based rating scale designed for use in evaluating psychiatric problems of children and adolescents
Clinical Global Impressions Scale[b]	A primary outcome frequently used in medical care and clinical research to measure in studies evaluating the efficacy of treatments
Children's Global Impressions Scale[b]	An adaptation of the Clinical Global Impressions Scale for children
Bunny-Hamburg Global Ratings Psychosis subscale[b] Depression subscale[b]	Two subscales that, when used together, best exclude COS as a viable diagnosis (62% accuracy at screening, 85% accuracy at the medication-free period)[34]
Simpson-Angus Scale	An established instrument for neuroleptic-induced parkinsonism
Abnormal Involuntary Movement Scale	12-item clinician administered and scored anchored scale used to detect and follow the occurrence of tardive dyskinesia in patients receiving neuroleptic medications

[a] Used as indicated by the results of the K-SADS-PL.
[b] Available in the *Handbook of Psychiatric Measures* (book with CD-ROM for Windows) by the American Psychiatric Association.

Using the results from the Psychiatric Genomic Consortium analysis of genome-wide association study data for schizophrenia, an association test was created using a set of 80 single nucleotide polymorphisms and 108 schizophrenia risk loci. The COS probands had higher polygenic risk scores compared with their siblings, and the polygenetic risk scores effectively predict COS. The risk score for autism was also calculated and was higher for the probands compared with their siblings.[54]

Many studies have shown that there are large and rare copy number variants (CNVs) associated with schizophrenia. The CNV burden was increased for genes controlling synaptic function and neurobehavior. Those with COS have a higher rate of common and rare CNVs compared with both their healthy siblings and AOS patients.[54,56]

Although a deletion at 15q13.3 has been shown to be an etiologic factor in psychiatric disorders, there were 2 patients with COS who had duplications at 15q13.3. The rate of this duplication is higher than what is seen in AOS, AOS controls, intellectual disability (ID) controls, and ASD controls. The rate of the duplication, however, was not significantly higher than what is seen in COS siblings, attention deficit hyperactivity disorder (ADHD), ADHD controls, ID, and ADHD.[55]

Despite these research findings, as well as the increased incidence of 22q11.2 deletion syndrome in individuals with schizophrenia versus the general population,[54,55,60–63] the American Academy of Child and Adolescent Psychiatry Treatment Guidelines do not recommend routine genetic screening for the evaluation of individuals with COS or EOS, unless there are phenotypic indicators of an underlying or comorbid genetic abnormality.[65]

Imaging

Structural brain abnormalities are an established feature of schizophrenia, characterized by decreased total gray matter (GM) volume reduction in cortex, hippocampus, and amygdala.[54,55,60–66] COS patients present with smaller brain volume and a progressive decline over adolescence.[67,68] They also have been shown to have larger ventricles with a greater progressive increase in ventricular size, with a particular difference in the lateral ventricles.[69]

The number of imaging studies of childhood and EOS is growing, with most them coming from the NIMH cohort. Advances in computational image analysis permit regional GM density, or cortical thickness measurements, which, when automated, can be applied to large samples, increasing statistical power,[56–59,60] which provides unprecedented anatomic detail of cortical GM change across both the entire cortex and the age (**Fig. 1**).[59,64] Prospective longitudinal brain magnetic resonance imaging rescan measures for the NIMH COS sample show progressive changes in COS, particularly during adolescence, and slowing as these COS patients reach age 20,[70–72] highlighting this period as critical and particularly vulnerable to treatment influences. As it is, the GM volume of COS is 8% to 10% less than that of age-matched controls. The result is a fixed volume deficit of 6% to 7% bilaterally.[73] There is no gender influence on the degree of cortical thinning seen in COS, but, for all subcortical structures, male patients had more volume than female patients.[74] These changes occur only during a limited period because the rate and degree of cortical loss if continued would resemble the extreme loss seen in some dementias.[59,64] These studies also support the previous findings that, although representing a more severe form, COS is continuous with its adult-onset counterpart. The total, frontal, temporal, and parietal GM loss, not seen in healthy children and adolescents or in those with atypical psychosis, seems to be diagnostically specific for COS.[70]

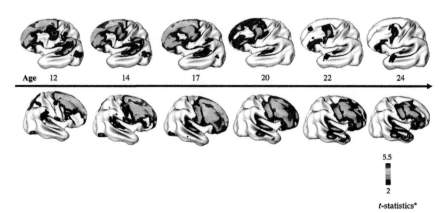

Fig. 1. Progression of cortical GM loss in COS (n = 70, 162 scans) relative to age-matched, sex-matched, and scan interval–matched healthy controls (n = 72, 168 scans) from adolescence to young adulthood (ages, 12–24 years).[67,69] Analyses were performed using mixed-model regression statistics and covaried from mean cortical thickness. Side bar shows *t*-statistic with threshold to control for multiple comparisons using the false discovery rate procedure with q = 0.05. Differences are from mixed model regression with age centered at approximately 3-year intervals for middle 80% of the age range; colors represent areas of statistically significant thinning in COS.[64]

Bilateral deficits in hippocampal volume are an established neurobiological difference seen in schizophrenia, and first-degree relatives of patients share hippocampal volume deficits.[75,76]

COS patients show fixed volumetric differences with inward deformities bilaterally at the anterior hippocampus compared with controls.[73,75–77] For COS patients, the degree of deformities correlates with symptom severity,[75,76] specifically positive symptoms.[73] Additionally, healthy siblings of COS patients also have an initially decreased cortical thickness, which lends support to the notion that this is a heritable risk factor rather than a marker of illness.[78]

The cerebellum is a particularly important anatomic structure because its development is highly heritable.[79] There is decreased cerebellar volume in the vermis, midsagittal inferior posterior lobe, and the surrounding area in COS.[79] COS patients also have smaller bilateral anterior lobes and smaller volumes of the anterior and total vermis.[80] Additionally, cerebellar deficits emerge over time in the healthy siblings of COS patients.[80]

The insula has been investigated for its potential etiologic role in positive symptoms due its role in discriminating between the self and nonself. There is evidence that the insula is activated during auditory hallucinations, and, in COS, there are more positive symptoms.[81] COS patients exhibit lower left, right, and total insula volumes compared with their healthy siblings and in total volume compared with controls. These volumetric differences are steady over time and correlate positively with global functioning and negatively with hallucinations.[82]

PATHOLOGIC CONDITION

Identifying the neurobiological basis and pathophysiology of schizophrenia is an essential future goal for establishing its diagnostic validity, delineating meaningful subtypes or alternate diagnoses, and finding causative mechanisms and novel targets for drug development.[83,84] To date, the cause of schizophrenia is unknown. There is general agreement that this is a brain disease, with alterations of white matter and gray matter, disconnectivity, and in vivo brain function. Research measures, such as neural synchrony, sleep architecture, smooth pursuit eye movements, and prepulse inhibition, all reflect widespread disorder.

The general model of schizophrenia as a neurodevelopmental disorder is widely held. One version focused on schizophrenia as a static lesion, occurring during fetal brain development,[85] whereas others argued that schizophrenia occurs as a result of a second hit in the form of abnormal brain development during adolescence, such as excessive synaptic and/or dendritic elimination resulting in aberrant neuronal connectivity.[9,86,87]

Altered connectivity that correlates with symptom severity in COS patients has been demonstrated in 26 brain regions in 2 key areas: the social and cognitive association areas (posterior cingulate, medial prefrontal cortex, and temporal regions) and the somatosensory and motor areas (precentral and postcentral gyri, supplementary motor area, and motor regions of the putamen and cerebellum).[88] Also, reduced connectivity between the frontal and temporal cortices in psychotic children 11 years old to 13 years old may explain why negative symptoms often emerge before positive symptoms.[89]

These theories have merged and it is now generally understood that COS is a multifactorial illness, characterized by multiple genetic elements, each contributing a modest degree of risk[90] and interacting with the environment. There also are various other hypotheses focused on the cortical amino acid neurotransmitter systems (ie, dopamine, glutamate, γ-aminobutyric acid [GABA], and serotonin).[91,92]

Alterations in genetics, neurodevelopment, and neurotransmitter systems[93] remain among the most promising directions for further research. Schizophrenia risk genes are associated with transcripts that are enriched in, or unique to, the human brain. Some also show preferential expression in the fetal brain.[94] Studies have revealed aberrant neuronal development, specifically localized to prefrontal and temporal cortices.[86] Alterations in timing of developmental disruption of GABAergic interneurons as the basis for several different neurodevelopmental disorders are gaining increasing support.[78] It is almost certain that both dopamine and glutamate transmission are abnormal in this disorder[73,74,95] and striatal dopamine overactivity may be critical to conversion to psychosis or psychotic symptoms generally.[8,75,86]

Not only are the causes of COS elusive bus also several roadblocks to progress toward finding the cause remain. First, the phenotypic, biologic, and etiologic heterogeneity of schizophrenia may account for the effect size of these individual risks not supporting any single neurobiological finding as a core deficit in the illness.[73,77,84] Second, the difficulty in studying the human brain and the lack of good animal models continue to be a handicap. Recent postmortem studies indicate time-specific developmental genetic effects. It remains clear, however, that schizophrenia, including COS, has no clearly definable neuropathologic markers (eg, demyelinated neurons in multiple sclerosis).[84] Although the study of COS suggests it may have more salient genetic effects,[79] there is no finding of even a rare form of genetic dominant transmission for COS.

DIAGNOSTIC DILEMMAS

The diagnosis of COS is a difficult, time-consuming process. Although early developmental abnormalities in social, motor, and language domains in COS are more striking compared with the later-onset cases,[22–24,28,80] they are not diagnostic and do not cumulatively represent a reliable premorbid phenotype. In addition, not only do healthy children experience hallucinations but also children with various other psychiatric and behavioral disturbances present with positive symptoms.[81,82] Pressure from families, the severity of the clinical picture, and time limitations placed on providers coalesce to make a diagnosis of COS a tedious process fraught with pitfalls. The most common disorders misdiagnosed as COS are affective disorders, organic psychosis, pervasive developmental disorders, and a group referred to as having atypical psychosis or as multidimensionally impaired (MDI). Details regarding these disorders, the last of which is an important differential, will be described in detail later, and achieving diagnostic clarity are described elsewhere in this issue.

The NIMH study was conducted from 1990 to 2017 and used nationwide recruitment. More than 3000 referrals were screened during this period. Of these, 90% were rejected from further consideration because they failed to meet the criteria for COS. More than 300 children were screened in person, of whom approximately 60% received other psychiatric diagnoses, such as affective disorders, anxiety, or behavioral disorders. More than 200 children who seemed likely to meet criteria for COS were admitted to the research unit and underwent an initial observation period followed by complete medication washout. After being observed off medications for up to 3 weeks, an additional 20% of children did not meet criteria for COS and received an alternative diagnosis. A 4-year to 6-year follow-up study of the ruled-out cases indicated good stability of the alternative diagnoses and nonschizophrenic status.[76] The most frequent alternative diagnoses have been affective disorders and anxiety disorders. A subgroup of children has also shown a form of atypical psychosis provisionally labeled MDI[28,96,97] based on a unique set of features, which warrants further description.

THE MULTIDIMENSIONALLY IMPAIRED GROUP

Thirty three children have been given the provisional diagnosis of MDI after the medication washout period and have been followed prospectively along with the COS children. This heterogeneous group of children, in general, has severe functional impairment associated with transient psychotic symptoms, multiple developmental abnormalities, abnormal neuropsychological test profiles, eye movement abnormalities, and familial risk factors that are not adequately characterized by existing *Diagnostic and Statistical Manual of Mental Disorders* (Fourth Edition) (*DSM-IV*) categories.[96,98,99] Despite the presence of overlapping symptoms with childhood and EOS, there are distinct features that have been used as operational diagnostic criteria by the NIMH group to distinguish these individuals[96,98]:

1. Brief, transient episodes of psychosis and perceptual disturbance, typically in response to stress
2. Nearly daily periods of emotional lability disproportionate to precipitants
3. Impaired interpersonal skills despite the desire to initiate peer friendships (distinction from COS)
4. Cognitive deficits as indicated by multiple deficits in information processing
5. No clear thought disorder (clinically can be difficult to define, especially in the presence of communication disorder)

ADHD is highly comorbid in the MDI group.

At first glance, the symptom cluster these patients present suggests these children will likely progress to develop schizophrenia spectrum disorders; in the

DSM-IV-TR, these patients could be considered psychotic disorder not otherwise specified. These children are similar in some way to some of the other syndromes described, such as the multiple complex developmental disorder, borderline syndrome of childhood, or other borderline disorders of childhood.[99–102] Contrary to MDI, however, these other syndromes have more predominant symptoms of pervasive developmental disorder, greater evidence of formal thought disorder, and onset before age 5.[99,103,104] The MDI group seems to have a distinct course, with none progressing to schizophrenia at long-term follow-up,[105] but strikingly, 38% developing bipolar disorder, type I.[88] These long-term data emphasize that when diagnosing a child with schizophrenia, there are significant short-term and long-term implications, including the potential for neglecting other disorders, because psychosis often becomes the primary focus.

PROCESS OF ELIMINATION

It has long been known that hallucinations, delusions, and disordered thoughts can occur in healthy nonpsychotic children[106] but usually diminish after age 6.[89] Transient anxiety-related and stress-related visual hallucinations also are occasionally reported in preschool children,[107] and the prognosis of these phenomena is benign. When psychotic phenomena occur in school-aged children, however, they generally tend to be more persistent and associated with drug toxicity or more significant mental illness.[1,108–110]

COMORBIDITIES

COS is highly correlated with other illnesses and disorders (**Box 1**).[24] During the evaluation of children with suspected COS, it is imperative they are screened, with a high index of suspicion, for other comorbid illnesses and disorders, both psychiatric[18] and medical[112] (see **Table 4**),[111] the latter of which accounts for almost 60% of premature deaths not related to suicide in adult schizophrenia patients.[112,113]

Box 1
Select comorbidities for childhood-onset schizophrenia

Psychiatric comorbidities
- Obsessive-compulsive disorder
- ADHD
- Expressive language disorders
- Receptive language disorders
- Auditory processing deficits
- Executive functioning deficits
- Mood disorder, primarily major depressive disorder

Medical comorbidities associated with treatment
- Diabetes[a]
- Hyperlipidemia[a]
- Cardiovascular disease[a]
- Obesity[a]
- Hyperprolactinemia[a]
- Dyskinesia

[a] Highly correlated with the treatment of schizophrenia.[111]

TREATMENT

Given the developmental impact of a diagnosis of COS or EOS, it is imperative that any treatment plan consists of both pharmacologic and nonpharmacologic interventions. Once the diagnosis is established, treatment planning should encompass aggressive psychopharmacologic, psychotherapeutic, and psychosocial interventions.

Two treatment trials were conducted in the NIMH COS cohort that demonstrated the superiority of clozapine over haloperidol and olanzapine as a third-line treatment of COS.[114] A review of the NIMH cohort also showed that COS patients have a greater degree of response to clozapine than do AOS patients.[115–122] This could be related to numerous variables, to include diagnostic validity, compliance, homogeneity of the sample, and management of side effects.

Asenapine and ziprasidone were not superior to placebo, and ziprasidone showed inferiority in a meta-analysis looking at seven second-generation antipsychotics (aripiprazole, asenapine, olanzapine, paliperidone, quetiapine, risperidone, and ziprasidone) and 1 first-generation antipsychotic (molindone).[123]

Although showing promise as a method to reduce the symptom exacerbations and increase compliance, to date, there have been no noteworthy or definitive studies on the use of long-acting injectables in the COS or EOS populations.

SUMMARY: IMPLICATIONS FOR CLINICAL PRACTICE

Schizophrenia is a devastating illness, particularly when presenting in childhood or adolescence. Despite the presence of premorbid characteristics, a reliable premorbid phenotype has not been defined, and research into the pathophysiology of the syndrome remains ongoing without a substantial target demonstrated in a systematic way. The frequency and duration of psychotic episodes have deleterious neuropsychological, neurophysiologic, and neurostructural effects,[124–128] making prompt, aggressive treatment an important component of care. Once a diagnosis is established and other comorbid conditions are adequately assessed, clinicians should treat this illness aggressively. Treatment planning should encompass psychopharmacologic, psychotherapeutic, and early psychosocial interventions, such as support and education of the family about the disorder, particularly during the first years of the evolution of the disease, because these can actually improve the course of illness.[129–136] In addition, clinicians should not avoid using clozapine, as evidenced by the epidemiologic studies demonstrating that its use occurs even much later than that recommended by the clinical guidelines.[129]

REFERENCES

1. Schreier HA. Hallucinations in nonpsychotic children: more common than we think? J Am Acad Child Adolesc Psychiatry 1999;38(5):623–5.

2. Childs B, Scriver CR. Age at onset and causes of disease. Perspect Biol Med 1986;29(3 Pt 1):437–60.

3. Kelleher I, Cannon M. Psychotic-like experiences in the general population: characterizing a high-risk group for psychosis. Psychol Med 2011;41(1):1–6.

4. Kelleher I, Connor D, Clarke MC, et al. Prevalence of psychotic symptoms in childhood and adolescence: a systematic review and meta-analysis of population-based studies. Psychol Med 2012;42(9):1857–63.

5. Werry JS. Child and adolescent (early onset) schizophrenia: a review in light of DSM-III-R. J Autism Dev Disord 1992;22(4):601–24.
6. McKenna K, Gordon CT, Rapoport JL. Childhood-onset schizophrenia: timely neurobiological research. J Am Acad Child Adolesc Psychiatry 1994;33(6): 771–81.
7. Gordon CT, Frazier JA, McKenna K, et al. Childhood-onset schizophrenia: an NIMH study in progress. Schizophr Bull 1994;20(4):697–712.
8. Gogtay N, Weisinger B, Bakalar JL, et al. Psychotic symptoms and gray matter deficits in clinical pediatric populations. Schizophr Res 2012;140(1–3):149–54.
9. Rapoport JL, Gogtay N. Childhood onset schizophrenia: support for a progressive neurodevelopmental disorder. Int J Dev Neurosci 2011;29(3):251–8.
10. Nicolson R, Malaspina D, Giedd JN, et al. Obstetrical complications and childhood-onset schizophrenia. Am J Psychiatry 1999;156(10):1650–2.
11. Nicolson R, Giedd JN, Lenane M, et al. Clinical and neurobiological correlates of cytogenetic abnormalities in childhood-onset schizophrenia. Am J Psychiatry 1999;156(10):1575–9.
12. De Hert M, Dobbelaere M, Sheridan EM, et al. Metabolic and endocrine adverse effects of second-generation antipsychotics in children and adolescents: a systematic review of randomized, placebo controlled trials and guidelines for clinical practice. Eur Psychiatry 2011;26(3):144–58.
13. Large M, Nielssen O, Slade T, et al. Measurement and reporting of the duration of untreated psychosis. Early Interv Psychiatry 2008;2(4):201–11.
14. Singh SP. Outcome measures in early psychosis; relevance of duration of untreated psychosis. Br J Psychiatry Suppl 2007;50:s58–63.
15. Schimmelman BG, Conus P, Cotton SM, et al. Pre-treatment, baseline, and outcome differences between early-onset and adult-onset psychosis in an epidemiological cohort of 636 first-episode patients. Schizophr Res 2017; 95:1–8.
16. Stentebjerg-Olesen M, Pagsberg AK, Fink-Jensen A, et al. Clinical characteristics and predictors of outcome of schizophrenia-spectrum psychosis in children and adolescents: a systematic review. J Child Adolesc Psychopharmacol 2016; 26(5):410–27.
17. Jones HJ, Stergiakouli E, Tansey KE, et al. Phenotypic manifestation of genetic risk for schizophrenia during adolescence in the general population. JAMA Psychiatry 2016;73:221–8.
18. Riglin L, Collishaw S, Richards A, et al. Schizophrenia risk alleles and neurodevelopmental outcomes in childhood: a population-based cohort study. Lancet Psychiatry 2017;4(1):57–62.
19. Black K, Peters L, Rui Q, et al. Duration of untreated psychosis predicts treatment outcome in an early psychosis program. Schizophr Res 2001;47(2–3): 215–22.
20. Done DJ, Crow TJ, Johnstone EC, et al. Childhood antecedents of schizophrenia and affective illness: social adjustment at ages 7 and 11. BMJ 1994; 309(6956):699–703.
21. Jones P, Rodgers B, Murray R, et al. Child development risk factors for adult schizophrenia in the British 1946 birth cohort. Lancet 1994;344(8934): 1398–402.
22. Rapoport J, Chavez A, Greenstein D, et al. Autism spectrum disorders and childhood-onset schizophrenia: clinical and biological contributions to a relation revisited. J Am Acad Child Adolesc Psychiatry 2009;48(1):10–8.

23. Gupta S, Rajaprabhakaran R, Arndt S, et al. Premorbid adjustment as a predictor of phenomenological and neurobiological indices in schizophrenia. Schizophr Res 1995;16(3):189–97.

24. Gupta S, Andreasen NC, Arndt S, et al. Neurological soft signs in neuroleptic-naive and neuroleptic-treated schizophrenic patients and in normal comparison subjects. Am J Psychiatry 1995;152(2):191–6.

25. Gupta SK, Kunka RL, Metz A, et al. Effect of alosetron (a new 5-HT3 receptor antagonist) on the pharmacokinetics of haloperidol in schizophrenic patients. J Clin Pharmacol 1995;35(2):202–7.

26. Hollis C. Child and adolescent (juvenile onset) schizophrenia. A case control study of premorbid developmental impairments. Br J Psychiatry 1995;166(4):489–95.

27. Alaghband-Rad J, McKenna K, Gordon CT, et al. Childhood-onset schizo- phrenia: the severity of premorbid course. J Am Acad Child Adolesc Psychiatry 1995;34(10):1273–83.

28. Nicolson R, Lenane M, Singaracharlu S, et al. Premorbid speech and language impairments in childhood-onset schizophrenia: association with risk factors. Am J Psychiatry 2000;157(5):794–800.

29. Kolvin I. Studies in the childhood psychoses. I. Diagnostic criteria and classification. Br J Psychiatry 1971;118(545):381–4.

30. Asarnow JR, Ben-Meir S. Children with schizophrenia spectrum and depressive disorders: a comparative study of premorbid adjustment, onset pattern and severity of impairment. J Child Psychol Psychiatry 1988;29(4):477–88.

31. Russell A, Bott L, Sammons C. The phenomena of schizophrenia occurring in childhood. J Am Acad Child Adolesc Psychiatry 1989;28:399–407.

32. Watkins JM, Asarnow RF, Tanguay PE. Symptom development in childhood onset schizophrenia. J Child Psychol Psychiatry 1988;29(6):865–78.

33. Nicolson R, Rapoport JL. Childhood-onset schizophrenia: rare but worth studying. Biol Psychiatry 1999;46(10):1418–28.

34. Association AP. Recent updates to proposed revisions for DSM-5. 2012. Available at: http://www.dsm5.org/Pages/RecentUpdates.aspx. Accessed November 28, 2012.

35. Greenstein D, Kataria R, Gochman P, et al. Looking for childhood-onset schizophrenia: diagnostic algorithms for classifying children and adolescents with psychosis. J Child Adolesc Psychopharmacol 2014;24(7):366–73.

36. Kumra S, Jacobsen LK, Lenane M, et al. Multidimensionally impaired disorder": is it a variant of very early-onset schizophrenia? J Am Acad Child Adolesc Psychiatry 1998;37(1):91–9.

37. Towbin KE, Dykens EM, Pearson GS, et al. Conceptualizing "borderline syndrome of childhood" and "childhood schizophrenia" as a developmental disorder. J Am Acad Child Adolesc Psychiatry 1993;32(4):775–82.

38. Dahl EK, Cohen DJ, Provence S. Clinical and multivariate approaches to the nosology of pervasive developmental disorders. J Am Acad Child Psychiatry 1986;25(2):170–80.

39. Petti TA, Vela RM. Borderline disorders of childhood: an overview. J Am Acad Child Adolesc Psychiatry 1990;29(3):327–37.

40. Van der Gaag RJ, Buitelaar J, Van den Ban E, et al. A controlled multivariate chart review of multiple complex developmental disorder. J Am Acad Child Adolesc Psychiatry 1995;34(8):1096–106.

41. Cohen DJ, Paul R, Volkmar FR. Issues in the classification of pervasive and other developmental disorders: toward DSM-IV. J Am Acad Child Psychiatry 1986; 25(2):213–20.

42. Ad-Dab'bagh Y, Greenfield B. Multiple complex developmental disorder: the "multiple and complex" evolution of the "childhood borderline syndrome" construct. J Am Acad Child Adolesc Psychiatry 2001;40(8):954–64.

43. Nicolson R, Lenane M, Brookner F, et al. Children and adolescents with psychotic disorder not otherwise specified: a 2- to 8-year follow-up study. Compr Psychiatry 2001;42(4):319–25.

44. Gogtay N, Ordonez A, Herman DH, et al. Dynamic mapping of cortical development before and after the onset of pediatric bipolar illness. J Child Psychol Psychiatry 2007;48(9):852–62.

45. Lukianowicz N. Hallucinations in non-psychotic children. Psychiatr Clin (Basel) 1969;2(6):321–37.

46. Caplan R. Thought disorder in childhood. J Am Acad Child Adolesc Psychiatry 1994;33(5):605–15.

47. Rothstein A. Hallucinatory phenomena in childhood. A critique of the literature. J Am Acad Child Psychiatry 1981;20(3):623–35.

48. Abramowicz M. Drugs that cause psychiatric symptoms. Med Lett Drugs Ther 1993;35:65–70.

49. Davison K. Schizophrenia-like psychoses associated with organic cerebral disorders: a review. Psychiatr Dev 1983;1(1):1–33.

50. McGee R, Williams S, Poulton R. Hallucinations in nonpsychotic children. J Am Acad Child Adolesc Psychiatry 2000;39(1):12–3.

51. Lambert TJ, Velakoulis D, Pantelis C. Medical comorbidity in schizophrenia. Med J Aust 2003;178(Suppl):S67–70.

52. Colton CW, Manderscheid RW. Congruencies in increased mortality rates, years of potential life lost, and causes of death among public mental health clients in eight states. Prev Chronic Dis 2006;3(2):A42.

53. Goff DC, Cather C, Evins AE, et al. Medical morbidity and mortality in schizophrenia: guidelines for psychiatrists. J Clin Psychiatry 2005;66(2):183–94 [quiz: 147]. 273–4.

54. Ahn K, An SS, Shugart YY, et al. Common polygenic variation and risk for childhood-onset schizophrenia. Mol Psychiatry 2016;21(1):94–6.

55. Zhou D, Gochman P, Broadnax DD, et al. 15q13.3 duplication in two patients with childhood-onset schizophrenia. Am J Med Genet B Neuropsychiatr Genet 2016;171(6):777–83.

56. Hoffmann A, Ziller M, Spengler D. Childhood-onset schizophrenia: insights from induced pluripotent stem cells. Int J Mol Sci 2018;19(12) [pii:E3829].

57. Curie A, Lesca G, Bussy G, et al. Asperger syndrome and early-onset schizophrenia associated with a novel MECP2 deleterious missense variant. Psychiatr Genet 2017;27(3):105–9.

58. Jolly LA, Homan CC, Jacob R, et al. The UPF3B gene, implicated in intellectual disability, autism, ADHD and childhood onset schizophrenia regulates neural progenitor cell behaviour and neuronal outgrowth. Hum Mol Genet 2013; 22(23):4673–87.

59. Ambalavanan A, Girard SL, Ahn K, et al. De novo variants in sporadic cases of childhood onset schizophrenia. Eur J Hum Genet 2016;24(6):944–8.

60. Arinami T, Ohtsuki T, Takase K, et al. Screening for 22q11 deletions in a schizophrenia population. Schizophr Res 2001;52(3):167–70.

61. Green T, Gothelf D, Glaser B, et al. Psychiatric disorders and intellectual functioning throughout development in velocardiofacial (22q11.2 deletion) syndrome. J Am Acad Child Adolesc Psychiatry 2009;48(11):1060–8.

62. Monteiro FP, Vieira TP, Sgardioli IC, et al. Defining new guidelines for screening the 22q11.2 deletion based on a clinical and dysmorphologic evaluation of 194 individuals and review of the literature. Eur J Pediatr 2013;172(7):927–45.

63. Ahn K, Gotay N, Andersen TM, et al. High rate of disease-related copy number variations in childhood onset schizophrenia. Mol Psychiatry 2014;19(5):568–72.

64. McClellan J, Stock S, American Academy of Child and Adolescent Psychiatry (AACAP) Committee on Quality Issues (CQI). Practice parameter for the assessment and treatment of children and adolescents with schizophrenia. J Am Acad Child Adolesc Psychiatry 2013;52(9):976–90.

65. Murphy KC, Jones LA, Owen MJ. High rates of schizophrenia in adults with velocardio-facial syndrome. Arch Gen Psychiatry 1999;56(10):940–5.

66. Gochman P, Miller R, Rapoport JL. Childhood-onset schizophrenia: the challenge of diagnosis. Curr Psychiatry Rep 2011;13(5):321–2.

67. Giedd JN, Jeffries NO, Blumenthal J, et al. Childhood-onset schizophrenia: progressive brain changes during adolescence. Biol Psychiatry 1999;46(7):892–8.

68. Giedd JN, Raznahan A, Alexander-Bloch A, et al. Child psychiatry branch of the National Institute of Mental Health longitudinal structural magnetic resonance imaging study of human brain development. Neuropsychopharmacology 2015;40(1):43–9.

69. Rapoport JL, Giedd J, Kumra S, et al. Childhood-onset schizophrenia. progressive ventricular change during adolescence. Arch Gen Psychiatry 1997;54(10):897–903.

70. Lawrie SM, Abukmeil SS. Brain abnormality in schizophrenia. A systematic and quantitative review of volumetric magnetic resonance imaging studies. Br J Psychiatry 1998;172:110–20.

71. Wright IC, Rabe-Hesketh S, Woodruff PW, et al. Meta-analysis of regional brain volumes in schizophrenia. Am J Psychiatry 2000;157(1):16–25.

72. Shenton ME, Dickey CC, Frumin M, et al. A review of MRI findings in schizophrenia. Schizophr Res 2001;49(1–2):1–52.

73. Anvari AA, Friedman LA, Greenstein D, et al. Hippocampal volume change relates to clinical outcome in childhood-onset schizophrenia. Psychol Med 2015;45(12):2667–74.

74. Weisinger B, Greenstein D, Mattai A, et al. Lack of gender influence on cortical and subcortical gray matter development in childhood-onset schizophrenia. Schizophr Bull 2013;39(1):52–8.

75. Johnson SL, Wang L, Alpert KI, et al. Hippocampal shape abnormalities of patients with childhood-onset schizophrenia and their unaffected siblings. J Am Acad Child Adolesc Psychiatry 2013;52(5):527–36.e2.

76. Johnson SL, Greenstein D, Clasen L, et al. Absence of anatomic corpus callosal abnormalities in childhood-onset schizophrenia patients and healthy siblings. Psychiatry Res 2013;211(1):11–6.

77. Mattai A, Hosanagar A, Weisinger B, et al. Hippocampal volume development in healthy siblings of childhood-onset schizophrenia patients. Am J Psychiatry 2011;168(4):427–35.

78. Ordóñez AE, Luscher ZI, Gogtay N. Neuroimaging findings from childhood onset schizophrenia patients and their non-psychotic siblings. Schizophr Res 2016;173(3):124–31.

79. Jacobsen LK, Giedd JN, Berquin PC, et al. Quantitative morphology of the cerebellum and fourth ventricle in childhood onset schizophrenia. Am J Psychiatry 1997;154(12):1663–9.
80. Greenstein D, Lenroot R, Clasen L, et al. Cerebellar development in childhood onset schizophrenia and non-psychotic siblings. Psychiatry Res 2011;193(3): 131–7.
81. Jardri R, Pouchet A, Pins D, et al. Cortical activations during auditory verbal hallucinations in schizophrenia: a coordinate based meta-analysis. Am J Psychiatry 2011;168:73–81.
82. Moran ME, Weisinger B, Ludovici K, et al. At the boundary of the self: the insular cortex in patients with childhood-onset schizophrenia, their healthy siblings, and normal volunteers. Int J Dev Neurosci 2014;32:58–63.
83. Pantelis C, Yucel M, Wood SJ, et al. Structural brain imaging evidence for multiple pathological processes at different stages of brain development in schizophrenia. Schizophr Bull 2005;31(3):672–96.
84. Mathalon DH, Sullivan EV, Lim KO, et al. Progressive brain volume changes and the clinical course of schizophrenia in men: a longitudinal magnetic resonance imaging study. Arch Gen Psychiatry 2001;58(2):148–57.
85. Gur RE, Cowell P, Turetsky BI, et al. A follow-up magnetic resonance imaging study of schizophrenia. Relationship of neuroanatomical changes to clinical and neurobehavioral measures. Arch Gen Psychiatry 1998;55(2):145–52.
86. Lieberman J, Chakos M, Wu H, et al. Longitudinal study of brain morphology in first episode schizophrenia. Biol Psychiatry 2001;49(6):487–99.
87. DeLisi LE. Regional brain volume change over the life-time course of schizophrenia. J Psychiatr Res 1999;33(6):535–41.
88. Berman RA, Gotts SJ, McAdams HM, et al. Disrupted sensorimotor and social-cognitive networks underlie symptoms in childhood-onset schizophrenia. Brain 2016;139(Pt 1):276–91.
89. Jacobson S, Kelleher I, Harley M, et al. Structural and functional brain correlates of subclinical psychotic symptoms in 11-13 year old school children. Neuroimage 2010;49:1875–88.
90. Gogtay N. Cortical brain development in schizophrenia: insights from neuroimaging studies in childhood-onset schizophrenia. Schizophr Bull 2008; 34(1):30–6.
91. Luders E, Narr KL, Thompson PM, et al. Mapping cortical gray matter in the young adult brain: effects of gender. Neuroimage 2005;26(2):493–501.
92. Thompson PM, Mega MS, Vidal C, et al. Detecting disease specific patterns of brain structure using cortical pattern matching and a population-based probabilistic brain Atlas, IEEE conference on information processing in medical imaging (IPMI), UC Davis 2001. In: Insana M, Leahy RM, editors. Lecture notes in Computer Science (LNCS), vol. 2082. Berlin: Springer-Verlag; 2001. p. 488–501.
93. Thompson PM, Giedd JN, Woods RP, et al. Growth patterns in the developing brain detected by using continuum mechanical tensor maps. Nature 2000; 404(6774):190–3.
94. Gogtay N, Giedd JN, Lusk L, et al. Dynamic mapping of human cortical development during childhood through early adulthood. Proc Natl Acad Sci U S A 2004;101(21):8174–9.
95. Watsky RE, Pollard KL, Greenstein D, et al. Severity of cortical thinning correlates with schizophrenia spectrum symptoms. J Am Acad Child Adolesc Psychiatry 2016;55(2):130–6.

96. Greenstein D, Lerch J, Shaw P, et al. Childhood onset schizophrenia: cortical brain abnormalities as young adults. J Child Psychol Psychiatry 2006;47(10): 1003–12.

97. Gogtay N, Greenstein D, Lenane M, et al. Cortical brain development in nonpsychotic siblings of patients with childhood-onset schizophrenia. Arch Gen Psychiatry 2007;64(7):772–80.

98. Gogtay N, Sporn A, Clasen LS, et al. Comparison of progressive cortical gray matter loss in childhood-onset schizophrenia with that in childhood-onset atyp- ical psychoses. Arch Gen Psychiatry 2004;61(1):17–22.

99. Sporn AL, Greenstein DK, Gogtay N, et al. Progressive brain volume loss during adolescence in childhood-onset schizophrenia. Am J Psychiatry 2003;160(12): 2181–9.

100. Gogtay N, Sporn A, Clasen LS, et al. Structural brain MRI abnormalities in healthy siblings of patients with childhood-onset schizophrenia. Am J Psychiatry 2003;160(3):569–71.

101. Keshavan MS, Berger G, Zipursky RB, et al. Neurobiology of early psychosis. Br J Psychiatry Suppl 2005;48:s8–18.

102. Keshavan MS, Tandon R, Boutros NN, et al. Schizophrenia, "just the facts": what we know in 2008. Part 3: neurobiology. Schizophr Res 2008;106(2–3): 89–107.

103. Weinberger DR. Implications of normal brain development for the pathogenesis of schizophrenia. Arch Gen Psychiatry 1987;44(7):660–9.

104. Rapoport JL, Giedd JN, Gogtay N. Neurodevelopmental model of schizo- phrenia: update 2012. Mol Psychiatry 2012;17(12):1228–38.

105. Feinberg I. Schizophrenia: caused by a fault in programmed synaptic elimination during adolescence? J Psychiatr Res 1982;17(4):319–34.

106. Yang Z, Xu Y, Xu T, et al. Brain network informed subject community detection in early-onset schizophrenia. Sci Rep 2014;4:5549.

107. Gogos JA, Gerber DJ. Schizophrenia susceptibility genes: emergence of positional candidates and future directions. Trends Pharmacol Sci 2006;27(4): 226–33.

108. Miyamoto S, LaMantia AS, Duncan GE, et al. Recent advances in the neurobiology of schizophrenia. Mol Interv 2003;3(1):27–39.

109. Weinberger DR. The biological basis of schizophrenia: new directions. J Clin Psychiatry 1997;58(Suppl 10):22–7.

110. Sawa A, Snyder SH. Schizophrenia: diverse approaches to a complex disease. Science 2002;296(5568):692–5.

111. Marin O. Interneuron dysfunction in psychiatric disorders. Nat Rev Neurosci 2012;13(2):107–20.

112. Kleinman JE, Law AJ, Lipska BK, et al. Genetic neuropathology of schizo- phrenia: new approaches to an old question and new uses for postmortem hu- man brains. Biol Psychiatry 2011;69(2):140–5.

113. Henn FA. Dopamine: a marker of psychosis and final common driver of schizophrenia psychosis. Am J Psychiatry 2011;168(12):1239–40.

114. Gogtay N, Rapoport JL. Clozapine use in children and adolescents. Expert Opin Pharmacother 2008;9(3):459–65.

115. Kasoff LI, Ahn K, Gochman P, et al. Strong treatment response and high maintenance rates of clozapine in childhood-onset schizophrenia. J Child Adolesc Psychopharmacol 2016;26(5):428–35.

116. Al-Dhaher Z, Kapoor S, Saito E, et al. Activating and tranquilizing effects of first-time treatment with aripiprazole, olanzapine, quetiapine, and risperidone in youth. J Child Adolesc Psychopharmacol 2016;26(5):458–70.

117. Ienciu M, Romosan F, Bredicean C, et al. First episode psychosis and treatment delay–causes and consequences. Psychiatr Danub 2010;22(4):540–3.

118. Franz L, Carter T, Leiner AS, et al. Stigma and treatment delay in first-episode psychosis: a grounded theory study. Early Interv Psychiatry 2010; 4(1):47–56.

119. Norman RM, Mallal AK, Manchanda R, et al. Does treatment delay predict occupational functioning in first-episode psychosis? Schizophr Res 2007;91(1–3): 259–62.

120. Compton MT, Esterberg ML. Treatment delay in first-episode nonaffective psychosis: a pilot study with African American family members and the theory of planned behavior. Compr Psychiatry 2005;46(4):291–5.

121. Harrigan SM, McGorry PD, Krstev H. Does treatment delay in first-episode psychosis really matter? Psychol Med 2003;33(1):97–110.

122. Vera I, Rezende L, Molina V, et al. Clozapine as treatment of first choice in first psychotic episodes. What do we know? Actas Esp Psiquiatr 2012;40(5):281–9.

123. Pagsberg AK, Tarp S, Glintborg D, et al. Acute antipsychotic treatment of children and adolescents with schizophrenia spectrum disorders: a systematic review and network meta-analysis. J Am Acad Child Adolesc Psychiatry 2017; 56(3):191–202.

124. Lewis DA, Gonzalez-Burgos G. Neuroplasticity of neocortical circuits in schizophrenia. Neuropsychopharmacology 2008;33(1):141–65.

125. Beneyto M, Lewis DA. Insights into the neurodevelopmental origin of schizophrenia from postmortem studies of prefrontal cortical circuitry. Int J Dev Neurosci 2011;29(3):295–304.

126. Howes OD, Bose SK, Turkheimer F, et al. Dopamine synthesis capacity before onset of psychosis: a prospective [18F]-DOPA PET imaging study. Am J Psychiatry 2011;168(12):1311–7.

127. Howes OD, Kapur S. The dopamine hypothesis of schizophrenia: version III–the final common pathway. Schizophr Bull 2009;35(3):549–62.

128. Tandon R, Keshavan MS, Nasrallah HA. Schizophrenia, "just the facts" what we know in 2008. 2. Epidemiology and etiology. Schizophr Res 2008; 102(1–3):1–18.

129. Tsuang MT, Faraone SV. The case for heterogeneity in the etiology of schizophrenia. Schizophr Res 1995;17(2):161–75.

130. Walsh T, McClellan JM, McCarthy SE, et al. Rare structural variants disrupt multiple genes in neurodevelopmental pathways in schizophrenia. Science 2008; 320(5875):539–43.

131. Green WH, Padron-Gayol M, Hardesty AS, et al. Schizophrenia with childhood onset: a phenomenological study of 38 cases. J Am Acad Child Adolesc Psychiatry 1992;31(5):968–76.

132. Garralda ME. Hallucinations in children with conduct and emotional disorders:II. The follow-up study. Psychol Med 1984;14(3):597–604.

133. Garralda ME. Hallucinations in children with conduct and emotional disorders: I. The clinical phenomena. Psychol Med 1984;14(3):589–96.

134. Calderoni D, Wudarsky M, Bhangoo R, et al. Differentiating childhood-onset schizophrenia from psychotic mood disorders. J Am Acad Child Adolesc Psychiatry 2001;40(10):1190–6.

135. McKenna K, Gordon CT, Lenane M, et al. Looking for childhood-onset schizo-phrenia: the first 71 cases screened. J Am Acad Child Adolesc Psychiatry 1994;33(5):636–44.
136. Kumra S, Briguglio C, Lenane M, et al. Including children and adolescents with schizophrenia in medication-free research. Am J Psychiatry 1999;156(7): 1065–8.

Affective Disorders with Psychosis in Youth
An Update

Gabrielle A. Carlson, MD[a], Caroly Pataki, MD[b],*

KEYWORDS

- Mania • Depression • Bipolar • Psychosis • Mood congruent/incongruent

KEY POINTS

- Studies in adults and youth of mood disorders with psychosis have been complicated by misunderstanding the state versus trait aspect of the psychosis.
- It is important, especially in children, to distinguish between true psychosis and nonspecific odd beliefs and transitory hallucinations. This is true even in high-risk samples.
- Mood-related psychotic symptoms are more likely to occur in the context of a severe mood disorder; however, some individuals with severe mood disorders do not experience psychotic symptoms.
- Psychotic symptoms seem to be strongly associated with childhood adversity, especially abuse, and may occur in the absence of a major depressive disorder or bipolar disorder.
- Eliciting psychotic symptoms in youth requires experience. There are a number of structured assessments that help word the questions.

HISTORY

Although manic depression was considered a "psychosis" in the *Diagnostic and Statistical Manual of Mental Disorders* (DSM) I and II, for all intents and purposes, severe psychosis was mostly associated with schizophrenia rather than mood disorders in both adults and youth until the 1980s. Three somewhat related events elevated the importance of psychosis in depression and mania. First, there was a growing

Disclosures: Research funding from NIMH, PCORI. Dr G.A. Carlson's husband is on the data safety monitoring board for Pfizer (ziprasidone) and Lundbeck (vortioxetine).
[a] Child and Adolescent Psychiatry, Stony Brook University School of Medicine, Putnam Hall – South Campus, 101 Nichols Road, Stony Brook, NY 11794, USA; [b] Department of Psychiatry and Biobehavioral Sciences, David Geffen School of Medicine, University of California Los Angeles, 546 16th Street, Los Angeles, CA 90402, USA
* Corresponding author.
E-mail address: CPataki@mednet.ucla.edu

Abbreviations	
CI	confidence interval
DSM	diagnostic and statistical manual of mental disorders
KSADS	schedule for affective disorders and schizophrenia for school aged children present and lifetime version
MDD	major depressive disorder

realization in the 1960s that psychiatric diagnoses were very unreliable. The "cross-national study of diagnosis of mental disorders: hospital diagnoses and hospital patients in New York and London" established that although symptoms of patients admitted to psychiatric hospitals in the United States and UK were very similar, the proportion of patients given a diagnosis of schizophrenia was nearly twice as high in the United States as the UK.[1] The US concept of schizophrenia was very broad and encompassed patients who in the UK were regarded as suffering from depression, mania (sometimes with psychosis), or personality disorder. Shortly after this, the International Pilot Study of Schizophrenia confirmed that psychiatrists in the United States (and also in Moscow) had a broader concept of the disorder than other countries.[2]

A second relevant contribution came from Washington University of St. Louis's Department of Psychiatry where 2 important publications, the 1973 "Feighner criteria,"[3] and a book on *Manic-depressive Illness* by Winokur and associates[4] that delineated the phenomenology of manic-depression. The goal to revolutionize psychiatric diagnoses, which led to the DSM III, emerged from this renewed interest in phenomenology, and the definition of schizophrenia became more narrowly defined, and the symptoms of mania and depression with psychosis were also spelled out more clearly.

The final important influence resulted from the approval of lithium carbonate for the acute and prophylactic treatment of mania in 1970. That made the task of recognizing manic depression and differentiating it from schizophrenia of great clinical importance.[5] A number of studies were published highlighting the fact that there could be periods during an affective psychosis in which symptoms seemed to be indistinguishable from schizophrenia[6,7] and that proper diagnosis of what we now call bipolar disorder could be life changing for patients.[5]

Child and adolescent psychiatrists ultimately embraced the fact that mood disorders were common at least in adolescents and that distinguishing schizophrenia from serious mood disorders where both mania and depression could emerge with extreme psychosis could be achieved by obtaining more systematic information on patient history, phenomenology and family history.[8–11] Severe psychosis, however, had not been a problem in prepubertal children diagnosed with bipolar disorder.

ISSUES COMPLICATING THE STUDY OF AFFECTIVE PSYCHOSIS

Several issues complicate the interpretation of studies of affective psychosis. By definition, in mood disorder with psychosis, psychosis should occur only within a mood episode. However, mood episodes are often recurrent, so patients can be psychotic within one episode and not another.[12] For instance, in a county-wide sample of patients with a first hospitalization for psychosis,[13] 37% of the sample had subsequent mood episodes but no further psychosis over the next 48 months. Thus, it is important to understand whether a study was done on a patient with a lifetime psychosis (which has long since remitted) or a current psychosis.

The significance of psychosis also is not clear.[14] Although it could be a severity marker,[15] patients with equally severe mood symptoms by other criteria are not necessarily psychotic.[16,17] Relatedly, psychosis is more common in mania than depression, but bipolar depression with psychosis is not rare and in an adolescent, may be the harbinger of a future bipolar course (see[18,19] for review).

In addition, the term bipolar disorder with psychosis does not tell us whether the patient had mania, depression, or both with psychosis. Some studies indicate that psychosis during mania worsens the prognosis, including more frequent relapses, greater chronicity, and less complete remission between episodes, whereas other studies have found no difference in outcome.[13,20] In young people, a first episode of psychotic depression may portend a bipolar course while psychotic symptoms in a nonbipolar depression may portend a schizophrenic course.[21]

There is a spectrum of psychosis that includes nondiagnostic phenomena (eg, brief hallucinations) that occur in up to 10% of the general population[22] and are even more common in children, with 17% of 9- to 12-year-olds and 7.5% of 13- to 18-year-olds reporting symptoms.[23] Factors distinguishing psychotic-like experiences are symptom frequency, distress, help seeking, degree of negative content of hallucinations, and the overall impairment conferred by voices with negative content.[24]

Finally, psychotic symptoms that are very detailed or overly dramatic, or where content is associated with past traumatic experiences, or only present when the person is angry, or presented for some gain, are likely to be transient, and probably do not represent true affective disorder psychosis.[25]

RATES OF PSYCHOSIS IN CLINIC SAMPLES

Rates of psychosis in youth with affective disorder depend on where the sample is obtained (research or clinic sample), the age of the child (child or adolescent), and the type interview used to elicit psychotic symptoms (eg,[26–30]). In a large clinical sample (n = 2031 of youths ages 5–21), the Schedule for Affective Disorders and Schizophrenia for School Aged Children Present and Lifetime Version (KSADS–PL)[26] revealed 91 (4.5%) with definite psychotic symptoms, 95 (4.7%) with probable psychotic symptoms, and 1845 (90.8%) without psychotic symptoms.[27] Among those with definite psychosis, 44% had major depressive disorder (MDD), 22% had bipolar disorder (presumably mania, but this was not specified), and the rest had assorted other disorders, with conduct disorder (16.5%) being the largest residual category. Factor analysis of the psychotic symptoms indicated that hallucinations explained most of the variance (21%), followed by thought disorder (11%), delusions (6%), and manic thought disorder (6%). However, the factor analysis was for all psychotic symptoms, not specifically for mood-related psychosis.

Bipolar disorder, which has been studied much more frequently than nonbipolar major depression, can be divided into those that examine lifetime versus current psychosis. In mania, lifetime psychotic symptoms vary considerably from a low of about 16%[28,29] to a high of 60%.[30–33] Kowatch and colleagues[34] summed this up with a meta-analysis of studies, deriving a weighted rate of psychosis of 42% (95% confidence interval [CI], 24%–62%) but with statistically significant differences in rates among the samples. The range of psychosis in adults with bipolar disorder is somewhat higher with a weighted mean of 62% and range from 47% to 90%.[35(p53)]

Rates of current manic symptoms are more difficult to glean from reported studies and are best obtained from drug studies, where current mood episode is being rated and treated. These rates are much lower.[36] In studies of 10- to 17-year-olds with acute or mixed manic symptoms, rates of psychosis ranged from 8.6% in the study of lithium and divalproex,[37] 5.2% in the aripiprazole versus placebo study,[38] 11% in the divalproex-ER study,[39] and 27.3% in the study of 13- to 17-year-olds with olanzapine.[40] This contrasts with adult drug studies where rates of psychosis ranged from 27.7%[41] to 55.6%.[42]

Comparisons of samples of youth bipolar patients with and without lifetime psychosis suggest that psychosis in probands predicted a greater likelihood of a family history of anxiety disorders and suicide attempts,[43,44] more psychiatric hospitalizations, higher rates of comorbidity, worse cognitive functioning and worse global functioning than bipolar patients without psychosis.[44,45]

Psychotic symptoms have been subtyped into mood congruent and mood incongruent. Mood-congruent delusions and hallucinations in depression contain themes of nihilism, guilt, deserved punishment, or personal failures that are consistent with depression. Those symptoms that involve inflated self-worth, extraordinary powers, knowledge, or relationship to a deity or famous person are consistent with mania. Persecutory delusions or paranoia may be mood congruent in the context of severe depression or mania (one is being persecuted because of terrible failings, or because one has some very valuable power). Mood-incongruent delusions include Schneiderian symptoms as well as certain delusions of persecution.

If psychosis is unstable across episodes, so is mood congruence. Whereas 66% of a cohort of adult bipolar patients had lifetime mood incongruent psychosis, only one-third (32%) of their 1539 episodes demonstrated mood incongruence. In other words, people had more episodes without than with mood-incongruent psychosis.[46] Also, the type of mood incongruence may be important. Schneiderian symptoms were associated with lower global functioning and more time ill over follow-up, but paranoia was not associated with poor outcome (see[13] for a review).

PSYCHOTIC SYMPTOMS: DEFINITIONS AND PREVALENCE IN MANIA

A hallucination is "a sensory perception that has the compelling sense of reality of a true perception but that occurs without external stimulation of the relevant sensory organ."[47(p823)] The patient's state of alertness, age and cognitive development, ability to express his or her internal state, and interviewer bias and conviction help determine whether to count a phenomenon as a true hallucination. In 91 youth with psychosis described by Ulloa and colleagues,[27] 73% had auditory hallucinations, 38.5% visual, and 26.2% olfactory hallucinations. Goodwin and Jamison[35] provide a weighted mean frequency of hallucinations in mania of 23% for a current episode. Child bipolar studies report hallucinations that range from 22% auditory and 18% visual[44] to 37.4% (pathologic hallucinations including visual).[31]

Delusions are false beliefs, not culturally accepted, and firmly held despite incontrovertible evidence to the contrary. Again, a spectrum exists between overvalued ideas and actual delusions.[47(p821)] Judgment is required in ascertaining the impact of development on cultural acceptance: Convictions of a monster in one's closet is not considered delusional in a young child, but would be considered delusional in a teen. Finally, the boundary between an obsession and a delusion is not always clear.

Grandiose delusions ("delusions of inflated worth, power, knowledge, identity or special relationship to a deity or famous person")[47] are common in mania, but can also occur in schizophrenia. Grandiosity occurs very often in mania (87%), but actual delusions occurred in about 31% of manic adults.[35] In children and adolescents, lifetime grandiosity occurred in more than 70% of participants in 3 large studies of mania (86%,[31] 83%,[29] 75.5%[32]), although grandiose delusions were less common. The Washington University Kiddie Schedule for Affective Disorders and Schizophrenia provided rates of 67% of respondents with grandiose delusions.[31] Geller and colleagues[30] describe a grandiose child: An 8-year-old girl, failing at school, met the mayor; she stated that she spent her evenings practicing for when she would be the first female president. She was also planning how to train her husband to be the First Gentleman. When asked how she could fail school and still be president, she said she just knew.[30]

Additional examples of grandiose delusions in adolescents include a 13-year-old manic girl who believed she was having labor pains from being pregnant and would give birth to Moses; a 14½-year-old boy who stated he is the Messiah (he feared he was going to die because he had seen God); and a 16 ½-year-old girl who felt she was the reincarnation of Newton or Jesus.[8]

Persecutory or paranoid delusions include feelings that one is being attacked, harassed, cheated, persecuted, or conspired against. Almost 40% of adults with mania were paranoid,[35] but paranoia occurred in only 8.2% of 1 sample of children and adolescents.[31] Delusions in teens with psychosis were[8]: "claims the staff and patients are purposely making toilets flush louder than normal, changing the water temperature in the shower, and pressurizing the room to wake her up." Another was "I'm being watched by everyone—they have a special plan for me." Paranoia in young adults with mania was associated with a greater number of psychotic episodes over 4 years of follow-up, but not with poorer function per se.[13]

Delusions of reference are defined as the conviction that "events, objects or other persons in one's immediate environment have a particular and unusual significance." Tillman and associates[31] reported rates of 5.8% in children and 8% in teens.

Mood-incongruent delusions are those of being controlled ("feelings, impulses, thoughts or actions …are under the control of some external force"), thought broadcasting ("one's thoughts are being broadcast out loud so that they can be perceived by others"), thought insertion ("one's thoughts are not one's own, but rather are inserted into one's mind"), and bizarre delusions (other delusions that are totally implausible).[47] Considered first-rank symptoms of schizophrenia as originally delineated by Schneider (see[48] for a review), they can occasionally occur in mood disorders and usually portend lower global functioning and more time ill.[13] They were rare in the sample of children described by Tillman and colleagues.[31]

Positive formal thought disorder, known in DSM-IV as disorganized speech, has been operationalized in the Scale for the Assessment of Positive Symptoms,[49] as follows

Fluent speech that tends to communicate poorly for a variety of reasons. The subject tends to skip from topic to topic without warning, to be distracted by events in the nearby environment, to join words together because they are semantically or phonologically alike, even though they make no sense, or to ignore the question and ask another. This type of speech may be rapid, and it frequently seems quite disjointed. Unlike alogia (negative formal thought disorder), a wealth of detail is provided, and the flow of speech tends to have an energetic, rather than an apathetic quality to it.[49]

In adults, rates disorganized speech were 84%[7]; 44% in hospitalized manic teens and in a meta-analysis by Kowatch and coworkers,[34] rates of flight of ideas ranged from 44% to 69% with a weighted percent of 56%. On the Young Mania Rating Scale,[50] language/thought disorder anchors are 0 (absent), 1 (circumstantial; mild distractibility; quick thoughts); 2 (distractible; loses goal of thought; changes topics frequently; racing thoughts); 3 (flight of ideas; tangentiality; difficult to follow; rhyming; echolalia); and 4 (incoherent; communication impossible). The pooled item score from 457 youth (mean age, 14.2 years) was 2.2 ± 0.7. The comparable score in 649 adults was 2.2 ± 1.0.[36]

PSYCHOTIC SYMPTOMS IN DEPRESSION

In a population study of almost 20,000 people age 15 and older, 16.5% of the sample reported at least 1 depressive symptom on a questionnaire. However, the prevalence of major depressive episode with psychotic features was 0.4% (95% CI, = 0.35%-0.54%) and without psychotic features was 2.0% (95% CI, 1.9%-2.1%); 18.5% of the participants who fulfilled the criteria for a major depressive episode had psychotic features. Treatment seeking was higher in depressed subjects with psychotic features.[51]

Major depression with psychosis is understudied in youth outside of its predictive relationship to the development of bipolar disorder[18,19] and is usually an exclusionary criterion for antidepressant studies. Among Ulloa's depression and anxiety clinic patients, 44% with psychotic symptoms had a major depressive episode.[27] In older studies of prepubertal major depression with the KSADS,[52] 38% of 58 children with MDD had psychopathologically meaningful hallucinations, 36% of which were auditory (mostly command), 16% nonauditory, mostly visual. This was considerably higher than found in teens (10%). Delusions were found in only 7% of the sample.[52] Comparing prepubertal, adolescent, and adult patients with major depression,[53] depressive hallucinations seemed to decrease with age (22% hallucinations in children, 14.1% in adolescents, and 9% in adults). By contrast, depressive delusions increased with age (4.2% in children and adolescents, 9% in adults). Chambers and colleagues[52] concluded that the precise psychopathologic meaning of psychotic symptoms in prepubertal children was unclear.

In a young adult first admission for psychosis sample, diagnostic stability is much less certain than in older samples later in course. In the 104 participants who had been assessed 4 times over 48 months (71% of the sample), only 31% had MDD with psychosis diagnosed at all 4 time points.[54] This may have some implications for children and adolescents with psychotic depression because of their early age of onset.

PSYCHOTIC SYMPTOMS AND CHILDREN AT RISK FOR MOOD DISORDERS

The Pittsburgh Bipolar Offspring study examined the relevance of psychotic symptoms in 235 offspring of bipolar I, II, or not otherwise specified parents and 140 controls, with a mean age of 11.9 ± 3.6 years. They reported that 16.9% of bipolar offspring and 11.7% of controls had definite or probable hallucinations or delusions, although the rates of actual psychotic disorders was lower (2.5% in both groups). The psychotic symptoms were associated with psychopathology in general, poor psychosocial functioning, and exposure to physical or sexual abuse. In other words, high-risk offspring were similar to those in the general population.[55]

In a somewhat older sample (about 16 years at intake and 23 years at follow-up), Duffy and colleagues[56] divided the parent bipolar probands into those who were lithium responsive and those who were not. A cumulative incidence of psychotic spectrum disorders of 1% in lithium responders' offspring versus 20.22% of lithium nonresponders' offspring (P = .025) was reported with rates of subthreshold psychotic symptoms were around 15%.

IMPACT OF CHILDHOOD ADVERSE EVENTS ON AFFECTIVE DISORDERS AND PSYCHOSIS IN YOUTH

Childhood adverse events, especially when recurrent over a long period of time, are well-known to be associated with a variety of mood and behavioral disturbances in youth and often into adulthood. For instance, in the Generation R Study of almost 4000 children of mean age of 10, psychotic-like experiences are consistently associated with early childhood adversities for example, greater than 2 adversities: adjusted odds ratio, 2.24; 95% (CI, 1.72–2.92), which remained significant after adjustment for comorbid psychiatric problems.[57]

Child and adolescent sexual abuse was a significant risk factor for psychotic symptoms in a community sample of adolescents and young adults with MDD,[58] and in people with bipolar disorder, a significant association was found between childhood abuse and mood-congruent and abusive auditory hallucinations in 2000 participants.[59] Studies of the relationship between childhood abuse and subsequent psychosis have found associations between adverse events and both hallucinations and delusions within psychotic illness in a meta-analysis,[60] and an association of child abuse with specific psychotic symptoms such as mood congruent auditory hallucinations among those with depressive disorder and bipolar disorder.[58] A retrospective chart review of 250 former psychiatric inpatients with psychosis found a correlation between the number of reported childhood adverse events and the total number of emergent psychotic symptoms.[61] A meta-analysis of childhood adverse events and psychosis concluded that childhood adversities may contribute to the earlier onset of psychotic symptoms and disorders.[62]

Neurobiology research of the adolescent brain highlights a vulnerability for the emergence of psychotic symptoms based in part on the changes taking place in the refinement of synaptic structures and the increasing social and cognitive demands in adolescence.[63]

Clearly, childhood adverse events, including sexual abuse, physical abuse, and neglect, have far-reaching long-term impacts on the development of psychiatric and physical illness in youth and adults.[64] There are strong associations between childhood adverse events and both severity and earlier onset of both affective disorders and psychotic symptoms and disorders.[58] It is always important for clinicians to ask about past and present experiences of sexual abuse, physical abuse, and emotional and physical neglect, not only to understand their potential contributions to an individual's development of affective and psychotic symptom disorders, but also to potentially recommend therapeutic interventions to ameliorate the effects of trauma on other areas of development and functioning.

ASSESSMENT OF PSYCHOSIS IN MOOD DISORDERS

A good history requires tracking the onset and polarity of episodes, whether and in which episode psychosis occurred, and whether it occurred outside of the mood symptoms, which would suggest a schizoaffective state. As we noted at the start of this article, hallucinatory phenomena are not rare in children. The question is whether the phenomena elicited mean anything diagnostically. Most structured interviews take the examiner through a list of questions that become increasingly more specific.[26,65–68] They start with questions like "do you ever feel your ears are playing tricks on you?", and progress through "do you hear sounds and realize there was probably nothing there?", "Do you ever hear a voice that others do not seem to or cannot hear?", "Does it sound clear like the way I'm sounding?", and "What is it saying?"

Mood-related hallucinations are most often auditory. If they are mood congruent, and depressive, voices heard will be telling the person that he or she is bad, ugly, evil, nasty, and so on. The clinician should ask, therefore, if the child or adolescent has described symptoms of depression, and if he or she has ever felt so down and depressed that their imagination started to play tricks on them? Did they hear something or someone saying insulting or bad things about them? Conversely during mania, one should ask if the person ever felt so good that they started to experience something really special? Hear from God, or hear beautiful music, or see mystical things?

Rating scales, for example, the Brief Psychiatric Rating Scale for Children[69] help to anchor the severity of what is being elicited. In the case of auditory hallucinations, they are rated as not present, mild (hears name called), moderate to severe (definite voices, comment or command), and extremely severe (eg, constantly commanding voices).

If hallucinations are tricky to elicit, delusions are even trickier. Three levels of misunderstanding can occur with ascertaining delusions in general and grandiosity in particular.[69] The first occurs because children may be unable to accurately self-evaluate and distinguish between pretend and reality. Another source of misunderstanding comes from misinterpreting the question. Finally, it is also possible that what an adult thinks is delusional is either the child not interpreting things the way the parent wants or it may be true. A child told this author that he pitched the fastest ball on the east coast. It sounded grandiose. It turned out to be true. Parents often feel their child is delusional when the child says he does not have to study for a test because he knows it all, or that she will get into the college of her choice even with grades that are failing.[70] Most of the time the child knows full well that what he or she is saying is not true but will not give the parent the satisfaction of admitting it. Usually the examiner can ascertain this by asking, "is this really true, or do you just wish it were true?"

Examples of items from the Structured Interview for Prodromal Symptoms,[71] which address grandiosity, for instance, ask "Do you feel you have special gifts or talents? Do people ever tell you that your plans or goals are unrealistic? Do you ever think of yourself as a famous or important person? Or chosen by God for a special role?"

Questions eliciting paranoid feelings include, "Do you feel people around you are thinking of you in a negative way? Are you mistrustful or suspicious of other people? Do feel you have to pay close attention to what's going on in order to feel safe? Do you feel like you are being singled out or watched? Or that people might be intending to harm you?"

The Brief Psychiatric Rating Scale for Children anchors delusions as follows: not present; mild (occasionally feels strangers may be looking/talking or laughing at them); moderate to severe (frequent distortion of thinking, mistrust, suspicious); extremely severe (mistrusts everything); and cannot distinguish from reality. Until the clinician is well-versed in the ascertainment of delusions, it is wise to use anchors to help determine severity.

SUMMARY

Mood disorders in youth, as in adults, are episodic and often serious. Psychosis adds another layer of severity and complexity. Clinicians must separate insignificant from significant psychotic symptoms, judge whether they represent part of a manic or depressive episode or are part of another disorder like schizophrenia. A good mental status examination and clinical history require close questioning to make sure the informants understand the questions being asked regarding mood episodes and psychosis and the clinician must synthesize the information into a developmentally appropriate clinical narrative.

REFERENCES

1. Cooper JE, Kendall RE, Gurland BJ, et al. Psychiatric diagnosis in New York and London: a comparative study of mental hospital admissions. Oxford: Oxford U. Press, Institute of Psychiatry, Maudsley Monographs; 1972.

2. World Health Organisation. Report of the international pilot study of schizophrenia. Geneva (Switzerland): WHO; 1973.
3. Feighner JP, Robins E, Guze SB, et al. Diagnostic criteria for use in psychiatric research. Arch Gen Psychiatry 1972;26(1):57–63.
4. Winokur G, Clayton P, Reich T. Manic depressive illness. St Louis (MO): C.V. Mosby Press; 1969.
5. Goodwin FK, Ghaemi SN. The impact of the discovery of lithium on psychiatric thought and practice in the USA and Europe. Aust N Z J Psychiatry 1999; 33(Suppl):S54–64.
6. Carlson GA, Goodwin FK. The stages of mania. A longitudinal analysis of the manic episode. Arch Gen Psychiatry 1973;28(2):221–8.
7. Abrams R, Taylor MA. Importance of schizophrenic symptoms in the diagnosis of mania. Am J Psychiatry 1981;138(5):658–61.
8. Carlson GA, Strober M. Manic-depressive illness in early adolescence. A study of clinical and diagnostic characteristics in six cases. J Am Acad Child Psychiatry 1978;17(1):138–53.
9. Carlson GA, Strober M. Affective disorder in adolescence: issues in misdiagnosis. J Clin Psychiatry 1978;39(1):59–66.
10. Joyce PR. Age of onset in bipolar affective disorder and misdiagnosis as schizophrenia. Psychol Med 1984;14(1):145–9.
11. Carlson GA, Fennig S, Bromet EJ. The confusion between bipolar disorder and schizophrenia in youth: where does it stand in the 1990s? J Am Acad Child Adolesc Psychiatry 1994;33(4):453–60.
12. Winokur G, Scharfetter C, Angst J. Stability of psychotic symptomatology (delusions, hallucinations), affective syndromes, and schizophrenic symptoms (thought disorder, incongruent affect) over episodes in remitting psychoses. Eur Arch Psychiatry Neurol Sci 1985;234(5):303–7.
13. Carlson GA, Kotov R, Chang SW, et al. Early determinants of four-year clinical outcomes in bipolar disorder with psychosis. Bipolar Disord 2012;14(1):19–30.
14. Dunayevich E, Keck PE Jr. Prevalence and description of psychotic features in bipolar mania. Curr Psychiatry Rep 2000;2(4):286–90.
15. Coryell W, Leon A, Winokur G, et al. Importance of psychotic features to long-term course in major depressive disorder. Am J Psychiatry 1996;153(4):483–9.
16. Coryell W, Leon AC, Turvey C, et al. The significance of psychotic features in manic episodes: a report from the NIMH collaborative study. J Affect Disord 2001;67(1–3):79–88.
17. Forty L, Jones L, Jones I, et al. Is depression severity the sole cause of psychotic symptoms during an episode of unipolar major depression? A study both between and within subjects. J Affect Disord 2009;114(1–3):103–9.
18. Strober M, Carlson G. Bipolar illness in adolescents with major depression: clinical, genetic, and psychopharmacologic predictors in a three- to four-year prospective follow-up investigation. Arch Gen Psychiatry 1982;39(5):549–55.
19. DelBello MP, Carlson GA, Tohen M, et al. Rates and predictors of developing a manic or hypomanic episode 1 to 2 years following a first hospitalization for major depression with psychotic features. J Child Adolesc Psychopharmacol 2003; 13(2):173–85.
20. Coryell W, Winokur G, Shea T, et al. Long term stability of depressive subtypes. Am J Psychiatry 1994;151:199–204.
21. Bromet EJ, Kotov R, Fochtmann LJ, et al. Diagnostic shifts during the decade following first admission for psychosis. Am J Psychiatry 2011;168(11):1186–94.

22. van Os J, Linscott RJ, Myin-Germeys I, et al. A systematic review and meta-analysis of the psychosis continuum: evidence for a psychosis-proneness-persistence-impairment model of psychotic disorder. Psychol Med 2008;8:1–17.
23. Kelleher I, Cannon M. Psychotic-like experiences in the general population: characterizing a high-risk group for psychosis. Psychol Med 2011;41(1):1–6.
24. Daalman K, Boks MP, Diederen KM, et al. The same or different? A phenomenological comparison of auditory verbal hallucinations in healthy and psychotic individuals. J Clin Psychiatry 2011;72(3):320–5.
25. Hlastala SA, McClellan J. Phenomenology and diagnostic stability of youths with atypical psychotic symptoms. J Child Adolesc Psychopharmacol 2005;15(3): 497–509.
26. Kaufman J, Birmaher B, Brent D, et al. Schedule for affective Disorders and schizophrenia for School-Age Children-Present and Lifetime version (K-SADS-PL): initial reliability and validity data. J Am Acad Child Adolesc Psychiatry 1997;36:980–8.
27. Ulloa RE, Birmaher B, Axelson D, et al. Psychosis in a pediatric mood and anxiety disorders clinic: phenomenology and correlates. J Am Acad Child Adolesc Psychiatry 2000;39(3):337–45.
28. Wozniak J, Biederman J, Kiely K, et al. Mania-like symptoms suggestive of childhood-onset bipolar disorder in clinically referred children. J Am Acad Child Adolesc Psychiatry 1995;34:867–76.
29. Findling RL, Gracious BL, McNamara NK, et al. Rapid, continuous cycling and psychiatric co-morbidity in pediatric bipolar I disorder. Bipolar Disord 2001;3: 202–10.
30. Geller B, Zimerman B, Williams M, et al. Phenomenology of prepubertal and early adolescent bipolar disorder: examples of elated mood, grandiose behaviors, decreased need for sleep, racing thoughts and hypersexuality. J Child Adolesc Psychopharmacol 2002;12(1):3–9.
31. Tillman R, Geller B, Klages T, et al. Psychotic phenomena in 257 young children and adolescents with bipolar I disorder: delusions and hallucinations (benign and pathological). Bipolar Disord 2008;10(1):45–55.
32. Axelson D, Birmaher B, Strober M, et al. Phenomenology of children and adolescents with bipolar spectrum disorders. Arch Gen Psychiatry 2006;63(10): 1139–48.
33. Topor DR, Swenson L, Hunt JI, et al. Manic symptoms in youth with bipolar disorder: factor analysis by age of symptom onset and current age. J Affect Disord 2013;145(3):409–12.
34. Kowatch RA, Youngstrom EA, Danielyan A, et al. Review and meta-analysis of the phenomenology and clinical characteristics of mania in children and adolescents. Bipolar Disord 2005;7(6):483–96.
35. Goodwin FK, Jamison KR. Manic-depressive illness: bipolar disorders and recurrent depression. New York: Oxford University Press; 2007.
36. Safer DJ, Zito JM, Safer AM. Age-grouped differences in bipolar mania. Compr Psychiatry 2012;53(8):1110–7.
37. Findling RL, McNamara NK, Youngstrom EA, et al. Double-blind 18-month trial of lithium versus divalproex maintenance treatment in pediatric bipolar disorder. J Am Acad Child Adolesc Psychiatry 2005;44(5):409–17.
38. Mankoski R, Zhao J, Carson WH, et al. Young mania rating scale line item analysis in pediatric subjects with bipolar I disorder treated with aripiprazole in a short-term, double-blind, randomized study. J Child Adolesc Psychopharmacol 2011;21:359–64.

39. Wagner KD, Redden L, Kowatch RA, et al. A double-blind, placebo-controlled trial of divalproex extended release in the treatment of bipolar disorder in children and adolescents. J Am Acad Child Adolesc Psychiatry 2009;48:519–32.
40. Tohen M, Krzyhanovskaya L, Carlson G, et al. Olanzapine versus placebo in the treatment of adolescents with bipolar mania. Am J Psychiatry 2007;164:1547–56.
41. Tohen M, Sanger TM, McElroy SL, et al. Olanzapine versus placebo in the treatment of acute mania. Am J Psychiatry 1999;156:702–9.
42. Bowden CL, Mosolov S, Hranov L, et al. Efficacy of valproate versus lithium in mania or mixed mania: a randomized, open 12-week trial. Int Clin Psychopharmacol 2010;28:60–7.
43. Rende R, Birmaher B, Axelson D, et al. Psychotic symptoms in pediatric bipolar disorder and family history of psychiatric illness. J Affect Disord 2006;96(1–2): 127–31.
44. Hua LL, Wilens TE, Martelon M, et al. Psychosocial functioning, familiarity, and psychiatric comorbidity in bipolar youth with and without psychotic features. J Clin Psychiatry 2011;72(3):397–405.
45. Caetano SC, Olvera RL, Hunter K, et al. Association of psychosis with suicidality in pediatric bipolar I, II and bipolar NOS patients. J Affect Disord 2006; 91(1):33–7.
46. Marneros A, Röttig S, Röttig D, et al. Bipolar I disorder with mood-incongruent psychotic symptoms: a comparative longitudinal study. Eur Arch Psychiatry Clin Neurosci 2009;259(3):131–6.
47. American Psychiatric Association. Diagnostic and statistical manual of mental disorders. 4th edition. Washington, DC; 2000.
48. Tanenberg-Karant M, Fennig S, Ram R, et al. Bizarre delusions and first-rank symptoms in a first-admission sample: a preliminary analysis of prevalence and correlates. Compr Psychiatry 1995;36(6):428–34.
49. Andreasen NC. Scale for the assessment of positive symptoms (SAPS); scale for the assessment of negative symptoms (SANS). Iowa City (IA): University of Iowa; 1984.
50. Young RC, Biggs JT, Ziegler VE, et al. A rating scale for mania; reliability, validity and sensitivity. Br J Psychiatry 1978;133:429–35.
51. Ohayon MM, Schatzberg AF. Prevalence of depressive episodes with psychotic features in the general population. Am J Psychiatry 2002;159(11):1855–61.
52. Chambers WJ, Puig-Antich J, Tabrizi MA, et al. Psychotic symptoms in prepubertal major depressive disorder. Arch Gen Psychiatry 1982;39(8):921–7.
53. Carlson GA, Kashani JH. Phenomenology of major depression from childhood through adulthood: analysis of three studies. Am J Psychiatry 1988;145(10): 1222–5.
54. Ruggero CJ, Kotov R, Carlson GA, et al. Diagnostic consistency of major depression with psychosis across 10 years. J Clin Psychiatry 2011;72(9):1207–13.
55. Mendez I, Axelson D, Castro-Fornieles J, et al. Psychotic-like experiences in offspring of parents with bipolar disorder and community controls: a longitudinal study. J Am Acad Child Adolesc Psychiatry 2019;58(5):534–43.
56. Duffy A, Goodday S, Keown-Stoneman C, et al. The emergent course of bipolar disorder: observations over two decades from the Canadian High-Risk Offspring Cohort. Am J Psychiatry 2019;176(9):720–9.
57. Bolhuis K, Koopman-Verhoeff ME, Blanken LME, et al. Psychotic-like experiences in pre-adolescence: what precedes the antecedent symptoms of severe mental illness? Acta Psychiatr Scand 2018;138(1):15–25.

58. Holshasen K, Bowie CR, Harkness KL. The relation of child maltreatment to psychotic symptoms in adolescents and young adults with depression. J Clin Child Adolesc Psychol 2016;45(3):241–7.

59. Upthegrove R, Chard C, Jones L, et al. Adverse childhood events and psychosis in bipolar disorder. Br J Psychiatry 2015;206:191–7.

60. Bailey T, Alvarez-Jimenez M, Garcia-Sanchez AM, et al. Childhood trauma is associated with severity of hallucinations and delusions in psychotic disorders: a systematic review and meta-analysis. Schizophr Bull 2018;44(5):1111–22.

61. Longden E, Sampson M, Read J. Childhood adversity and psychosis: generalized or specific effects? Epidemiol Psychiatr Sci 2016;25:349–59.

62. Morgan C, Gayer-Anderson C. Childhood adversities and psychosis: evidence, challenges, implications. World Psychiatry 2016;15:93–102.

63. Keshavan MS, Giedd J, Lau JYF, et al. Changes in the adolescent brain and the pathophysiology of psychotic disorders. Lancet Psychiatry 2014;1:549–58.

64. Hughes K, Bellis MA, Hardcastle KA, et al. The effect of multiple adverse childhood experiences on health: a systematic review and meta-analysis. Lancet Public Health 2017;2(8):e356–66.

65. Geller B, Williams M, Zimerman B, et al. Washington University in St. Louis Kiddie Schedule for affective disorders and schizophrenia (WASH-U-KSADS). St Louis (MO): Washington University; 1996.

66. Angold A, Cox A, Prendergast M, et al. The child and adolescent psychiatric assessment (CAPA). Durham (NC): Duke University; 1998.

67. the NIMH DISC Editorial Board. In: Shaffer D, Fisher P, Lucas C, editors. Diagnostic interview schedule for children (DISC-IV), parent version. New York: Columbia University/New York State Psychiatric Institute; 1998.

68. Spitzer RL, Williams J, Gibbon M, et al. The Structured Clinical Interview for DSM-III-R (SCID).I: history, rationale, and description. Arch Gen Psychiatry 1992;49:624–9.

69. Hughes CW, Rintelmann J, Emslie GJ, et al. A revised anchored version of the BPRS-C for childhood psychiatric disorders. J Child Adolesc Psychopharmacol 2001;11(1):77–93.

70. Carlson GA, Meyer SE. Phenomenology and diagnosis of bipolar disorder in children, adolescents, and adults: complexities and developmental issues. Dev Psychopathol 2006;18(4):939–69.

71. Miller TJ, McGlashan TH, Rosen JL, et al. Prospective diagnosis of the initial prodrome for schizophrenia based on the Structured Interview for Prodromal Syndromes: preliminary evidence of interrater reliability and predictive validity. Am J Psychiatry 2002;159(5):863–5.

Autism, Psychosis, or Both? Unraveling Complex Patient Presentations

Tara Chandrasekhar, MD[a],*, John Nathan Copeland, MD[a],
Marina Spanos, PhD[b], Linmarie Sikich, MD[a]

KEYWORDS

- Autism spectrum disorders • Schizophrenia spectrum disorders • Psychosis
- 22q11.2 deletion syndrome

KEY POINTS

- Autism spectrum disorders (ASDs) and schizophrenia spectrum disorders (SSDs) co-occur at elevated rates, likely in part due to shared genetic risk factors.
- Although many core features of ASD may seem similar to symptoms of psychosis, a thorough diagnostic assessment is key to differentiating features of each disorder.
- Individuals with both ASDs and SSDs may experience more severe symptoms and may be more likely to experience lack of response from multiple antipsychotic medications.
- Catatonia is a frequently overlooked psychomotor syndrome that may occur with both ASDs and SSDs. Affected individuals may require electroconvulsive therapy if they do not improve with benzodiazepines.

INTRODUCTION

Autism spectrum disorders (ASDs) are characterized by deficits in social communication and social interaction, restricted interests, repetitive behaviors, and sensory hypo- or hyperresponsivity. These features vary substantially in severity and functional impact across individuals and must be present from early childhood. Schizophrenia spectrum disorders (SSDs), which often manifest in adolescence or young adulthood, also range in severity and include positive symptoms (eg, delusions and

Disclosure Statement: Disclosures since 2015. Dr J.N. Copeland has nothing to disclose. Dr T. Chandrasekhar, Dr M. Spanos, and Dr L. Sikich have participated in clinical trials with Curemark Biopharmaceutical Developments, Roche Pharmaceuticals, and Sunovion. Dr T. Chandrasekhar and Dr L. Sikich have received research funding from NICHD.
a Department of Psychiatry and Behavioral Sciences, Duke University School of Medicine, 2608 Erwin Road, Suite 300, Durham, NC 27705, USA; b Department of Psychiatry and Behavioral Sciences, Duke University Medical Center, 2608 Erwin Road, Suite 300, Durham, NC 27705, USA
* Corresponding author.
E-mail address: tara.chandrasekhar@duke.edu

hallucinations), negative symptoms (eg, flattened affect, withdrawal), and disorganized speech or behavior. As diagnostically distinct conditions, ASDs and SSDs share multiple clinical features and genetic risk factors and seem to co-occur at elevated rates. Shared clinical features include social-emotional challenges (eg, alexithymia, theory of mind deficits), executive functioning deficits, and catatonia. Further, symptoms of one disorder may mimic the other, as illustrated by phenotypic similarities between negative psychotic symptoms (eg, social withdrawal) and reduced social-emotional reciprocity in ASD. Although presentations of comorbid ASD and psychosis pose challenges to the modern-day clinician, such dilemmas have their roots in the historical context of both disorders.

The term "autism" is credited to Swiss psychiatrist Eugen Bleuler, who described it in the early 1900s as a preoccupation with inner life while actively avoiding the external world.[1–3] Contemporaneously, German psychiatrist Emil Kraepelin described autistic-like behavior as evidence of early onset schizophrenia, writing, "we are dealing with children who have always shown a quiet, shy, withdrawn nature, engaged in no friendships and only lived for themselves."[4] Autistic features were integrated into descriptions of schizoid personality disorder by luminaries such as Ernst Kretschmer[4] and described in association with catatonia in the 1920s by Russian pediatric neurologist G. Ewa Ssucharewa.[5] Early versions of the Diagnostic and Statistical Manual (DSM) made no distinction between ASD and childhood schizophrenia, stating that latter may be characterized by "autistic, atypical, and withdrawn behavior."[6] It was not until the 1970s that ASD and childhood schizophrenia were reconsidered and redefined as separate conditions by Rutter[7] and Kolvin,[8] leading to the characterization of pervasive developmental disorders (PDD) in DSM-III.[9] Further evolution of diagnostic criteria has led to the present iteration of ASD in DSM-5, which emphasizes deficits in social communication and restricted, repetitive behaviors and interests, although ASDs and SSDs continue to be considered closely related as evidenced by their neighboring sections in the manual.[10] This historical framework provides context for the following discussion of the overlaps and distinctions between ASDs and SSDs, which will include genetic factors, affected brain regions, epidemiologic features, clinical assessment, and treatment considerations for individuals with both comorbid conditions.

SHARED GENETIC VULNERABILITY

Genetics play a significant role in both ASD and schizophrenia with heritability estimated at about 80% for both conditions.[11] Given the overlap of ASDs and SSDs, one could hypothesize that these conditions share common genetic risk factors. Indeed, Sullivan and colleagues[12] demonstrated in a Swedish cohort that presence of schizophrenia in parents significantly increased risk for ASD (odds ratio [OR] 2.9; 95% confidence interval [CI] 2.5–3.4). Studies have implicated single genes that share overlapping dysregulation in ASD and schizophrenia,[13] common single nucleotide polymorphisms,[14] and genomic regions or genes associated with both conditions.[15,16] Copy number variant (CNV) loci, in which sections of the genome are duplicated or deleted, have also demonstrated risk for development of ASDs and SSDs. Many of the identified CNV duplication or deletion syndromes (eg, 16p11.2,[17] 22q13.3 [SHANK3][18]), while clinically relevant, only account for about 1% of cases.

ASDs and SSDs may share a reciprocal genetic relationship, in which deletions predispose an individual to one disorder and duplications to the other. Indeed,

ASDs tend to be associated with upregulation of pathways from loss of function of negative regulators, and SSDs tend to occur due to reduced pathway activation.[19] The 22q11.2 deletion syndrome (22q11.2DS), the most common chromosomal microdeletion disorder (1 in 2000–4000 live births[20]), illustrates this reciprocal genetic relationship as well as the range of clinical manifestation in individuals at risk for both ASDs and SSDs.

22q11.2 Deletion Syndrome

22q11.2DS is associated with a spectrum of neuropsychiatric conditions including intellectual disability, schizophrenia, and ASD.[21] Historically these symptoms have been known as DiGeorge or velocardiofacial syndrome, but this nomenclature is now reserved for those who present with the above symptoms but do not have a 22q11.2deletion.[21] Approximately 25% of patients are diagnosed with schizophrenia, and as many as 50% of individuals will receive a diagnosis of ASD.[21,22] Critical regions of the 22q11.2 gene are associated with ASDs,[22,23] whereas others are associated with SSDs.[19] Some studies that examine the correlation between childhood autism symptoms and later psychosis show that subgroups of patients with ASD do not develop schizophrenia in adulthood. This suggests that in some individuals ASD and SSD associated with 22q11.2DS may be considered 2 unrelated phenomena associated with a single genetic variant.[24,25] The complexities of shared genetic risk are illustrated by the varied manifestations of neuropsychiatric disorders in individuals with 22q11.2DS. Further study of shared genetic markers may shed light on the causes of both ASDs and SSDs.

BRAIN REGIONS IMPLICATED IN AUTISM AND SCHIZOPHRENIA

Although common genetic regions provide insight into the underlying cause of both ASDs and SSDs, brain imaging studies have implicated specific regions of the brain in these disorders. Areas of the brain that demonstrate overlap in ASD and schizophrenia include the corpus callosum,[26,27] fusiform gyrus,[28,29] and amygdala.[30] The amygdala represents a characteristic example of how brain region dysfunction may manifest in each condition. In ASD populations, some studies suggest that amygdala hypoactivity is implicated in theory of mind tasks,[30,31] whereas others suggest that amygdala hyperactivation may occur during facial discrimination, eye gaze,[32] and other socially and emotionally salient situations.[33] This hyperactivation is hypothesized to contribute to anxiety and rigidity commonly seen in ASDs.[34]

Similar to ASDs, studies in individuals with SSDs have shown both hypoactivation and hyperactivation of the amygdala compared with controls, and this difference seems to occur based on the social-emotional stimuli presented.[35] However, somewhat contrary to what was seen in ASD, neutral stimuli (eg, neutral facial expressions) have been found to produce hyperactivation of the amygdala[36] while there is hypoactivity in more socially salient stimuli (eg, fearful faces) compared with neutral stimuli.[37,38]

The possibility of shared etiologic mechanisms is further suggested by a 2010 brain imaging study of 660 participants that revealed lower gray matter volumes within the limbic-striato-thalamic circuitry in both individuals with ASD and schizophrenia, compared with 801 controls.[39] Brain imaging studies will likely be an increasingly valuable research tool to increase our insight into the etiology of both disorders, and more studies are needed to characterize functional connectivity patterns and the neuroanatomical basis of symptoms in patients with comorbid ASDs and SSDs.

EPIDEMIOLOGIC FEATURES OF COMORBID AUTISM AND PSYCHOSIS

Genetic and neurocircuitry overlap provide a neurobiological basis for recent studies that indicate elevated risk for ASD in those with SSDs and vice versa. The prevalence of psychotic features in ASD populations as well as the prevalence of autistic-like traits in individuals with a diagnosis of a psychotic disorder is reviewed later.

Epidemiologic Features of Psychosis in Individuals with Autism

Recent studies suggest that individuals with ASD are at elevated risk for SSDs, with prevalence rates as high as 34.8%.[40] The likelihood that an individual with ASD will develop a psychotic illness was assessed in a large nested Swedish case-control study in which researchers determined that the odds ratio for experiencing a comorbid nonaffective psychotic disorder was 5.6 (95% CI, 3.3–8.5) for individuals with ASD without intellectual disability and 3.5 (95% CI, 2.0–6.0) for individuals with ASD and intellectual disability.[41] Danish researchers estimated a similar adjusted odds ratio for schizophrenia (OR 3.3, 95% CI, 0.8–11.8) in a population of 414 ASD cases, although their results lacked statistical significance.[42] Findings from the Avon Longitudinal Study of Parents and Children (ALSPC), a large and ongoing British cohort study, similarly indicated elevated risk of psychosis in youth with ASD as well as identified risk factors for later psychotic symptoms. A study based on 8253 individuals in the ALSPC cohort showed that children diagnosed with PDD at age 8 years seemed at heightened risk (OR 8.0; 95% CI, 2.2–30.0) for later psychotic experiences, although the study suffered from low statistical power due to a relatively small number of participants meeting criteria for this diagnosis. However, of those who did meet criteria for PDD, more than half of the children reported psychotic experiences at age 13 years.[43] Potential risk factors for later psychotic symptoms were suggested by other studies of the ASPLC cohort, including an association between greater risk for psychosis and poorer early pragmatic language[44] and maternal concern regarding speech development and excessive rituals or habits.[45] In summary, these studies imply that rates of comorbidity of psychosis in ASD populations are elevated, and communication or language delays are associated with later psychotic symptoms.

Epidemiologic Features of Autism in Individuals with Schizophrenia

Schizophrenia, which may be considered a developmental disorder in its own right, has been associated with a history of developmental delay since the 1990s.[46–48] Longitudinal studies of children with childhood schizophrenia (onset before age 13 years)[49] suggest high rates of comorbid ASD or other developmental delay. A 2004 National Institutes of Mental Health longitudinal cohort study indicated that of a sample of 75 children with childhood schizophrenia, 25% (n = 19) had a lifetime diagnosis of an ASD, although the majority (n = 16) met criteria for PDD rather than autistic disorder or Asperger disorder using DSM-IV-TR criteria.[50] Similarly, Rapoport and colleagues[16] characterized 97 children with childhood schizophrenia and found that a comparable proportion (28%) met criteria for a lifetime diagnosis of ASD.

Studies of adolescents and young adults with SSDs have yielded lower rates of ASD, although this is an area that requires further study. Researchers from Sweden obtained rates of comorbid diagnoses of neurodevelopmental disorders in a large cohort (n = 2091) of individuals hospitalized for first-episode psychosis between ages 16 and 25 years. They found that 5% of the individuals had a diagnosis of autism and that delusional disorder was more commonly found in the autism group (OR = 2.3, P<.05). The ASD group was more likely than the rest of the cohort to be taking antipsychotic medication 2 years later, potentially suggesting that the ASD group experienced a more severe or chronic psychotic illness.[51] Taken together, these studies indicate that individuals with early onset SSDs are more likely to have a history of developmental delay or features of ASD, whereas rates of meeting full ASD criteria are mixed.

CLINICAL PRESENTATION AND ASSESSMENT OF PSYCHOSIS IN INDIVIDUALS WITH AUTISM

Clinicians often struggle with diagnostic assessment in individuals with possible comorbid ASDs and SSDs, particularly in cases that are complex. Clinicians may be faced with the dilemma of unraveling symptoms of both conditions or ruling one condition out in favor of another one. The components of a thorough diagnostic assessment as well as potential ASD features that may be mistaken for psychosis are discussed later. Catatonia, a frequently underdiagnosed syndrome that occurs in both ASDs and SSDs is a complex condition that warrants special consideration.

Red Flags for Psychosis in Autism: Diagnostic Assessment

A clinician should consider a comorbid diagnosis of a psychotic disorder in an individual with ASD who reports perceptual abnormalities or beliefs and exhibits behaviors that seem different from baseline. These symptoms, as well as a change in social, cognitive, or adaptive functioning from baseline should lead to further inquiry. Collateral information from parents, caregivers, or teachers is often crucial to sorting out what features may or may not be due to psychosis. Parents and caregivers can often identify changes in behavior from baseline, even if they are unsure of how to understand what they are observing. The value of collateral information becomes apparent, for example, during an assessment for thought disorder in a child with ASD whose verbalizations are primarily repetitive or scripted. Although scripted speech may itself seem idiosyncratic or nonsensical, often when provided with context and interpretation by others, clinicians realize that such verbalizations are a feature of ASD rather than disorganized thinking. However, if a parent or a caregiver is unable to decipher the underlying meaning of a child's thoughts and verbalizations, then concern for psychosis should increase. Similarly, monitoring for psychosis should occur, with evidence of a change in baseline social interactions, increased withdrawal, or presence of odd or unusual behaviors that do not fit with an individual's typical interests or rituals.

In addition to collateral information, a careful developmental, behavioral, medical, and psychiatric history is necessary for diagnostic clarity, as there are currently no biomarkers available to distinguish between ASDs and SSDs. A longitudinal assessment of symptoms and mental status is often helpful in clarifying the diagnosis. Appropriate diagnostic and laboratory testing to rule out a medical condition as the cause for psychosis should be obtained.[52] Genetic testing should be completed in individuals in which both conditions are suspected, starting with a microarray and then proceeding to a whole genome sequence and later whole exome sequence if indicated. A family history of psychotic symptoms may provide information regarding heritable genetic risk factors.[53]

Autism Spectrum Disorder Traits that Resemble Psychosis

Core features of ASD may be mistaken for psychosis if the clinician lacks relevant clinical history or information regarding baseline functioning. The following examples illustrate potential mischaracterizations of ASD features:

- A teenager with ASD and a history of being bullied voices distrust and negative beliefs about a group of people who he feels resembles his bullies. Rigid perseverative thoughts, limited perspective taking, and difficulty reading emotions may lead to concerns that the individual is paranoid or delusional, rather than struggling with core social skills. History from family members about his social relatedness and past experience with peers, as well as reality testing and attempts to understand his fearful thoughts, may reveal that these challenges are consistent with his baseline rather than psychotic symptoms.
- A child who is highly focused on sensory input (eg, sounds) and experiences auditory hypersensitivity may seem to be preoccupied with internal stimuli when she suddenly pauses, seems to stare in the distance, and seems more disconnected and inattentive than usual. Observation when this occurs, history from others who also hear the sensory input, and careful assessment to rule out other medical causes of potential staring spells may clarify that this behavior is a feature of ASD.

The prodromal or attenuated psychosis period may present several features that overlap with ASD (eg, social withdrawal, reduced emotional expression, executive functioning difficulties),[54] leading to questions and potentially false-positive diagnoses of autism before the onset of hallucinations or delusions.[55] This underscores the need for a careful history that establishes the individual's baseline functioning while evaluating for a psychotic illness.

Table 1 illustrates the potential overlap that may occur between ASD features and psychotic symptoms, in terms of social-emotional and communication domains, thought content, and behaviors.

Catatonia

Catatonia, an underrecognized psychomotor syndrome characterized by several signs and symptoms, occurs with multiple neuropsychiatric and medical causes, including ASDs and SSDs. Diagnosis is based on the assessment of fluctuations in activity level (eg, excitement, unresponsiveness, staring, withdrawal) as well as behavior and motor changes (eg, catalepsy, echopraxia, negativism, posturing, echolalia).[10] Catatonia is a DSM-5 specifier for both autism and schizophrenia, potentially creating

Table 1
Overlap between core autism features and psychosis

	Autism	Psychosis
Social-Emotional Challenges	• Lack of social-emotional reciprocity • Misreading social queues • Restricted or flattened affect	• Social withdrawal • Blunted affect • Paranoia • Low mood • Alexithymia
Communication Challenges	• Language delay • Echolalia	• Poverty of speech • Unusual or bizarre speech
Unusual Thought Content	• Restricted interests • Perseveration • Concrete thinking • Problems with perceptual processing	• Perseveration • Delusions • Disorganization • Hallucinations
Behavioral Features	• Repetitive movements	• Posturing and stereotypies during catatonia

confusion to the diagnostician when a child or adolescent with ASD develops catatonic features. Indeed, many catatonia symptoms overlap with ASD features, including mutism, stereotypic speech, repetitive speech, and seemingly purposeless activity,[56] further contributing to risk of underdiagnoses. Prevalence estimates in children vary greatly (0.6%–17%), and catatonia is also likely underrecognized and undertreated in the general child and adolescent population.[57] Two systematic studies estimate the prevalence of catatonia in ASD to be 12% to 17%.[58,59] Of note, all patients in these studies were diagnosed with comorbid catatonia after adolescence. Shorter and Wachtel have suggested that the triad of autism, psychosis, and catatonia (a so-called Iron Triangle) may encompass 3 different manifestations of the same underlying brain disorder rather than separate conditions,[4] underscoring the complex genetic relationship, pathophysiology, and treatment. The authors are not aware of large systematic treatment studies for catatonia in individuals with the comorbid psychosis and autism, although Fink and colleagues[60] proposed a medication treatment algorithm in 2006 that suggested initial use of high-dose lorazepam (6–24 mg/d) followed by electroconvulsive therapy (ECT) if there is lack of response. The literature also contains case reports that suggest the utility of a more rapid initiation of ECT over benzodiazepines.[61,62]

TREATMENT OF PSYCHOSIS IN AUTISM SPECTRUM DISORDER POPULATIONS

The authors are not aware of large treatment studies that address medication efficacy or safety in populations of patients with comorbid autism and schizophrenia. Individuals with comorbid ASD and SSDs may be less likely to experience benefit from antipsychotics, as suggested by a 2017 study in which comorbid ASDs were significantly associated with failure of multiple (>2) antipsychotics.[63] The authors' clinical experiences suggest that earlier use of clozapine may be helpful to reduce psychotic symptoms and improve functional outcomes. There is one case report and recent small Turkish retrospective review that indicated that patients with ASD and schizophrenia experienced a reduction in psychotic symptoms with clozapine treatment.[64] Further, the authors recommend a family centered approach that includes psychoeducation, supportive therapy, and focus on functional outcomes and symptom reduction, as well as carefully monitored psychopharmacologic interventions when treating patients with comorbid ASDs and SSDs.

FUTURE DIRECTIONS

Although there is increasing recognition of the co-occurrence of ASDs and SSDs, there have been few systematic studies of outcomes for individuals with both conditions. There is a critical need for better characterization of strategies to ensure safety, given the increased overall risk of suicidal behavior in individuals with ASDs[65] as well as a growing evidence base to suggest higher rates of depression and suicidal thinking in those with autism spectrum traits experiencing first episode psychosis.[66] In addition, better characterization of the range of clinical presentations and better recognition of catatonia will likely lead to reduced morbidity in this population.

Studies that explore the cause and genetic risk factors for individuals with comorbid ASD and SSD may lead to novel treatment approaches and improved functional outcomes given the elevated rates of co-occurrence of these conditions.

REFERENCES

1. McNally K. Eugene Bleuler's four As. Hist Psychol 2009;12(2):43–59.

2. Peralta V, Cuesta MJ. EugenBleuler and the schizophrenias: 100 Years after. Schizophr Bull 2011;37(6):1118–20.

3. Volkmar FR, Cohen DJ. Comorbid association of autism and schizophrenia. Am J Psychiatry 1991;148(12):1705–7.

4. Wachtel LE, Schuldt S, Ghaziuddin N, et al. The potential role of electroconvulsive therapy in the 'Iron Triangle' of pediatric catatonia, autism, and psychosis. ActaPsychiatrScand 2013;128(5):408–9.

5. Wolff S. The first account of the syndrome Asperger described? Eur Child AdolescPsychiatry 1996;5(3):119–32.

6. Association AP. Diagnostic and statistical manual of mental disorders (DSM II). 2nd edition. Washington, DC: American Psychiatric Association; 1968.

7. Rutter M. Childhood schizophrenia reconsidered. JAutism Child Schizophr 1972; 2(4):315–37.

8. Kolvin I, Ounsted C, Humphrey M, et al. The phenomenology of childhood psychoses. Br J Psychiatry 1971;118(545):385–95.

9. American Psychiatric Association. DSM-III: diagnostic and statistical manual of mental disorders. 3rd edition. Washington, DC: American Psychiatric Association; 1980.

10. American Psychiatric Association. Diagnostic and statistical manual of mental disorders. 5th edition. Arlington (VA): American Psychiatric Association; 2013.

11. Carroll LS, Owen MJ. Genetic overlap between autism, schizophrenia and bipolar disorder. Genome Med 2009;1(10):102.

12. Sullivan PF, Magnusson C, Reichenberg A, et al. Family history of schizophrenia and bipolar disorder as risk factors for autism. Arch Gen Psychiatry 2012;69(11): 1099–103.

13. Guan J, Cai JJ, Ji G, et al. Commonality in dysregulated expression of gene sets in cortical brains of individuals with autism, schizophrenia, and bipolar disorder. Transl Psychiatry 2019;9(1):152.

14. Cross-Disorder Group of the Psychiatric Genomics Consortium, Lee SH, Ripke S, Neale BM, et al, International Inflammatory Bowel Disease Genetics Consortium (IIBDGC). Genetic relationship between five psychiatric disorders estimated from genome-wide SNPs. Nat Genet 2013;45(9):984–94.

15. King BH, Lord C. Is schizophrenia on the autism spectrum? Brain Res 2011;1380: 34–41.

16. Rapoport J, Chavez A, Greenstein D, et al. Autism spectrum disorders and childhood-onset schizophrenia: clinical and biological contributions to a relation revisited. J Am Acad Child AdolescPsychiatry 2009;48(1):10–8.

17. McCarthy SE, Gillis J, Kramer M, et al. De novo mutations in schizophrenia implicate chromatin remodeling and support a genetic overlap with autism and intellectual disability. Mol Psychiatry 2014;19(6):652–8.

18. Gauthier J, Champagne N, Lafrenière RG, et al. De novo mutations in the gene encoding the synaptic scaffolding proteinSHANK3in patients ascertained for schizophrenia. ProcNatlAcadSci U S A 2010;107(17):7863–8.

19. Crespi B, Stead P, Elliot M. Comparative genomics of autism and schizophrenia. ProcNatlAcadSci U S A 2010;107(suppl_1):1736–41.

20. Grati FR, Molina Gomes D, Ferreira JCPB, et al. Prevalence of recurrent pathogenic microdeletions and microduplications in over 9500 pregnancies. Prenatal Diagn 2015;35(8):801–9.

21. McDonald-Mcginn DM, Sullivan KE, Marino B, et al. 22q11.2 deletion syndrome. Nat Rev Dis Primers 2015;1:15071.

22. Clements CC, Wenger TL, Zoltowski AR, et al. Critical region within 22q11.2 linked to higher rate of autism spectrum disorder. MolAutism 2017;8:58.

23. Fiksinski AM, Breetvelt EJ, Duijff SN, et al. Autism Spectrum and psychosis risk in the 22q11.2 deletion syndrome. Findings from a prospective longitudinal study. Schizophr Res 2017;188:59–62.

24. Bearden C. Same DNA deletion paves paths to autism, schizophrenia. Spectrum 2016.

25. Vorstman JAS, Breetvelt EJ, Thode KI, et al. Expression of autism spectrum and schizophrenia in patients with a 22q11.2 deletion. Schizophr Res 2013; 143(1):55–9.

26. Koshiyama D, Fukunaga M, Okada N, et al. Role of frontal white matter and corpus callosum on social function in schizophrenia. Schizophr Res 2018;202: 180–7.

27. Just MA, Cherkassky VL, Keller TA, et al. Functional and anatomical cortical underconnectivity in autism: evidence from an fMRI study of an executive function task and corpus callosum morphometry. CerebCortex 2007;17(4):951–61.

28. Toal F, Bloemen OJ, Deeley Q, et al. Psychosis and autism: magnetic resonance imaging study of brain anatomy. Br J Psychiatry 2009;194(5):418–25.

29. Belger A, Carpenter KLH, Yucel GH, et al. The neural circuitry of autism. Neurotox Res 2011;20(3):201–14.

30. Sugranyes G, Kyriakopoulos M, Corrigall R, et al. Autism spectrum disorders and schizophrenia: meta-analysis of the neural correlates of social cognition. PLoSOne 2011;6(10):e25322.

31. Wang AT, Dapretto M, Hariri AR, et al. Neural correlates of facial affect processing in children and adolescents with autism spectrum disorder. J Am Acad Child AdolescPsychiatry 2004;43(4):481–90.

32. Dalton KM, Nacewicz BM, Johnstone T, et al. Gaze fixation and the neural circuitry of face processing in autism. Nat Neurosci 2005;8(4):519–26.

33. Tottenham N, Hertzig ME, Gillespie-Lynch K, et al. Elevated amygdala response to faces and gaze aversion in autism spectrum disorder. SocCogn Affect Neurosci 2014;9(1):106–17.

34. Hariri AR. Looking inside the disordered brain: an introduction to the functional neuroanatomy of psychopathology. Sunderland (MA): Sinauer Associates, Inc; 2015.

35. Mier D, Lis S, Zygrodnik K, et al. Evidence for altered amygdala activation in schizophrenia in an adaptive emotion recognition task. Psychiatry Res 2014; 221(3):195–203.

36. Mier D, Sauer C, Lis S, et al. Neuronal correlates of affective theory of mind in schizophrenia out-patients: evidence for a baseline deficit. Psychol Med 2010; 40(10):1607–17.

37. Hall J, Whalley HC, McKirdy JW, et al. Overactivation of fear systems to neutral faces in schizophrenia. Biol Psychiatry 2008;64(1):70–3.

38. Pinkham AE, Loughead J, Ruparel K, et al. Abnormal modulation of amygdala activity in schizophrenia in response to direct- and averted-gaze threat-related facial expressions. Am J Psychiatry 2011;168(3):293–301.

39. Cheung C, Yu K, Fung G, et al. Autistic disorders and schizophrenia: related or remote? An anatomical likelihood estimation. PLoSOne 2010;5(8):e12233.

40. Chisholm K, Lin A, Abu-Akel A, et al. The association between autism and schizophrenia spectrum disorders: a review of eight alternate models of co-occurrence. NeurosciBiobehav Rev 2015;55:173–83.

41. Selten J-P, Lundberg M, Rai D, et al. Risks for nonaffective psychotic disorder and bipolar disorder in young people with autism spectrum disorder. JAMA Psychiatry 2015;72(5):483.
42. Abdallah MW, Greaves-Lord K, Grove J, et al. Psychiatric comorbidities in autism spectrum disorders: findings from a Danish Historic Birth Cohort. Eur Child AdolescPsychiatry 2011;20(11–12):599–601.
43. Siebald C, Khandaker GM, Zammit S, et al. Association between childhood psychiatric disorders and psychotic experiences in adolescence: a population-based longitudinal study. Compr Psychiatry 2016;69:45–52.
44. Sullivan SA, Hollen L, Wren Y, et al. A longitudinal investigation of childhood communication ability and adolescent psychotic experiences in a community sample. Schizophr Res 2016;173(1–2):54–61.
45. Bevan Jones R, Thapar A, Lewis G, et al. The association between early autistic traits and psychotic experiences in adolescence. Schizophr Res 2012;135(1–3): 164–9.
46. Isohanni M, Jones P, Kemppainen L, et al. Childhood and adolescent predictors of schizophrenia in the Northern Finland 1966 birth cohort–a descriptive life-span model. Eur Arch Psychiatry ClinNeurosci 2000;250(6):311–9.
47. Jones P, Rodgers B, Murray R, et al. Child development risk factors for adult schizophrenia in the British 1946 birth cohort. Lancet 1994;344(8934):1398–402.
48. Done DJ, Crow TJ, Johnstone EC, et al. Childhood antecedents of schizophrenia and affective illness: social adjustment at ages 7 and 11. BMJ 1994;309(6956): 699–703.
49. McClellan J, Stock S. Practice parameter for the assessment and treatment of children and adolescents with schizophrenia. J Am Acad Child AdolescPsychiatry 2013;52(9):976–90.
50. Sporn AL, Addington AM, Gogtay N, et al. Pervasive developmental disorder and childhood-onset schizophrenia: comorbid disorder or a phenotypic variant of a very early onset illness? Biol Psychiatry 2004;55(10):989–94.
51. Stralin P, Hetta J. First episode psychosis and comorbid ADHD, autism and intellectual disability. Eur Psychiatry 2019;55:18–22.
52. Sikich L. Diagnosis and evaluation of hallucinations and other psychotic symptoms in children and adolescents. Child AdolescPsychiatrClin N Am 2013; 22(4):655–73.
53. Cochran DM, Dvir Y, Frazier JA. "Autism-plus" spectrum disorders: intersection with psychosis and the schizophrenia spectrum. Child AdolescPsychiatrClin N Am 2013;22(4):609–27.
54. Addington J. The prodromal stage of psychotic illness: observation, detection or intervention? J PsychiatryNeurosci 2003;28(2):93–7.
55. Ross CA. Problems with autism, catatonia and schizophrenia in DSM-5. Schizophr Res 2014;158(1–3):264–5.
56. Mazzone L, Postorino V, Valeri G, et al. Catatonia in patients with autism: prevalence and management. CNS Drugs 2014;28(3):205–15.
57. Hauptman AJ, Benjamin S. The differential diagnosis and treatment of catatonia in children and adolescents. Harv Rev Psychiatry 2016;24(6):379–95.
58. Billstedt E, Gillberg IC, Gillberg C. Autism after adolescence: population-based 13- to 22-year follow-up study of 120 individuals with autism diagnosed in childhood. J AutismDevDisord 2005;35(3):351–60.
59. Wing L, Shah A. Catatonia in autistic spectrum disorders. Br J Psychiatry 2000; 176(4):357–62.

60. Fink M, Taylor MA, Ghaziuddin N. Catatonia in autistic spectrum disorders: a medical treatment algorithm. Int Rev Neurobiol 2006;72:233–44.
61. Shorter E, Wachtel LE. Childhood catatonia, autism and psychosis past and present: is there an 'iron triangle'? ActaPsychiatrScand 2013;128(1):21–33.
62. Zaw FK, Bates GD, Murali V, et al. Catatonia, autism, and ECT. Dev Med Child Neurol 1999;41(12):843–5.
63. Downs JM, Lechler S, Dean H, et al. The association between comorbid autism spectrum disorders and antipsychotic treatment failure in early-onset psychosis. J ClinPsychiatry 2017;78(9):e1233–41.
64. Sahoo S, Padhy SK, Singla N, et al. Effectiveness of clozapine for the treatment of psychosis and disruptive behaviour in a child with Atypical Autism: a case report and a brief review of the evidence. Asian J Psychiatry 2017;29:194–5.
65. Chen MH, Pan TL, Lan WH, et al. Risk of suicide attempts among adolescents and young adults with autism spectrum disorder: a nationwide longitudinal follow-up study. J ClinPsychiatry 2017;78(9):e1174–9.
66. Upthegrove R, Abu-Akel A, Chisholm K, et al. Autism and psychosis: clinical implications for depression and suicide. Schizophr Res 2018;195:80–5.

Childhood Trauma and Psychosis: An Updated Review

Kate J. Stanton, MD[a], Brian Denietolis, PsyD[a],
Brien J. Goodwin, MS[b], Yael Dvir, MD[a],*

KEYWORDS

- Childhood trauma • Childhood adversity • Childhood abuse • Psychosis

KEY POINTS

- Growing evidence supports the links between childhood trauma and psychosis, which include higher risk for psychosis, increased severity of psychotic symptoms, increased frequency of affective symptoms and substance use, and worse functional impairment.
- Biological factors explaining this link include gender, brain-derived neurotrophic factor, and other inflammatory markers.
- Psychological mechanisms explaining this link include dysfunctional cognitive schemas and affective dysregulation.
- Evidence supports the use of cognitive behavioral therapies in the treatment of trauma and posttraumatic stress disorder in youth as well as in adults with cooccurring trauma and psychotic illnesses.

INTRODUCTION

The Link Between Childhood Trauma and Psychosis

Evidence for the association between childhood trauma and psychosis is well supported and continues to grow. In a recent sample of more than 4000 children, Croft and colleagues[1] assessed for psychotic symptoms and trauma history, using the Psychosis-Like symptoms Semi-Structured Interview at ages 12 and 18 years, and a parent-completed 121-question assessment about traumatic events. They found that at age 18, 83.8% of those with psychotic symptoms had traumatic experiences, compared with 62.6% of those without psychotic symptoms. Youth who experienced trauma in the first 17 years of life were 2.91 times more likely to have psychotic symptoms at 18 years of age, and those who experienced 3 or more types of childhood trauma were 4.7 times more likely to have psychotic symptoms. In a sample of 101 first

The authors have no disclosures.
[a] Department of Psychiatry, University of Massachusetts Medical School, 55 Lake Avenue North, Worcester, MA 01655, USA; [b] Department of Psychological and Brain Sciences, University of Massachusetts Amherst, 135 Hicks Way/Tobin Hall, Amherst, MA 01003, USA
* Corresponding author.
E-mail address: yael.dvir@umassmed.edu

Abbreviations	
BDNF	Brain-derived neurotrophic factor
CBT	Cognitive behavioral therapy
CECA-Q	Childhood Experiences of Care and Abuse Questionnaire
CHR	Clinically high risk
CI	Confidence interval
COMT	Catechol-o-methyl-transferase
CT	Cognitive therapy
EMDR	Eye movement desensitization and reprocessing
FEP	First episode psychosis
OR	Odds ratio
PANSS	Positive and negative syndrome scale
PE	Prolonged exposure
PTSD	Posttraumatic stress disorder
PTSS	Posttraumatic stress symptoms
RCT	Randomized controlled trial
TF-CBT	Trauma-focused cognitive behavioral therapy
TSCC	Trauma symptom checklist for children
UCLA-PTSD-RI	University of California, Los Angeleschild/adolescent posttraumatic stress disorder reaction index for *Diagnostic and Statistical Manual of Mental Disorders* (Fifth Edition)

episode psychosis (FEP) patients aged 18 to 35 years, Trauelsen and colleagues[2] had similar findings, with 89% of FEP patients reporting a history of childhood trauma, compared with 37% of matched controls. Psychosis risk was magnified by 2.5 times for every additional trauma, and the risk for psychosis increased by 5 for those who experienced 3 or more traumatic events.

Systematic reviews of the literature and metaanalyses have demonstrated a clear relationship between childhood trauma and the severity of psychotic symptom presentation. There is now considerable empirical evidence that exposure to childhood physical abuse, sexual abuse, emotional abuse, and neglect increases risk for developing psychosis.[3] Within adolescent populations considered clinically high risk (CHR) for psychosis, Loewy and colleagues[4] found that CHR adolescents with cooccurring trauma had significantly more severe perceptual disturbances and affective symptoms when compared with CHR adolescents without trauma. In addition, the number of traumatic events endorsed was associated with more severe suspiciousness, perceptual abnormalities, and general affective instability. In similar studies, childhood trauma was associated with more severe positive symptoms of psychosis,[5] pronounced comorbid affective disturbances,[6,7] and diminished neuropsychological performance within domains of attention, working memory, and cognitive flexibility.[8] In a study of 361 individuals aged 18 years and older diagnosed with schizophrenia or schizoaffective disorder, those who had experienced emotional neglect were more likely to experience a major depressive episode; those who had experienced physical neglect were more likely to be diagnosed with posttraumatic stress disorder (PTSD), and individuals with any type of trauma history had higher scores on the Beck Hopelessness Scale.[9] Severity of childhood trauma in adolescents considered ultrahigh risk for psychosis was also associated with greater rates of suicidality and nonsuicidal self-harm, poorer clinical outcomes, and poorer adaptive functioning.[10] In 1 metaanalysis, Bailey and colleagues[11] discovered that the severity of positive symptoms of psychosis, including hallucinations and delusions, was most associated with the total number of traumatic events experienced as well as exposure to childhood sexual and physical abuse. Negative symptom severity, in contrast, was most significantly associated with childhood neglect.

There is an increased prevalence of substance use in individuals with psychosis who have a history of childhood trauma. Tomassi and colleagues[12] conducted a multicenter randomized control study of individuals with FEP aged 18 to 54 years and collected data regarding childhood trauma history and substance use history using the Childhood Experiences of Care and Abuse Questionnaire (CECA-Q) and Cannabis Experiences Questionnaire, respectively. They found that severe childhood sexual abuse was associated with increased lifetime cannabis use; both sexual and physical abuse were associated with lifetime heroin use, and that severe physical abuse was associated with lifetime cocaine use. The investigators concluded that because individuals with FEP who were severely sexually abused were 5 times more likely to receive a diagnosis of affective psychosis, mood symptoms, such as depression, may precede substance use.

Last, studies point to a more refractory and prolonged illness course in patients with psychotic illness and a childhood trauma history. In a study of 96 FEP patients aged 18 to 65 years, Aas and colleagues[13] found that a childhood trauma history affected both illness course and functioning. Those with a childhood trauma history had lower Global Assessment of Functioning scores at baseline and less improvement over time; this was especially significant for emotional neglect, although this trend was also present for physical and sexual abuse. Individuals with higher childhood trauma scores also had significantly lower premorbid adjustment and longer duration of untreated psychosis. Trotta and colleagues[14] followed 285 patients aged 18 to 65 years first presenting for psychosis and found that physical abuse was associated with not being in a relationship, and parental separation was associated with longer hospitalizations and medication nonadherence at 1-year follow-up.

Gender Differences in Effects of Childhood Trauma

In recent years, there has been considerable research investigating gender differences in the link between childhood trauma and psychosis. Gender differences in schizophrenia have been well explored, and many sources point toward a slightly later age of onset in girls, more positive symptoms, less negative symptoms, and a less severe course, particularly in premenopausal girls, compared with their male counterparts.[15] Research has suggested that gender may affect children's susceptibility to certain types of abuse, and that they also may also respond to trauma exposure differently based on gender, affecting psychosis course. In 2009, Fisher and colleagues[16] investigated gender differences in the effects of childhood sexual and physical abuse in 181 individuals with FEP aged 16 to 64 years and 246 healthy controls, using the CECA-Q to collect trauma history and the Schedules for Clinical Assessment in Neuropsychiatry to assess psychotic symptoms. The investigators found that girls with FEP were twice as likely to have experienced childhood physical or sexual abuse compared with female healthy controls; no significant difference was found for boys. Comacchio and colleagues[17] found that although childhood sexual and physical abuse were correlated with increased negative symptoms in both genders, a younger age of psychotic illness onset was seen in girls only. Similarly, in a study of 102 individuals aged 18 to 69 years diagnosed with schizophrenia and schizoaffective disorder, childhood physical abuse was found to predict a younger age of onset in girls only.[18]

Childhood trauma is also found to have effects on symptoms in psychosis, particularly in girls. Garcia and colleagues[19] found that women with psychotic disorders and a higher Childhood Trauma Questionnaire score, especially emotional and physical neglect, had worse positive and negative symptoms, general psychopathology, depressive symptoms, and social functioning. In a study of 94 adults with first episode schizophrenia, Misiak and colleagues[20] investigated the effects of trauma on lifetime psychotic symptoms with the Operational Criteria for Psychotic Illness checklist, and acute symptoms with the Positive and Negative Syndrome Scale (PANSS). Their findings revealed that the number of auditory verbal hallucination types (third-person auditory hallucinations and abusive/accusatory/persecutory voices) and "hallucinatory behavior" (as measured by PANSS) were predicted by childhood trauma, especially sexual abuse, in girls only, even after accounting for confounders (antipsychotic treatment, duration of untreated illness, and PANSS depression factor score). There is evidence that women suffering from psychosis who experienced trauma have a greater severity of depressive symptoms.[21,22] These gender differences in the manifestations of childhood trauma and psychosis may be explained by gender differences in the effects of trauma on the hypothalamic-pituitary-adrenal axis activity and neurotransmitter release, and on prefrontal-hippocampal connectivity/prefrontal-amygdala pathway, potentially leading to increased risk of mood symptoms in women who have experienced trauma.[19,21]

Brain-Derived Neurotrophic Factor and Inflammatory Response in Childhood Trauma and Psychosis

Brain-derived neurotrophic factor (BDNF) is a protein important to neurogenesis and neuroplasticity, and neurotransmitter release within the brain, particularly within the hippocampus,[23] a structure significant in both schizophrenia and childhood trauma effects. It is considered to be a potential biomarker for schizophrenia given that multiple studies have found that low levels of BDNF are associated with psychosis risk.[23,24] A single nucleotide polymorphism within BDNF, Val66Met, in which a valine is substituted by a methionine, has been found to be somewhat common in individuals with schizophrenia and to affect the structure and availability of the protein.[23,24]

Reduced BDNF levels have also been associated with childhood trauma.[25] In a population of adults with FEP, Theleritis and colleagues[26] found that physical abuse predicted lower plasma levels of BDNF, and that sexual abuse, physical abuse, and separation from parents showed a trend toward lower BDNF levels that was not measured in healthy controls. These findings held true even when controlling for treatment with antipsychotics, which have been found to have an effect on BDNF levels. Similarly, in a study population of 249 patients with psychotic disorders (schizophrenia or bipolar spectrum disorders) and 476 healthy controls aged 18 to 65 years, Aas and colleagues[27] found evidence for a dose-relationship between the number of childhood trauma experiences and lower BDNF levels, with the most significant effects seen in those who had suffered sexual abuse. In this sample, reduced BDNF levels were also associated with increased affective episodes, and there were gender differences, with BDNF levels being the lowest in women who have been sexually abused. Brain MRIs showed that in *Met* carriers there was a relationship between abuse and smaller hippocampus volumes. *Met* carriers with a history of childhood trauma also demonstrated more significant cognitive impairments in executive function, working memory, and verbal abilities, compared with those who did not experience childhood trauma. This association was no longer significant when controlling for hippocampal volume, suggesting a potential shared mechanism.[27]

Bi and colleagues[28] found that the gene-environment interactions between Val66Met polymorphism and childhood trauma (physical neglect, physical abuse, and emotional neglect) jointly drove schizophrenia. Alemany and colleagues[29] demonstrated a similar gene-environment interaction in an adult general population sample demonstrating that those with Vall66Met polymorphism, reduced BDNF levels, and exposure to childhood abuse were more likely to have positive psychotic-like experiences compared with Val/Val homozygotes after correcting for several confounders, including age, gender, schizotypal personality, cannabis use, and anxiety. The catechol-o-methyl-transferase (COMT) gene, important in the metabolism of dopamine and norepinephrine, has also been of interest with some evidence for a gene-environment interaction in an adolescent general population sample, suggesting that those with COMT-Val158Met polymorphism and childhood abuse were more likely to have psychotic experiences $(P = .06)$.[30]

Other genetic changes associated with childhood trauma may also be important in the development of psychosis. Similar to other environmental factors, childhood trauma has been found to be linked with epigenetic changes, through transcription-altering methylation of genes. Misiak and colleagues[31] found that first-episode schizophrenia patients with a history of childhood trauma had significantly lower methylation of DNA repetitive sequences, predicted by emotional abuse and total trauma score on the Early Trauma Inventory Self Report–Short Form.

The links between childhood trauma and increased stress and inflammatory response have been well supported. It is possible that DNA hypomethylation occurring within genes related to inflammatory response is linked to this increased stress reactivity and psychosis risk.[32] Janusek and colleagues[33] measured the inflammatory and stress response by looking at interleukin-6 (IL-6; proinflammatory cytokine) and cortisol levels in adults' responses to acute stress using the Trier Social Stress Test and found that those who had experienced more childhood trauma had greater IL-6 responses. They also demonstrated that DNA hypomethylation of the IL-6 promoter was associated with increased childhood trauma.

Manifestation of Cooccurring Trauma and Psychosis in Adolescents

There have been several studies conducted to explore models explaining the connection between traumatic events and psychotic symptoms.[34] The primary psychological mechanisms proposed include dysfunctional cognitive schemas and affective dysregulation. Cognitive models suggest that traumatic events drastically alter core cognitive schemata in children and adolescents, promoting maladaptive beliefs of self, others, the world, and their future. Experiences of interpersonal trauma greatly affect the underlying schemata and cognitive appraisal systems of individuals, priming them to view the world as dangerous, the self as vulnerable, and others as threatening and potentially unsafe. These distortions of thought significantly influence the interpretation of internal and external experiences and arguably lay the foundation for persecutory delusions experienced by those struggling with psychosis.[34–36] Associations between paranoia and negative cognitions about self and others have been well established in clinical[37] and nonclinical samples.[34,38] In fact, these cognitive distortions may be one of the primary mediators in the relationship between psychosis and trauma.[36] Research by Kilcommons and Morrison[39] demonstrated a statistically significant correlation between negative attributional styles associated with trauma and positive symptoms of psychosis, most notably hallucinations. Results of their study demonstrated a salient relationship between the content of childhood trauma and the subsequent themes of delusions and hallucinations reported by the participants within their clinical sample.[39] Similar research conducted by Gracie and colleagues[36] on a fairly large nonclinical sample revealed statistically significant associations between negative schematic beliefs and a predisposition to both paranoia and hallucinations with negative beliefs about self and others being most strongly associated with a predisposition to paranoid thoughts.

Recent research has also proposed an affective model to describe the connection between trauma and psychosis.[34] The link between childhood traumatic events and affect dysregulation has been well established.[40] Emotion regulation is considered a developmental task highly influenced by a safe, emotionally attuned and regulated caregiving environment. Interpersonal trauma, especially those traumatic events occurring within the caregiving environment, greatly disrupts the development of adaptive emotion regulation strategies, resulting in increased risk for emotional dysregulation.[40,41] Children who have experienced interpersonal trauma within the caregiving environment have a decreased understanding of negative emotions and diminished emotion regulation strategies[42] as well as increased occurrences of emotional dysregulation,[41,43] especially for those who have PTSD.[40,44] These deficits in affect regulation have been shown to correlate with and even exacerbate symptoms of psychosis.[45] Research by Kramer and colleagues[46] revealed that affective dysregulation is strongly correlated with reality testing impairments and paranoia. Prolonged emotional dysregulation is associated with increased risk for psychosis as well.[47] Moreover, studies have demonstrated that individuals with psychosis exposed to adverse childhood experiences tend to react to normal, daily stressors with increased emotional sensitivity and with greater negative affect.[48,49] Thus, traumatic exposures in childhood appear to foster the emergence of affective sensitivity, subsequent emotional dysregulation, and marked cognitive distortions, all of which lay the foundation for a complex interaction between cognitive appraisal systems and affective instability that increases the risk for the emergence of psychotic processes.

Diagnostic comorbidities

It is well established through comprehensive epidemiologic research that childhood trauma has robust associations with several diagnostic comorbidities.[50] Recent metaanalyses link childhood trauma to anxiety disorders, mood disorders, including unipolar and bipolar depression, and psychosis. Through a recent comprehensive metaanalytic review, van Nierop and colleagues[51] examined diagnostic comorbidities in a large sample of adolescents and adults with psychosis (N = 6646; aged 16–65) who have histories of childhood trauma. Results revealed that childhood trauma was associated with struggles in multiple cooccurring symptom domains. In general, exposure to childhood trauma was associated with increased risk for comorbid challenges in anxiety, depression, mania, and psychosis. Results from this metaanalysis further demonstrated that those presenting with cooccurring trauma and psychosis presented with increased rates of comorbid symptoms of depression, anxiety, and mania, even when adjusting for substance use and educational level. Although childhood trauma was statistically associated with comorbid symptoms of depression, mania, and anxiety, greater diagnostic complexity and symptom endorsement were noted in those presenting with cooccurring psychosis and trauma exposure. In addition to these diagnostic cooccurrences, substance use disorders, disruptive behavior disorders, and other attention and executive functioning challenges were noted for individuals with PTSD and for individuals with psychotic disorders.[50]

Evidence-based assessment procedures

Assessment of trauma There are several evidence-based questionnaires and clinical assessments designed to measure the intensity of posttraumatic stress symptoms (PTSS) in children and adolescents (**Table 1**). The Clinician-Administered PTSD Scale for Children and Adolescents is arguably the most widely used semistructured clinical interview in research and clinical settings. It carefully assesses the frequency and intensity of 17 PTSD symptoms as well as the effects of posttraumatic stress on social,

Table 1
Evidence-based assessments for trauma and psychosis in adolescents

Name	Type of Instrument	Purpose	Age Range, y	Time, min	Cost
Clinician-Administered PTSD Scale for Children and Adolescents (CAPS-CA)	Semistructured clinical interview	Designed to assess the frequency and intensity of 17 PTSD symptoms as well as their effect on social, developmental, and academic functioning	8–18	*Administration:* 45 *Scoring:* 20–30	$146.00
University of California, Los Angeles Child/Adolescent PTSD Reaction Index for *DSM-5* (UCLA-PTSD-RI)	Self-report screening tool	Designed to efficiently screen for symptoms of PTSD	6–18	*Administration:* 15–25 *Scoring:* 10–15	Free
Child PTSD Symptom Scale for *DSM-5* (CPSS-SR-5)	Self-report screening tool	Designed to efficiently screen for symptoms of PTSD	8–18	*Administration:* 10 *Scoring:* 5–10	Free
Trauma Symptom Checklist for Children (TSCC)	Self-report diagnostic measure	Designed to assess symptoms of posttraumatic stress as well as general anxiety, depression, anger, sexual concerns, and dissociation	8–17	*Administration:* 15–20 *Scoring:* 10–15	$261.00
Positive and Negative Syndrome Scale (PANSS)	Clinician-rated diagnostic measure	Designed to assess positive and negative symptoms of psychosis	18 & older	*Administration:* 30–40 *Scoring:* 20	$330.00

developmental, and academic functioning. The University of California, Los Angeles (UCLA) Child/Adolescent PTSD Reaction Index for *Diagnostic and Statistical Manual of Mental Disorders* (Fifth Edition) *(DSM-5)*[52] is a self-report or parent-report measure designed to assess trauma exposure history and measure symptoms of PTSD in children and adolescents. The child-, adolescent-, and parent-report measures comprise 14 items assessing history of trauma exposure, 27 items to assess symptoms of PTSD, and 4 additional items to assess for dissociative symptoms. The Child PTSD Symptom Scale for *DSM-5* is a 27-item self-report measure assessing PTSD symptom severity in children and adolescents.[53] All items correspond with the *DSM-5* diagnostic criteria for PTSD. The Trauma symptom checklist for children (TSCC)[54] is a comprehensive standardized self-report measure designed to assess symptoms of posttraumatic stress and related psychological symptoms. The TSCC has been standardized on a socioeconomically diverse sample of more than 3000 children and adolescents from urban, suburban, and rural areas. The TSCC consists of 54 items that correspond with 6 clinical scales assessing symptoms of depression, posttraumatic stress, sexual concerns, anger, dissociation, and generalized anxiety, as well as validity scales measuring both underreporting and overreporting.

Assessment of psychosis The PANSS[55] is a 30-item diagnostic screening tool designed to assess a range of negative and positive symptoms of psychosis. The PANSS has been widely used in clinical outcome research for schizophrenia spectrum disorders, and it is considered the "gold standard" for assessment of pharmacologic and psychotherapeutic treatment efficacy.[56] The PANNS guides practitioners in evaluating a multidimensional array of symptoms, including positive symptoms, negative symptoms, neuromotor symptoms, and depressive symptoms. Although the PANSS is typically administered within adult populations, it has also been used in adolescent treatment studies, like the Treatment for Early Onset Schizophrenia Study, and there is burgeoning evidence of its reliability and validity within adolescent population.[57]

Evidence-Based Treatments for Trauma and Psychosis in Adolescents

Cognitive behavioral therapy for pediatric posttraumatic stress disorder
The authors are not aware of any empirical studies to date investigating the efficacy of psychotherapeutic interventions for the treatment of cooccurring trauma and psychosis in children and adolescents despite repeated calls from researchers and clinicians that highlight the need for the evaluation of such treatments and their implementation.[58,59] However, there exists an extensive research base examining psychological treatments for child and adolescent PTSD. Of the bona fide treatments for child and adolescent PTSD, cognitive behavioral therapy (CBT) interventions have received the most empirical examination, with recent metaanalyses indicating that CBT for child and adolescent PTSD is the gold-standard approach.[60,61]

Findings from a large metaanalysis of 135 studies (N = 9562) yielded the largest effect size (Hedge's g = 1.39, 95% confidence interval [CI] = 0.08, 1.69) for CBT treatments for pediatric PTSD (ie, trauma-focused CBT [TF-CBT]; prolonged exposure [PE]; cognitive therapy for PTSD [CT for PTSD]) compared with controls.[60] Moderator analyses yielded clinically relevant interactive effects, which may be useful for treatment planning and prognostication, with older children showing greater PTSD symptom reduction than younger children, and caretaker involvement in treatment demonstrating larger effects (g = 1.01 vs g = .81) than therapies with only youth involvement. In a similar vein, in a metaanalysis of 39 studies of psychotherapeutic interventions for pediatric PTSD, TF-CBT yielded robust effects after treatment compared with waitlist controls (g = 1.44, 95% CI = 1.02, 1.86) and to active control conditions (g = 0.56, 95% CI = 0.33, 0.80), including eye movement desensitization and reprocessing (EMDR), psychodynamic psychotherapy, multidisciplinary treatment, classroom-based intervention for students, and child-centered therapy.[61] Moreover, there is substantial evidence that ameliorating effects of bona fide treatments are maintained after treatment termination. For example, in their metaanalysis investigating the long-term effects of psychotherapy for pediatric PTSD, Gutermann and colleagues[62] reported large pre-follow-up effect sizes in pooled analysis of controlled and uncontrolled studies at both the less than 6-month (g = .99, 95% CI = 83, 1.16) and ≥6-month follow-up periods (g = 1.24, 95% CI = 1.04, 1.45). In contrast to Gutermann and colleagues,[60] findings regarding the superiority of treatments involving caretakers compared with youth-only discussed above, effect sizes did not differ during either follow-up periods. The investigators posit that it is possible that parent involvement is important for acute-treatment gains, but psychological processes at work following treatment termination are dependent on the individual youth.[62]

Turning to the specifics of one of the most researched treatments for pediatric PTSD, TF-CBT is a time-limited (12–16 sessions) treatment modality that addresses a wide range pediatric trauma experiences.[63] Specific interventions of this treatment modality are represented in the PRACTICE acronym: psychoeducation, relaxation skills, affect recognition and modulation, cognitive coping skills, trauma narrative, in vivo exposure, conjoint parent-child sessions, cognitive restructuring, and enhancing future safety.[63]

Other evidence-based CBT treatments for pediatric PTSD (eg, PE, CT for PTSD) include many of the same specific interventions as those described in TF-CBT, including psychoeducation, skills training, imaginal exposure, and cognitive restructuring. As Smith and colleagues[64] note, the primary differences between CBT treatments for pediatric PTSD is in the privileging of 1 specific intervention over the other. For example, CT for PTSD focuses on cognitive restructuring, whereas PE's focus is on exposure.

Although clearly effective, Neelakantan and colleagues[65] posit that 1 hurdle to implementation of TF-CBT in routine practice is clinician's concern regarding the patient's experience of this treatment modality. However, in addition to the burgeoning quantitative literature on TF-CBT, there have also been several qualitative studies on youth's experiences in treatment that speak to these concerns. In a recent metasynthesis of 8 qualitative investigations of patient experiences in TF-CBT, 3 broad thematic categories emerged: "Engagement in TF-CBT," "Experience of Treatment Components," and "Therapeutic Outcomes." In light of youth and caregiver reports, investigators highlight specific points of consideration for the TF-CBT therapist, including the need to provide a clear treatment rationale and foster positive outcome expectation at the onset of therapy, the importance of the therapeutic relationship, therapist credibility, and attunement in facilitating youth engagement and disclosure, the importance of completing a trauma-narrative, and the adaptive function of the therapist in facilitating open communication between youth and caregiver.

Noncognitive behavioral therapy interventions for pediatric posttraumatic stress disorder

Of the non-CBT treatment approaches for pediatric PTSD, EMDR has received much recent attention. Although the putative mechanism (bilateral sensory input like saccadic eye movements, tapping, or alternating tones in headphones vs imaginal exposure) of EMDR has long been debated, with some studies suggesting comparable effects with exposure modalities without bilateral stimulation,[66] there is emerging evidence that EMDR is an efficacious intervention for child and adolescent PTSD. For example, in a metaanalysis examining the efficacy of EMDR for pediatric PTSD, including 8 randomized controlled trials (RCTs), EMDR proved superior to waitlist condition in reducing both PTSD symptoms (Cohen's $d = -0.49$, 95% CI $= -0.87, -0.10$) and cooccurring symptoms of anxiety ($d = -0.49$, 95% CI $= -0.76, -0.13$), but did not significantly impact depressive symptoms.[67] Similarly, in a metaanalysis of 30 studies comparing the effectiveness of TF-CBT with EMDR in the treatment of PTSS in children and adolescents, Lewey and colleagues[68] found a small but significant effect size for EMDR and TF-CBT ($d = -0.359$) supporting the effectiveness of both treatments, with comparative findings marginally favoring TF-CBT over EMDR.

Cognitive behavioral interventions for adults with trauma and psychosis
As previously noted, there have been no empirical investigations to date of psychotherapeutic treatments for children and adolescents with cooccurring PTSD and psychosis. However, there is a small but growing literature on the feasibility and efficacy of psychotherapeutic treatment of comorbid PTSD and psychosis in adults. For example, in a single-blind RCT (N = 155) involving adult participants with psychosis and PTSD randomized to receive 8 weekly sessions of PE, EMDR, or waitlist, those in the active treatment conditions demonstrated greater PTSD symptom reduction than the waitlist controls.[69] Participants in the PE condition were 56% more likely, and those in the EMDR condition were 60% more likely to no longer meet diagnostic criteria for PTSD during acute treatment compared with controls. Treatment gains were maintained at 6-month follow-up. Regarding secondary outcomes of interest, there were no significant differences in reports of adverse events between the 3 conditions, and attrition was comparable between PE and EDMR groups. In a follow-up study of the aforementioned trial comparing 12-month follow-up and 6-month follow-up, van den Berg and colleagues[70] found that therapeutic gains were largely maintained. For example, there were no significant differences in clinician- or patient-rated PTSD symptom severity in either active treatment conditions between the 6-month and 12-month follow-up. However, participants in the PE condition had a continued reduction in the severity of PTSD cognitions ($t[41] = 2.14$, $P = .038$), whereas those receiving EMDR did not.

There appears to be substantial evidence that trauma-focused therapies are both feasible and efficacious in the treatment of cooccurring PTSD and psychosis, with treatment effects stable across 1-year follow-up. Addressing what the investigators identify as the primary deterrent for providing trauma-focused treatments in this population, namely concerns surrounding psychosis symptom exacerbation, van den Berg and colleagues[71] conducted a secondary analysis of the same trial data. Results indicate that trauma-focused treatments had no adverse effects on the outcomes of interest at either treatment termination or 6-month follow-up, with people receiving trauma-focused therapies reporting lesser symptom exacerbation and fewer experiences of adverse events (odds ratio [OR] = 0.48, $P = .32$). Moreover, those receiving trauma-focused therapies were less likely to be revictimized (OR = 0.40, $P = .035$).

Taken together, results of these treatment studies for adults with PTSD and psychosis, in conjunction with the robust empirical support for trauma-focused treatments for pediatric PTSD, point to the feasibility, safety, and efficacy of these treatments for children and adolescents with PTSD and psychosis. However, further research is needed to determine if the findings from the adult literature will hold for children and adolescents. In the meantime, clinicians working with youths with PTSD who are at risk of developing psychosis may pay special attention to potential mediators of the trauma-psychosis association. For example, in a recent systematic review of

37 studies examining potential mediators of the childhood adversity and psychosis link, researchers identified several types of potential mediators, including affective dysregulation, maladaptive cognitions, and PTSS.[72] The authors suggest that targeting these "families" of mediators in treatment may enhance treatment outcomes for those who have experienced childhood adversity and are at risk for developing psychosis.

SUMMARY

This article highlights recent advances in understanding the connections between childhood trauma experiences, psychotic symptoms, and the development and course of psychotic disorders. Cross-sectional and longitudinal studies have consistently demonstrated clear associations between traumatic life events in childhood and the development of psychosis in late adolescence.[1] Although there is more to be discovered about the relationship between childhood trauma and psychosis, there is an abundance of data to highlight the importance of this association. There is significant evidence to indicate that those who have experienced childhood adversity not only have an increased psychosis risk but also are at risk for a psychotic illness course that is worse in severity. Additional research into the causal links between childhood adversity and psychosis, especially gene-environment interactions, is required. Considerable data support gender differences in response to trauma, affecting psychotic illness course; women with a history of childhood trauma can have a more severe psychotic illness course (compared with men), including a younger age of onset, worsening symptoms, and worse overall functioning. There is also growing evidence supporting other biological markers, such as BDNF and gene-environment interactions.

The central psychological mechanisms explaining the relationship between childhood trauma and psychotic symptoms include changes to cognitive schemata, so that the world is seen as negative and threatening.[34–36] As such, experiencing childhood trauma affects the content and type of delusion. In addition, the link between childhood traumatic events and affect dysregulation[40] may explain the higher rates of comorbidity (in particular, anxiety, depression, and substance use) present in those who experienced childhood trauma with or without psychosis. Given this, using evidence-based assessments of trauma to help identify the impact of trauma is critical. An expanding body of literature supports the use of TF-CBT and other cognitive behavioral interventions, which include principles of affect recognition, modulation and regulation, cognitive restructuring, and enhancing future safety, in the treatment of traumatized youth. Although no research has been conducted to support the use of those interventions in youth with cooccurring trauma and psychosis, emerging evidence in adults is encouraging.

The authors urge clinicians to always assess for cooccurring trauma in youth with psychotic symptoms, because there are important implications to presentation, course, and treatment.

REFERENCES

1. Croft J, Heron J, Teufel C, et al. Association of trauma type, age of exposure, and frequency in childhood and adolescence with psychotic experiences in early adulthood. JAMA Psychiatry 2019;76(1):79–80.
2. Trauelsen AM, Bendall S, Jansen JE, et al. Childhood adversity specificity and dose-response effect in non-affective first-episode psychosis. Schizophr Res 2015;165(1):52–9.

3. Bentall R, de Sousa P, Varese F, et al. From adversity to psychosis: pathways and mechanisms from specific adversities to specific symptoms. Soc Psychiatry Psychiatr Epidemiol 2014;49(7):1011–22.

4. Loewy RL, Corey S, Amirfathi F, et al. Childhood trauma and clinical high risk for psychosis. Schizophr Res 2019;205:10–4.

5. Falukozi E, Addington J. Impact of trauma on attenuated psychotic symptoms. Psychosis 2012;4(3):203–12.

6. Kraan T, Velthorst E, Smit F, et al. Trauma and recent life events in individuals at ultra high risk for psychosis: review and meta-analysis. Schizophr Res 2014; 161(2–3):143–9.

7. Thompson A, Marwaha S, Nelson B, et al. Do affective or dissociative symptoms mediate the association between childhood sexual trauma and transition to psychosis in an ultra-high risk cohort? Psychiatry Res 2016;236:182–5.

8. Üçok A, Kaya H, Uğurpala C, et al. History of childhood physical trauma is related to cognitive decline in individuals with ultra-high risk for psychosis. Schizophr Res 2015;169(1):199–203.

9. Hassan AN, Stuart EA, De Luca V. Childhood maltreatment increases the risk of suicide attempt in schizophrenia. Schizophr Res 2016;176(2–3):572–7.

10. de Vos C, Thompson A, Amminger P, et al. The relationship between childhood trauma and clinical characteristics in ultra-high risk for psychosis youth. Psychosis 2019;11(1):28–41.

11. Bailey T, Alvarez-Jimenez M, Garcia-Sanchez AM, et al. Childhood trauma is associated with severity of hallucinations and delusions in psychotic disorders: a systematic review and meta-analysis. Schizophr Bull 2018;44(5):1111–22.

12. Tomassi S, Tosato S, Mondelli V, et al. Influence of childhood trauma on diagnosis and substance use in first-episode psychosis. Br J Psychiatry 2017;211(3): 151–6.

13. Aas M, Andreassen OA, Aminoff SR, et al. A history of childhood trauma is associated with slower improvement rates: findings from a one-year follow-up study of patients with a first-episode psychosis. BMC Psychiatry 2016;16(1):126.

14. Trotta A, Murray RM, David AS, et al. Impact of different childhood adversities on 1-year outcomes of psychotic disorder in the genetics and psychosis study. Schizophr Bull 2015;42(2):464–75.

15. Thorup A, Petersen L, Jeppesen P, et al. Gender differences in young adults with first-episode schizophrenia spectrum disorders at baseline in the Danish OPUS study. J Nerv Ment Dis 2007;195(5):396–405.

16. Fisher H, Morgan C, Dazzan P, et al. Gender differences in the association between childhood abuse and psychosis. Br J Psychiatry 2009;194(4):319–25.

17. Comacchio C, Howard LM, Bonetto C, et al. The impact of gender and childhood abuse on age of psychosis onset, psychopathology and needs for care in psychosis patients. Schizophr Res 2019;210:164–71.

18. Kocsis-Bogár K, Mészáros V, Perczel-Forintos D. Gender differences in the relationship of childhood trauma and the course of illness in schizophrenia. Compr Psychiatry 2018;82:84–8.

19. Garcia M, Montalvo I, Creus M, et al. Sex differences in the effect of childhood trauma on the clinical expression of early psychosis. Compr Psychiatry 2016; 68:86–96.

20. Misiak B, Moustafa AA, Kiejna A, et al. Childhood traumatic events and types of auditory verbal hallucinations in first-episode schizophrenia patients. Compr Psychiatry 2016;66:17–22.

21. Kelly DL, Rowland LM, Patchan KM, et al. Schizophrenia clinical symptom differences in women vs. men with and without a history of childhood physical abuse. Child Adolesc Psychiatry Ment Health 2016;10(1):5.

22. Pruessner M, King S, Vracotas N, et al. Gender differences in childhood trauma in first episode psychosis: association with symptom severity over two years. Schizophr Res 2019;205:30–7.

23. Sahu G, Malavade K, Jacob T. Cognitive impairment in schizophrenia: interplay of BDNF and childhood trauma? A review of literature. Psychiatr Q 2016;87(3): 559–69.

24. de Castro-Catala M, van Nierop M, Barrantes-Vidal N, et al. Childhood trauma, BDNF Val66Met and subclinical psychotic experiences. Attempt at replication in two independent samples. J Psychiatr Res 2016;83:121–9.

25. Mondelli V, Cattaneo A, Murri MB, et al. Stress and inflammation reduce BDNF expression in first-episode psychosis: a pathway to smaller hippocampal volume. J Clin Psychiatry 2011;72(12):1677.

26. Theleritis C, Fisher HL, Shäfer I, et al. Brain derived neurotropic factor (BDNF) is associated with childhood abuse but not cognitive domains in first episode psychosis. Schizophr Res 2014;159(1):56–61.

27. Aas M, Haukvik UK, Djurovic S, et al. BDNF val66met modulates the association between childhood trauma, cognitive and brain abnormalities in psychoses. Prog Neuropsychopharmacol Biol Psychiatry 2013;46:181–8.

28. Bi X, Lv X, Ai X, et al. Childhood trauma interacted with BDNF Val66Met influence schizophrenic symptoms. Medicine (Baltimore) 2018;97(13):e0160.

29. Alemany S, Arias B, Aguilera M, et al. Childhood abuse, the BDNF-Val66Met polymorphism and adult psychotic-like experiences. Br J Psychiatry 2011;199(1): 38–42.

30. Ramsay H, Kelleher I, Flannery P, et al. Relationship between the COMT-Val158Met and BDNF-Val66Met polymorphisms, childhood trauma and psychotic experiences in an adolescent general population sample. PLoS One 2013;8(11): e79741.

31. Misiak B, Szmida E, Karpiński P, et al. Lower LINE-1 methylation in first-episode schizophrenia patients with the history of childhood trauma. Epigenomics 2015; 7(8):1275–85.

32. Tomassi S, Tosato S. Epigenetics and gene expression profile in first-episode psychosis: the role of childhood trauma. Neurosci Biobehav Rev 2017;83:226–37.

33. Janusek LW, Tell D, Gaylord-Harden N, et al. Relationship of childhood adversity and neighborhood violence to a proinflammatory phenotype in emerging adult African American men: an epigenetic link. Brain Behav Immun 2017;60:126–35.

34. Misiak B, Krefft M, Bielawski T, et al. Toward a unified theory of childhood trauma and psychosis: a comprehensive review of epidemiological, clinical, neuropsychological and biological findings. Neurosci Biobehav Rev 2017;75:393–406.

35. Morrison AP. A cognitive behavioural perspective on the relationship between childhood trauma and psychosis. Epidemiol Psychiatr Sci 2009;18(4):294–8.

36. Gracie A, Freeman D, Green S, et al. The association between traumatic experience, paranoia and hallucinations: a test of the predictions of psychological models. Acta Psychiatr Scand 2007;116(4):280–9.

37. Smith B, Fowler DG, Freeman D, et al. Emotion and psychosis: links between depression, self-esteem, negative schematic beliefs and delusions and hallucinations. Schizophr Res 2006;86(1):181–8.

38. Fowler D, Freeman D, Smith B, et al. The brief core schema scales (BCSS): psychometric properties and associations with paranoia and grandiosity in non-clinical and psychosis samples. Psychol Med 2006;36(6):749–59.

39. Kilcommons AM, Morrison AP. Relationships between trauma and psychosis: an exploration of cognitive and dissociative factors. Acta Psychiatr Scand 2005; 112(5):351–9.

40. Dvir Y, Ford JD, Hill M, et al. Childhood maltreatment, emotional dysregulation, and psychiatric comorbidities. Harv Rev Psychiatry 2014;22(3):149–61.

41. Maughan A, Cicchetti D. Impact of child maltreatment and interadult violence on children's emotion regulation abilities and socioemotional adjustment. Child Dev 2002;73(5):1525–42.

42. Shipman K, Edwards A, Brown A, et al. Managing emotion in a maltreating context: a pilot study examining child neglect. Child Abuse Negl 2005;29(9): 1015–29.

43. Burns EE, Jackson JL, Harding HG. Child maltreatment, emotion regulation, and posttraumatic stress: the impact of emotional abuse. Journal of Aggression, Maltreatment & Trauma 2010;19(8):801–19.

44. Tull MT, Barrett HM, McMillan ES, et al. A preliminary investigation of the relationship between emotion regulation difficulties and posttraumatic stress symptoms. Behav Ther 2007;38(3):303–13.

45. Wigman JTW, van Nierop M, Vollebergh WAM, et al. Evidence that psychotic symptoms are prevalent in disorders of anxiety and depression, impacting on illness onset, risk, and severity-implications for diagnosis and ultra-high risk research. Schizophr Bull 2012;38(2):247–57.

46. Kramer I, Simons CJP, Wigman JTW, et al. Time-lagged moment-to-moment interplay between negative affect and paranoia: new insights in the affective pathway to psychosis. Schizophr Bull 2014;40(2):278–86.

47. van Rossum I, Dominguez M, Lieb R, et al. Affective dysregulation and reality distortion: a 10-year prospective study of their association and clinical relevance. Schizophr Bull 2011;37(3):561–71.

48. Lardinois M, Lataster T, Mengelers R, et al. Childhood trauma and increased stress sensitivity in psychosis. Acta Psychiatr Scand 2011;123(1):28–35.

49. Lataster T, Collip D, Lardinois M, et al. Evidence for a familial correlation between increased reactivity to stress and positive psychotic symptoms. Acta Psychiatr Scand 2010;122(5):395–404.

50. Kessler RC, Sonnega A, Bromet E, et al. Posttraumatic stress disorder in the national comorbidity survey. Arch Gen Psychiatry 1995;52(12):1048–60.

51. van Nierop M, Viechtbauer W, Gunther N, et al. Childhood trauma is associated with a specific admixture of affective, anxiety, and psychosis symptoms cutting across traditional diagnostic boundaries. Psychol Med 2015;45(6):1277–88.

52. Steinberg AM, Brymer MJ, Kim S, et al. Psychometric properties of the UCLA PTSD reaction index: part I. J Trauma Stress 2013;26(1):1–9.

53. Foa EB, Johnson KM, Feeny NC, et al. The child PTSD symptom scale: a preliminary examination of its psychometric properties. J Clin Child Psychol 2001;30(3): 376–84.

54. Briere J. Trauma symptom checklist for children (TSCC) professional manual. Odessa (FL): Psychological Assessment Resources; 1996.

55. Kay SR, Fiszbein A, Opler LA. The positive and negative syndrome scale (PANSS) for schizophrenia. Schizophr Bull 1987;13(2):261–76.

56. Opler MGA, Yavorsky C, Daniel DG. Positive and negative syndrome scale (PANSS) training: challenges, solutions, and future directions. Innov Clin Neurosci 2017;14(11–12):77.
57. Fields JH, Grochowski S, Lindenmayer JP, et al. Assessing positive and negative symptoms in children and adolescents. Am J Psychiatry 1994;151(2):249–53.
58. Dvir Y, Denietolis B, Frazier JA. Childhood trauma and psychosis. Child Adolesc Psychiatr Clin N Am 2013;22(4):629–41.
59. Schäfer I, Fisher H. Childhood trauma and posttraumatic stress disorder in patients with psychosis: clinical challenges and emerging treatments. Curr Opin Psychiatry 2011;24(6):514–8.
60. Gutermann J, Schreiber F, Matulis S, et al. Psychological treatments for symptoms of posttraumatic stress disorder in children, adolescents, and young adults: a meta-analysis. Clin Child Fam Psychol Rev 2016;19(2):77–93.
61. Morina N, Koerssen R, Pollet TV. Interventions for children and adolescents with posttraumatic stress disorder: a meta-analysis of comparative outcome studies. Clin Psychol Rev 2016;47:41–54.
62. Gutermann J, Schwartzkopff L, Steil R. Meta-analysis of the long-term treatment effects of psychological interventions in youth with PTSD symptoms. Clin Child Fam Psychol Rev 2017;20(4):422–34.
63. Cohen JA, Mannarino AP, Deblinger E. Treating trauma and traumatic grief in children and adolescents. New York: Guilford Press; 2006.
64. Smith P, Dalgleish T, Meiser-Stedman R. Practitioner review: posttraumatic stress disorder and its treatment in children and adolescents. J Child Psychol Psychiatry 2019;60(5):500–15.
65. Neelakantan L, Hetrick S, Michelson D. Users' experiences of trauma-focused cognitive behavioural therapy for children and adolescents: a systematic review and metasynthesis of qualitative research. Eur Child Adolesc Psychiatry 2019; 28(7):877–97.
66. Davidson PR, Parker KCH. Eye movement desensitization and reprocessing (EMDR): a meta-analysis. J Consult Clin Psychol 2001;69(2):305–16.
67. Moreno-Alcázar A, Treen D, Valiente-Gómez A, et al. Efficacy of eye movement desensitization and reprocessing in children and adolescent with posttraumatic stress disorder: a meta-analysis of randomized controlled trials. Front Psychol 2017;8:1750.
68. Lewey J, Smith C, Burcham B, et al. Comparing the effectiveness of EMDR and TF-CBT for children and adolescents: a meta-analysis. J Child Adolesc Trauma 2018;11(4):457–72.
69. van den Berg DP, de Bont PA, van der Vleugel BM, et al. Prolonged exposure vs eye movement desensitization and reprocessing vs waiting list for posttraumatic stress disorder in patients with a psychotic disorder: a randomized clinical trial. JAMA Psychiatry 2015;72(3):259.
70. van den Berg D, de Bont PAJM, van der Vleugel BM, et al. Long-term outcomes of trauma-focused treatment in psychosis. Br J Psychiatry 2018;212(3):180–2.
71. van den Berg DP, de Bont PA, van der Vleugel BM, et al. Trauma-focused treatment in PTSD patients with psychosis: symptom exacerbation, adverse events, and revictimization. Schizophr Bull 2016;42(3):693–702.
72. Williams J, Bucci S, Berry K, et al. Psychological mediators of the association between childhood adversities and psychosis: a systematic review. Clin Psychol Rev 2018;65:175–96.

Substance-induced Psychosis in Youth

David Beckmann, MD, MPH[a],*, Kelsey Leigh Lowman, AB[b], Jessica Nargiso, PhD[c], James McKowen, PhD[c], Lisa Watt, MSN[d], Amy M. Yule, MD[e]

KEYWORDS

- Substance-induced psychosis • Drug-induced psychosis • Adolescents • Cannabis
- Stimulants • Psychosis • Substance use disorder

KEY POINTS

- Substance-induced psychosis (SIP) is typically defined as hallucinations and/or delusions caused by intoxication or withdrawal from a substance, and it occurs in approximately 6.5 in 100,000 persons per year.
- Because primary psychotic disorders (PPDs) and substance use disorders are so frequently comorbid, SIP can be difficult to differentiate from PPD, although there can be some differences in the clinical presentation.
- Substances that are of particular clinical interest because of their risk of inducing psychosis are reviewed individually, including hallucinogens, cannabis, stimulants (particularly methamphetamine and cocaine), nicotine, research chemicals, and some commonly prescribed medications.
- Treatment of SIP ideally involves a comprehensive approach including psychosocial and pharmacologic treatment that simultaneously address psychosis and substance use. The most effective psychosocial interventions also involve parents or other supports of the youth experiencing psychosis.

Disclosures: Dr A.M. Yule has served as a consultant (clinical services) for Phoenix House (2015–2017) and Gavin House (2018 to present). She currently receives research funding from 5K12DA000357-17.

[a] Addiction Recovery Management Service, First Episode and Early Psychosis Program, Department of Psychiatry, Massachusetts General Hospital, Harvard Medical School, 55 Fruit Street WACC 812, Boston, MA 02114, USA; [b] Department of Psychiatry, Massachusetts General Hospital, 101 Merrimac Street, Suite 320, Boston, MA 02114, USA; [c] Addiction Recovery Management Service, Department of Psychiatry, Massachusetts General Hospital, Harvard Medical School, 55 Fruit Street WACC 812, Boston, MA 02114, USA; [d] Addiction Recovery Management Service, Department of Psychiatry, Massachusetts General Hospital, 15 Parkman Street YAW 6A, Boston, MA 02114, USA; [e] Addiction Recovery Management Service, Department of Psychiatry, Massachusetts General Hospital, Harvard Medical School, 15 Parkman Street YAW 6A, Boston, MA 02114, USA
* Corresponding author.
E-mail address: david.beckmann@mgh.harvard.edu

Child Adolesc Psychiatric Clin N Am 29 (2020) 131–143
https://doi.org/10.1016/j.chc.2019.08.006
childpsych.theclinics.com

INTRODUCTION

> *Kevin is a 16-year-old boy who recently finished the 11th grade of high school. He has attention-deficit/hyperactivity disorder (ADHD), which has been effectively treated by his pediatrician since the age of 7 years. Over the past 3 years he has taken mixed amphetamine salts, extended release 25 mg, in the morning and an additional 7.5 mg of immediate release after school. He has no other psychiatric history; neither his parents nor his pediatrician have ever been concerned about symptoms of a mood, anxiety, psychotic, or substance use disorder. He has no medical problems and does not take other medications.*
>
> *One evening in July, Kevin was brought to the emergency room by his parents for increasing concern about his behavior. Although he spent the first part of the summer with friends, he became increasingly withdrawn and isolated, and his parents thought he may be using cannabis after smelling this a few times. They also found his phone in a plastic bag in the refrigerator, and when they asked him about this, he replied, "It's just safer that way." On the night of presentation, his father had broken into Kevin's room; Kevin had locked himself in and could be heard repeatedly yelling, "Leave me alone!"*
>
> *In the emergency room, Kevin told staff that he was afraid of "shadow government agents." He described that they had been observing him through electronic devices for several weeks, and this evening he had seen shadowy figures in his home out of the corner of his eye. He was also able to hear them speaking to one another, and although he could not make out specific words, he felt certain they were conspiring to capture or kill him.*
>
> *His medical work-up was unremarkable except for a urine toxicology screen, which was positive for amphetamines and cannabinoids. He reported he had been smoking cannabis most days over the summer. He also reported that over the summer he was not taking the mixed amphetamine extended release because he often woke up late in the day. Instead he took the immediate release medication and occasionally took 3 to 4 times the prescribed dose when he was tired. He denied other substance use. The emergency room staff recommended voluntary hospitalization, which he and his parents declined. He was discharged to home with a plan to follow up in your clinic 3 days later. He was instructed to not use cannabis and to not take medication for his ADHD until he was evaluated further.*

This case is a common scenario for child and adolescent psychiatrists. This article reviews substance-induced psychosis (SIP), including the definition, epidemiology, causes, treatment, and prognosis.

DEFINITIONS AND EPIDEMIOLOGY

Clinicians face a key diagnostic challenge in the differentiation between SIP and a primary psychotic disorder (PPD). SIP is defined in the Diagnostic and Statistical Manual of Mental Disorders, Fifth Edition (DSM-5) by the presence of delusions and/or hallucinations that arise and persist in the context of acute intoxication or withdrawal from a substance and are not exclusively attributable to delirium.[1] A diagnosis of SIP also requires a lack of insight into the patient's symptoms and remission of symptoms within 1 month of sustained abstinence, although some studies suggest that psychosis can persist long after abstinence. Dawe and colleagues[2] (2011) interviewed 98 patients with a diagnosis of SIP (n = 47; 48%) or PPD (n = 51; 52%) within the first 2 days of admission to an acute psychiatric unit, with intermittent follow-up until discharge or day 51 of admission. Although patients with SIP showed similar positive symptom severity and more severely disturbed behavior at admission compared with patients with PPD, they also showed more rapid abatement in both symptom categories. However, Mauri and colleagues[3] (2017) found conflicting results in a follow-up study of 48 patients who initially presented to an inpatient psychiatric unit with SIP (n = 23; 48%) versus patients with PPD and concurrent substance misuse (n = 25; average of 4.96 years between baseline and follow-up). Their results suggested that following cessation of substance misuse, patients initially diagnosed with SIP did not experience more rapid symptom remission compared with patients with a PPD and concomitant substance use. Patients with SIP showed significantly less improvement of hallucinations from baseline to follow-up compared with patients with PPD.

Although epidemiologic research is scarce, 1 study estimates the incidence of SIP to be approximately 6.5 in 100,000 persons per year, compared with 9.7 with PPD and comorbid substance misuse, and 24.1 with PPD alone.[4] Among patients presenting to intervention services for first-episode psychosis (FEP), the proportion diagnosed with SIP as opposed to PPD or affective psychosis ranges between 6%[5] and 10%.[6] However, in studies examining an FEP cohort with past-month substance use, the prevalence of SIP increased dramatically, ranging from 44%[7] to 56%.[8] Although patients with SIP use substances at higher rates than patients with PPD,[6,7] substance use is still pervasive among patients with PPD, with reported rates varying from 35% to 61%.[6,8]

SUBSTANCE-SPECIFIC CONSIDERATIONS

Many substances, whether prescribed medically or used recreationally, are known to cause, exacerbate, or increase the likelihood of psychosis. Commonly used substances and substances associated with a high risk for psychosis are summarized here.

Cannabinoids

In 2017, 12.4% of youth aged 12 to 17 years used cannabis at least once that year, and for youth aged 18 to 25 years this number increased to 35%.[9] There is a growing body of literature supporting a strong link between the use of cannabis and psychosis.[10–12] There also seems to be a strong dose-response effect,[11] with daily use and the use of high-potency delta-9-tetrahydrocannabinol (THC) carrying the largest risk of psychosis.[10,11] THC potency in marijuana plants has increased dramatically over past 20 to 30 years. Specifically, the average potency of marijuana plants seized by the Drug Enforcement Administration was 4% in 1995 and increased to 12% in 2014.[13] In addition to the potency of marijuana plants continuing to increase, other products with even higher potency that are made by various processes of chemical extraction are now available. Examples of products with high levels of THC, often referred to as concentrates, include hash oil, wax, and edibles. In the state of Washington, where cannabis is legal, high-potency products, including marijuana plants with at least 20% THC content and concentrates with at least 60% THC content, make up the largest share of the cannabis market.[14] In 1 large study, individuals using high-potency cannabis (THC>10%) daily had a more than 4-fold risk of being diagnosed with a psychotic disorder compared with persons who do not use cannabis. Switching to cannabis with a lower THC content decreased this risk by half, even for people who continued to use cannabis daily.[10] This study provided the first direct evidence that cannabis use increased the incidence of psychotic disorders, suggesting that high-potency cannabis is responsible for the onset of FEP in a portion of individuals.[10]

Stimulants

Psychostimulants (often simply called stimulants) are commonly prescribed to treat ADHD and are commonly misused by youth (ie, taken at higher doses than prescribed, using stimulants that were prescribed to someone else, or crushing and insufflating these medications). In 2017, 1.8% of youth aged 12 to 17 years misused prescription stimulants, as did 7.5% of youth aged 18 to 25 years.[9] Each type of stimulant (a class that also includes cocaine and methamphetamines) has a unique profile with regard to the risk of psychosis, and, in general, there is a dose-response relationship with symptoms of psychosis.

Amphetamines

Use of amphetamines can result in acute psychosis. Otherwise healthy individuals in laboratory settings begin to experience symptoms of psychosis at doses between 100 and 300 mg.[15] SIP has been described in youth with ADHD being prescribed amphetamines, although this is rare when taken at prescribed doses.[16] Studies have found that between 8% and 46% of persons who regularly misuse amphetamines experience SIP, and a binge pattern of use may increase the likelihood of psychosis. The clinical presentation of amphetamine-induced psychosis is similar to schizophrenia spectrum illnesses, and can include disorganized thoughts, impaired concentration, delusional beliefs (often persecutory in nature), hallucinations, and hyperactivity.[15]

Methylphenidates

Rare cases of psychosis from the use of methylphenidates have been described,[17] with higher doses (>120 mg) likely carrying a higher risk. However, when the risk for SIP-associated prescription stimulant use was examined using a dataset derived from 2 US commercial insurance claims, methylphenidates were associated with a lower risk for SIP compared with amphetamines, although a causal relationship cannot be concluded.[18] Nevertheless, given their equal efficacy on average for the treatment of ADHD, there may be benefit in using methylphenidate products as first-line agents in treating youth with this condition.

Cocaine

Transitory paranoia resulting from acute effects of cocaine are one of the most common effects of cocaine use, occurring in about 90% of cases.[19] Common clinical characteristics of paranoia resulting from cocaine use include suspiciousness, distrust, compulsive behaviors, dysphoria, as well as aggressiveness and agitation. Most psychotic symptoms related to cocaine use remit within 24 to 28 hours.

Methamphetamines

Transient psychosis is one of the best-documented effects of heavy methamphetamine use. According to 1 study, methamphetamine-associated psychosis is experienced in about 23% of individuals who use methamphetamines.[20] Common clinical characteristics of methamphetamine-associated psychosis include persecutory delusions, auditory and visual hallucinations, hostility, anxiety, depression, cognitive disorganization, and hyperactivity.[21] There is inconsistent evidence whether negative symptoms of psychosis are associated with this phenomenon.[21] As with other substances, the risk of psychosis seems to be higher with increased drug potency and frequency of use.

Hallucinogens

Hallucinogens are a diverse group of both naturally occurring substances (such as psilocybin and mescaline) as well as synthetic lysergic acid diethylamide (LSD) and LSD-like substances. Because hallucinations are the intended toxidrome, these substances cause some psychosis by definition, but symptoms might persist beyond the initial period of intoxication.

Hallucinogen persisting perception disorder is characterized by spontaneous reoccurrence of perceptual disturbances, most commonly visual, that are similar to the individual's experience during acute intoxication. For people who use hallucinogens, the reported prevalence of flashbacks (reexperiencing of perceptual disturbances) ranges from 5% to 50%, with a smaller subset meeting criteria for hallucinogen persisting perception disorder.[22] Two different clinical syndromes for this disorder have been identified: type 1 usually reflects a short-term, reversible, benign course in which the individual experiences 1 or more perceptual symptoms, usually spontaneous visual images. Individuals experiencing type 1 generally do not experience significant impairment or distress from these experiences (and may even find the experience pleasurable), so psychiatric care is rarely sought. Hallucinogen persisting perception disorder type 2 typically reflects a more chronic, severe syndrome.[23] Individuals with type 2 reexperience 1 or more perceptual symptoms causing significant distress or functional impairment.

Symptoms related to hallucinogen persisting perception disorder usually include afterimages, halos, trails, or visual snows, without affecting other modalities (eg, auditory hallucinations). Prodromal symptoms are more often reported in cases of type 2. Type 1 episodes tend to occur less frequently, with shorter duration or intensity, following onset. In type 2, the frequency, duration, and intensity can increase over time,[23] and it has been suggested that this may convert into persistent psychotic illness. Most individuals experiencing hallucinogen persisting perception disorder do not report delusional beliefs related to perceptual disturbances, suggesting involvement of the primary visual cortex, and potentially distinguishing it from a schizophrenia spectrum disorder. A systematic review found very few well-designed studies examining hallucinogen persisting perception disorder,[22] making it difficult to summarize effective approaches for managing this condition.

Nicotine

Individuals who use cigarettes during adolescence have an increased risk for subsequent psychotic experiences. Daily tobacco use has been associated with an increased risk of psychosis and an earlier age at onset of psychotic illness.[24] Patients with FEP tend to have smoked for years before the onset of psychosis, have high prevalence of tobacco use at the time of treatment, and are more likely to smoke than age-matched controls.[25] Genetics may influence this association, because genes associated with psychosis have been shown to overlap with those for cigarette smoking.[26]

Research Chemicals and So-called Club Drugs

Research chemicals, also known as new psychoactive substances, include synthetic cannabinoids (spice, K2), synthetic cathinones (bath salts, flakka, methylone), psychedelics such as tryptamines (N,N-dimethyltryptamine [DMT], 5-methoxy-DMT), and phenethylamines (3,4-methylenedioxymethamphetamine [MDMA], ecstasy, Molly). Research on new psychoactive substances is limited. The prevalence and even the exact composition of these substances are rapidly changing as suppliers work to create new chemical variations to circumvent laws implemented to prevent their use. One case series describing psychosis associated with acute recreational drug toxicity found synthetic cannabinoids and tryptamines to be the most frequently involved substances.[27] Reviews on psychosis and synthetic cannabinoids suggested that these have stronger physiologic and psychological effects than THC and may either exacerbate previously stable psychotic symptoms or trigger new-onset psychosis.[28] Prolonged psychosis and the potential for violence have been reported with synthetic cathinones.[29] A case-control study also supported an association between ecstasy use, psychosis, aggression, and violent behaviors.[30]

Kratom

Kratom is a psychoactive plant preparation used medicinally for its stimulant effects, and as an opioid substitute.[31] Case reports have associated kratom exposure with psychosis, seizures, and death.[32] A study involving calls to US poison centers for kratom exposure over a 5-year period found close to 50% of callers reported moderate to severe adverse outcomes. Forty percent of callers described non–life-threatening outcomes but required treatment, and another 7% had life-threatening outcomes with some residual disability.[33] Adverse effects from chronic use of kratom include sleep and eating disorders, psychosis, and addiction[31]; the risk of psychosis seems to be much greater than in other opioids. Although the US Food and Drug Administration (FDA) has labeled kratom an opioid because it has activity at the opioid receptor and warned of its risk, kratom is currently not regulated at the federal level. The absence of federal regulation has raised concerns that exposure to kratom may increase amid the current opioid crisis.

Commonly Prescribed Medications

Steroids are commonly prescribed to reduce inflammation and immune activation in various diseases. This class of medications is known to have major systemic side effects, including fractures, infections, gastrointestinal bleeds, and cataracts.[34] Sometimes less appreciated are the neuropsychiatric side effects, which include affective, behavioral, and cognitive changes. These changes are often characterized as steroid psychosis, regardless of whether the patient truly experiences psychosis.[35] Symptoms tend to be mild and reversible and may include emotional lability, hypomania, mania, depression, psychosis, delirium, and confusion. Specifically, psychotic symptoms of hallucinations, delusions, and paranoid ideation have been documented.[35]

Antibiotics such as fluoroquinolones can also be associated with a variety of psychiatric and neurologic problems, including psychosis, as highlighted in a recent black box warning from the FDA. Specifically, psychotic symptoms of auditory and visual hallucinations as well as delusions have been documented.[36]

DIFFERENTIATING SUBSTANCE-INDUCED PSYCHOSIS FROM PRIMARY PSYCHOTIC DISORDER

Recent studies have strengthened the argument that at least some forms of SIP in adolescents and young adults, such as psychosis caused by daily use of high-potency cannabis, can convert to a PPD that otherwise would not have developed.[10] Nevertheless, the relationship between substance use and psychosis is complex, and how much of the correlation is causal remains controversial. Individuals predisposed to developing PPD might also have a predisposition to using substances and/or substance use may accelerate the course of an underlying psychotic disorder.

There is no single feature that differentiates SIP from PPD in a young patient using substances, and it is often only the presence or absence of psychotic symptoms during prolonged periods of abstinence, if this can be achieved, that definitively determines the need for ongoing treatment of psychosis. However, there are some clinical features that may point to 1 cause rather than another. SIP often features a later age of onset,[6,7] increased insight into symptoms of psychosis,[7] fewer or less severe negative symptoms,[2,7] and a weaker family history of psychosis compared with patients with a PPD.[8] Other characteristics of psychosis that have been examined to help differentiate SIP from PPD have shown inconsistent findings. For example, most of the evidence suggests that patients with SIP experience more positive symptoms,[4,7,37] but other findings have shown that positive symptom severity is similar between SIP and PPD.[2,6]

ASSESSING FOR SUBSTANCE USE DISORDERS

As outlined earlier, the prevalence of heavy substance use is high in adolescents with psychosis, whether the psychosis is primary or substance induced. Although the focus of this article is on psychosis, it is important to evaluate and treat any comorbid substance use disorder (SUD).

The description and classification of SUD changed substantially with the publication of the DSM-5. In place of the prior discrete categories of abuse and dependence, SUD is now classified by severity. Each SUD (alcohol use disorder, cannabis use disorder, and so forth) has 11 criteria, which differ little between different types of substances. If a patient meets 2 or 3 criteria, the SUD is classified as mild, 4 or 5 is classified as moderate, and the presence of 6 or more criteria is classified as severe. The 11 criteria are useful both in initially determining, and then following, the severity of illness in patients.

Despite the recognized importance of screening for and evaluating youth for SUD, there are few standards for how to do so in psychiatric settings. The most widely validated screening tool for adolescent SUD is the CRAFFT,[38] and although most of this evidence comes from primary care settings, the tool has been shown to have validity for screening in psychiatric patient populations.[39] There are several newer screeners that have promise as easier-to-use alternatives and are available free from the National Institute on Drug Abuse: in particular, Screening to Brief Intervention (S2BI); Brief Screener for Tobacco, Alcohol, and Other Drugs for adolescents; and the Tobacco, Alcohol, Prescription Medication, and Other Substance use (TAPS) tool for young adults.

Patients who screen positive for at-risk substance use should be further evaluated for an SUD, which assesses how the substance is affecting the patient's functioning, for each substance they are using, because polysubstance use is common in youth. Insight into SUD severity is often low, so collateral information from family and toxicology screening can be useful.

After his initial presentation to the emergency room, Kevin stopped smoking cannabis because he was worried about his symptoms and concerned that cannabis may be playing a role. His parents safely secured his medication for ADHD and stopped giving it to him. By the time you see him 3 days later, he is feeling a bit better. He seems to have improved insight into some of his symptoms, and no longer believes that there are intruders in his home. However, he has continued to largely isolate himself in his room, and although he has been using his phone and computer, he acknowledges avoiding certain sites because he "can't shake the feeling" that he, specifically, is being monitored in a nefarious way. His parents are very concerned about his prognosis, and you explain the ambiguity. Cannabis almost certainly contributed and abstinence from cannabis use will be important. His misuse of stimulants may have also played a role. You recommend treatment with a nonstimulant medication, atomoxetine, and start that medication now, because it takes a longer time to take effect and the new school year is a month away. You explain that these changes may be enough for all of his symptoms to resolve, or they may not.

You also assess his substance use further and determine that Kevin meets criteria for cannabis use disorder, moderate. You refer him to a colleague for SUD therapy and find a local resource that provides both group therapy and parent guidance for guardians of youth with SUD. Kevin declines to engage in these services, because he feels sufficiently motivated to stop using cannabis.

You continue to meet with him at short intervals for the rest of the summer to assess his symptoms of psychosis and his response to atomoxetine. Kevin seems to be doing well and by the beginning of his senior year he is feeling healthy and confident. He denies symptoms of psychosis as well as cannabis use, which is corroborated by urine toxicology screens that are negative for THC.

MANAGEMENT
Pharmacotherapy

If a young person is prescribed a medication that may have contributed to SIP, then this medication should be stopped. If continued pharmacotherapy is needed to treat an ongoing psychiatric or medical condition, an alternative medication should be prescribed if possible. If a young person with SIP has a co-occurring SUD, medication to treat the SUD should be discussed with the patient and family. There are several FDA-approved medications for adults with alcohol, nicotine, and opioid use disorders. Although there is limited research on the use of these medications in adolescents, there have been randomized controlled trials with positive findings for nicotine use disorder, as well as adolescents aged 16 years and older with an opioid use disorder.[40]

Antipsychotic medication is indicated for individuals with symptoms of psychosis that persist when they are not acutely intoxicated or withdrawing from substances, or individuals who are not able to establish periods of abstinence. To our knowledge, no clinical trials have been conducted in individuals with SIP, and the literature is limited on medication treatment of individuals with schizophrenia and a co-occurring SUD. Some small studies have suggested that treatment with atypical antipsychotic medications, including clozapine, is associated with decreased substance use.[41] When prescribing antipsychotic medications to individuals with SIP who also smoke tobacco regularly, clinicians should remember that smoking tobacco increases cytochrome P450 1A2 (CYP1A2) enzyme activity, which leads to increased metabolism and lower levels of clozapine, olanzapine, haloperidol, and fluphenazine.[42] CYP1A2 activity is affected by the products of tobacco smoke and not nicotine; therefore, if an individual begins nicotine replacement therapy and/or begins exclusively using an electronic cigarette, the dose of their medication will need to be decreased accordingly.

Psychosocial Interventions

Different approaches have been developed for the treatment of patients with an SUD and a psychotic disorder. One approach is referred to as parallel treatment, and involves simultaneous treatment of both disorders, but by different agencies or providers with expertise in their specific areas. An alternative approach is sequential treatment, in which a patient receives either psychosis-focused or substance use–focused treatment first, in isolation, based on the idea that resolving one problem allows the other to be more effectively treated. Kavanagh and Mueser[43] (2011) highlight concerns with both of these approaches given the risk of poor communication between providers; additional burden on the patient to see 2 clinicians or extend the time in care; and, most significantly, that the nuances of how substance use affects psychosis and vice versa may be ignored. Integrated care in which both disorders are addressed simultaneously by the same clinician has thus been identified as the gold standard for the treatment of SUD and comorbid psychiatric illness.

Regarding psychosis in the presence of substance use specifically, most studies on integrated psychosocial treatment have been conducted with (older) adults with schizophrenia and comorbid SUD.[44,45] Few studies have examined individuals identified as having SIP, and most studies with PPD and comorbid SUD do not distinguish between substances of use. Nevertheless, integrated motivational interviewing (MI) and cognitive behavior therapy (CBT), which combines MI techniques for addressing substance misuse and CBT for SUD and psychosis, is one intervention that has been associated with a reduction in substance use in persons with a co-occurring psychotic disorder and SUD compared with treatment as usual.[46] MI fosters a nonconfrontational, patient-centered approach that is inherently necessary when working with patients with SUD. Exploring ambivalence about substance use, the pros and cons of a substance, how use affects an individual's life goals (job, college, relationships), and potential long-term risks of use is key to exploring drivers of behavior. CBT for psychosis provides a theoretic model that is accessible for patients, explaining distal and proximal triggers to their psychotic thinking patterns (eg, how to understand the links between thoughts, feelings, and behaviors as they underpin, and potentially perpetuate, hallucinations and delusions). CBT for psychosis and SUD is designed to teach skills in managing stress, in managing unhelpful and unrealistic thinking patterns and behaviors, and to challenge cognitions that may support ongoing substance use, such as, "Marijuana is the only thing that calms my thoughts."

Other evidence-based treatments in addressing youth substance use, such as the Adolescent Community Reinforcement Approach,[47] can complement MI-CBT by enhancing motivation to engage in competing activities that do not involve substance use, improve communication and problem solving, and increase parental bonds. Involvement of parents is critical in working with youth, both for keeping youth engaged in care and also to enhance treatment gains by providing families with psychoeducation about addiction, psychosis, medication management, and recovery. Emerging data indicate that family-based treatments show promise for improving substance use in persons experiencing psychosis. Mueser and colleagues[48] (2009) developed a Family Intervention for Dual Diagnosis, which included family psychoeducation, communication and problem-solving skills training, and stress management, with improvements in both substance use and psychosis.

Effective integrated treatment programs for adults with schizophrenia and SUD highlight the importance of social support.[45] Leveraging prosocial connections may also be of benefit for youth with SIP and SUD. Identifying a relationship with an adult trusted by the adolescent, such as a teacher, coach, or work supervisor, might be helpful in monitoring the youth's symptoms, substance use, and functioning. Sometimes, having multiple community members identified as part of the team can be helpful, but alliance with the youth is likely best preserved if the youth feels involved in the selection of a limited number of adults.

PROGNOSIS

SIP is associated with the development of severe mental illness. Larger registry studies have found that 24% to 32% of patients with a diagnosis of SIP subsequently developed a schizophrenia spectrum disorder or bipolar disorder.[12]

Overall prognosis may be affected by the specific substance causing psychosis. Amphetamine-induced and other stimulant-induced psychoses tend to resolve within days, although some research suggests psychotic symptoms may persist for years.[15] Starzer and colleagues[12] (2018) found that 32.3% of individuals diagnosed with SIP related to amphetamine use were later diagnosed with either schizophrenia or bipolar disorder. The conversion rate for individuals experiencing SIP related to hallucinogen use to PPD was lower, at 24%. Cannabis-induced psychosis is associated with the highest risk for severe mental illness, with about 46% of patients subsequently developing schizophrenia.[12]

Several registry studies have found that patients converted from SIP to a serious mental illness within 2 to 3 years. Of relevance to clinicians working with young people, patients aged 16 to 25 years have been found to be at highest risk of converting from SIP to schizophrenia.[12]

Kevin returns to your office in the early fall and is very upset to have failed the first quiz of the year. You assess further and learn that he missed some classes because he believes that a government organization has infiltrated his school in an attempt to monitor and target him. When comparing this with his recent period without these beliefs, he reluctantly admits that he never stopped worrying about being monitored by the agency but did not want to admit this to you. He is also hesitant to provide a urine sample for toxicology testing, and when he does, acknowledges, "It's going to show weed. Wouldn't you smoke, too, if they were after you?" He does not appear depressed but demoralized from his situation.

In discussions with Kevin and his parents, everyone agrees to a trial of an antipsychotic medication to reduce his symptoms and optimize his functioning. His parents wonder whether this means he has schizophrenia, or whether he will have to be on medications for the rest of his life. You explain that it remains too early to know. It is also unclear how much cannabis may still be contributing to his symptoms. Depending on his response to treatment and the amount of cannabis he continues to use, it is reasonable to try without medication in the future.

In the meantime, you offer to continue to see Kevin regularly to try to minimize symptoms of psychosis and continue to address his substance use using MI. His parents agree to engage in parent guidance at the nearby adolescent SUD clinic to learn more about SUD and psychosis, as well as ways they can support Kevin's engagement in treatment. After a few more meetings with you and encouragement from his parents, Kevin agrees to attend individual and group sessions at the adolescent SUD clinic as well.

SUMMARY

Cases like Kevin's are common when working with youth. This complex presentation shows several of the ambiguities of these symptoms that cross diagnostic categories. Psychosis may be substance induced, or substance use may co-occur with PPD. Looking for patterns in symptoms, and how they do or do not track with substance use, might be helpful, as may looking at clues such as family history, age of onset, and prominence of negative symptoms, although none of these variables, alone or together, can conclusively differentiate the cause of psychosis. Removing agents that are likely to contribute to psychosis, such as cannabis, stimulants, and hallucinogens, is important, but this can be clinically difficult, and in some cases symptoms might persist for months.

A comprehensive approach is the best management for SIP, ideally including:

1. Medication management
2. Psychosocial treatment (individual and/or group therapy)
3. Engagement of family (and possibly other important social connections)

This combination of highly specific treatment can be difficult to find, even in resource-rich locations. Except in cases in which all symptoms of psychosis clearly resolve in the absence of the offending agent, treating psychosis and SUD simultaneously is more effective than trying to address these challenges sequentially.

In addition, these suggestions for clinical management are based on limited evidence, and further study of both pharmacologic and psychological interventions is needed to better understand how to provide the best care to vulnerable youth experiencing both symptoms of psychosis and substance use.

REFERENCES

1. American Psychiatric Association. Diagnostic and statistical manual of mental disorders. 5th edition. Washington, DC: American Psychiatric Publishing; 2013.

2. Dawe S, Geppert L, Occhipinti S, et al. A comparison of the symptoms and short-term clinical course in inpatients with substance-induced psychosis and primary psychosis. J Subst Abuse Treat 2011;40(1):95–101.
3. Mauri MC, Di Pace C, Reggiori A, et al. Primary psychosis with comorbid drug abuse and drug-induced psychosis: diagnostic and clinical evolution at follow up. Asian J Psychiatr 2017;29:117–22.
4. Weibell MA, Joa I, Bramness J, et al. Treated incidence and baseline characteristics of substance induced psychosis in a Norwegian catchment area. BMC Psychiatry 2013;13:319.
5. Thompson A, Marwaha S, Winsper C, et al. Short-term outcome of substance-induced psychotic disorder in a large UK first episode psychosis cohort. Acta Psychiatr Scand 2016;134(4):321–8.
6. O'Connell J, Sunwoo M, McGorry P, et al. Characteristics and outcomes of young people with substance induced psychotic disorder. Schizophr Res 2019;206: 257–62.
7. Caton CLM, Drake RE, Hasin DS, et al. Differences between early-phase primary psychotic disorders with concurrent substance use and substance-induced psychoses. Arch Gen Psychiatry 2005;62(2):137–45.
8. Fraser S, Hides L, Philips L, et al. Differentiating first episode substance induced and primary psychotic disorders with concurrent substance use in young people. Schizophr Res 2012;136(1–3):110–5.
9. Substance Abuse and Mental Health Services Administration. Key substance use and mental health indicators in the United States: results from the 2017 National Survey on Drug Use and Health. Rockville (MD): Center for Behavioral Health Statistics and Quality, Substance Abuse and Mental Health Services Administration; 2018. Available at: https://www.samhsa.gov/data/.
10. Di Forti M, Quattrone D, Freeman TP, et al. The contribution of cannabis use to variation in the incidence of psychotic disorder across Europe (EU-GEI): a multicentre case-control study. Lancet Psychiatry 2019;6(5):427–36.
11. Marconi A, Di Forti M, Lewis CM, et al. Meta-analysis of the association between the level of cannabis use and risk of psychosis. Schizophr Bull 2016;42(5): 1262–9.
12. Starzer MSK, Nordentoft M, Hjorthøj C. Rates and predictors of conversion to schizophrenia or bipolar disorder following substance-induced psychosis. Am J Psychiatry 2018;175(4):343–50.
13. ElSohly MA, Mehmedic Z, Foster S, et al. Changes in cannabis potency over the last 2 decades (1995-2014): analysis of current data in the United States. Biol Psychiatry 2016;79(7):613–9.
14. Smart R, Caulkins JP, Kilmer B, et al. Variation in cannabis potency and prices in a newly legal market: evidence from 30 million cannabis sales in Washington state. Addiction 2017;112(12):2167–77.
15. Bramness JG, Gundersen ØH, Guterstam J, et al. Amphetamine-induced psychosis–a separate diagnostic entity or primary psychosis triggered in the vulnerable? BMC Psychiatry 2012;12:221.
16. Calello DP, Osterhoudt KC. Acute psychosis associated with therapeutic use of dextroamphetamine. Pediatrics 2004;113(5):1466.
17. Kraemer M, Uekermann J, Wiltfang J, et al. Methylphenidate-induced psychosis in adult attention-deficit/hyperactivity disorder: report of 3 new cases and review of the literature. Clin Neuropharmacol 2010;33(4):204–6.
18. Moran LV, Ongur D, Hsu J, et al. Psychosis with methylphenidate or amphetamine in patients with ADHD. N Engl J Med 2019;380(12):1128–38.

19. Roncero C, Ros-Cucurull E, Daigre C, et al. Prevalence and risk factors of psychotic symptoms in cocaine-dependent patients. Actas Esp Psiquiatr 2012; 40(4):187–97.

20. McKetin R, McLaren J, Lubman DI, et al. The prevalence of psychotic symptoms among methamphetamine users. Addiction 2006;101(10):1473–8.

21. Voce A, McKetin R, Burns R, et al. The relationship between illicit amphetamine use and psychiatric symptom profiles in schizophrenia and affective psychoses. Psychiatry Res 2018;265:19–24.

22. Orsolini L, Papanti GD, De Berardis D, et al. The "endless trip" among the NPS users: psychopathology and psychopharmacology in the hallucinogen-persisting perception disorder. A systematic review. Front Psychiatry 2017;8:240.

23. G Lerner A, Rudinski D, Bor O, et al. Flashbacks and HPPD: a clinical-oriented concise review. Isr J Psychiatry Relat Sci 2014;51(4):296–301.

24. Gurillo P, Jauhar S, Murray RM, et al. Does tobacco use cause psychosis? Systematic review and meta-analysis. Lancet Psychiatry 2015;2(8):718–25.

25. Myles N, Newall HD, Curtis J, et al. Tobacco use before, at, and after first-episode psychosis: a systematic meta-analysis. J Clin Psychiatry 2012;73(4):468–75.

26. Gage SH, Munafò MR. Rethinking the association between smoking and schizophrenia. Lancet Psychiatry 2015;2(2):118–9.

27. Vallersnes OM, Dines AM, Wood DM, et al. Psychosis associated with acute recreational drug toxicity: a European case series. BMC Psychiatry 2016;16:293.

28. Fattore L. Synthetic cannabinoids-further evidence supporting the relationship between cannabinoids and psychosis. Biol Psychiatry 2016;79(7):539–48.

29. John ME, Thomas-Rozea C, Hahn D. Bath salts abuse leading to new-onset psychosis and potential for violence. Clin Schizophr Relat Psychoses 2017;11(2): 120–4.

30. Rugani F, Bacciardi S, Rovai L, et al. Symptomatological features of patients with and without Ecstasy use during their first psychotic episode. Int J Environ Res Public Health 2012;9(7):2283–92.

31. Cinosi E, Martinotti G, Simonato P, et al. Following "the roots" of kratom (Mitragyna speciosa): the evolution of an enhancer from a traditional use to increase work and productivity in Southeast Asia to a recreational psychoactive drug in Western countries. Biomed Res Int 2015;2015:968786.

32. Forrester MB. Kratom exposures reported to Texas poison centers. J Addict Dis 2013;32(4):396–400.

33. Anwar M, Law R, Schier J. Notes from the field: kratom (Mitragyna speciosa) exposures reported to poison centers - United States, 2010-2015. MMWR Morb Mortal Wkly Rep 2016;65(29):748–9.

34. Oray M, Abu Samra K, Ebrahimiadib N, et al. Long-term side effects of glucocorticoids. Expert Opin Drug Saf 2016;15(4):457–65.

35. Dubovsky AN, Arvikar S, Stern TA, et al. The neuropsychiatric complications of glucocorticoid use: steroid psychosis revisited. Psychosomatics 2012;53(2): 103–15.

36. Sellick J, Mergenhagen K, Morris L, et al. Fluoroquinolone-related neuropsychiatric events in hospitalized veterans. Psychosomatics 2018;59(3):259–66.

37. Fiorentini A, Volonteri LS, Dragogna F, et al. Substance-induced psychoses: a critical review of the literature. Curr Drug Abuse Rev 2011;4(4):228–40.

38. Knight JR, Sherritt L, Shrier LA, et al. Validity of the CRAFFT substance abuse screening test among adolescent clinic patients. Arch Pediatr Adolesc Med 2002;156(6):607–14.

39. Oesterle TS, Hitschfeld MJ, Lineberry TW, et al. CRAFFT as a substance use screening instrument for adolescent psychiatry admissions. J Psychiatr Pract 2015;21(4):259–66.
40. Hammond CJ. The role of pharmacotherapy in the treatment of adolescent substance use disorders. Child Adolesc Psychiatr Clin N Am 2016;25(4):685–711.
41. Brunette MF, Drake RE, Xie H, et al. Clozapine use and relapses of substance use disorder among patients with co-occurring schizophrenia and substance use disorders. Schizophr Bull 2006;32(4):637–43.
42. Cather C, Pachas GN, Cieslak KM, et al. Achieving smoking cessation in individuals with schizophrenia: special considerations. CNS Drugs 2017;31(6):471–81.
43. Kavanagh DJ, Mueser KT. The treatment of substance misuse in people with serious mental disorders. In: Hagan R, Turkington D, Berge T, et al, editors. CBT for psychosis: a symptom based approach. New York: Routledge; 2011. p. 161–74.
44. Hunt GE, Siegfried N, Morley K, et al. Psychosocial interventions for people with both severe mental illness and substance misuse. Cochrane Database Syst Rev 2013;(10):CD001088.
45. Drake RE, Essock SM, Shaner A, et al. Implementing dual diagnosis services for clients with severe mental illness. Psychiatr Serv 2001;52(4):469–76.
46. Barrowclough C, Haddock G, Wykes T, et al. Integrated motivational interviewing and cognitive behavioural therapy for people with psychosis and comorbid substance misuse: randomised controlled trial. BMJ 2010;341:c6325.
47. Meyers RJ, Smith JE, Serna B, et al. Community reinforcement approaches: CRA and CRAFT. In: Miller P, editor. Interventions for addiction: comprehensive addictive behaviors and disorders, vol. 3. Waltham (MA): Elsevier Inc.; 2013. p. 47–56.
48. Mueser KT, Glynn SM, Cather C, et al. Family intervention for co-occurring substance use and severe psychiatric disorders: participant characteristics and correlates of initial engagement and more extended exposure in a randomized controlled trial. Addict Behav 2009;34(10):867–77.

The Changing Legal Landscape of Cannabis Use and Its Role in Youth-onset Psychosis

Abigail Wright, PhD[a,b,]*, Corinne Cather, PhD[a,b],
Jodie Gilman, PhD[b,c], Anne Eden Evins, MD, MPH[b,c]

KEYWORDS

- First-episode psychosis • Schizophrenia • Cannabis use • Tetrahydrocannabinol
- THC • High potency • CBD

KEY POINTS

- The changing landscape of cannabis (eg, availability, potency, and risk perception) has contributed to an increase in cannabis use.
- Early and frequent cannabis use, and use of high-potency cannabis, may contribute to an increase in psychotic disorders.
- Prevention and treatment, including contingency management and first-episode psychosis programs, are becoming increasingly important to support youth mental health.

INCREASED AVAILABILITY, POTENCY, AND ROUTES OF ADMINISTRATION OF CANNABIS PRODUCTS

The *Cannabis sativa* plant has 2 primary cannabinoids: Δ^9-tetrahydrocannabinol (THC), the component of cannabis that produces intoxicating effects and is known to cause anxiety, euphoria, disrupted cognitive function, psychosislike (eg, suspiciousness, altered perception) and negative (eg, amotivation, apathy) symptoms[1]; and cannabidiol (CBD), which is not thought to lead to dependence and has been studied for potential antiinflammatory, anxiolytic, and antipsychotic effects.[2,3] Cannabis is the most commonly used illicit drug worldwide,[4] and its use has increased

---

Disclosure: The authors have no disclosures.
[a] Massachusetts General Hospital, Center of Excellence in Psychosocial and Systemic Research, 151 Merrimac Street, 6th Floor, Boston, MA 02114, USA; [b] Harvard Medical School, Boston, MA USA; [c] Massachusetts General Hospital, Center for Addiction Medicine, 101 Merrimac Street, Boston, MA 02114, USA
* Corresponding author.
E-mail address: AWRIGHT24@mgh.harvard.edu

over the last few decades,[5] with 18.4% of adolescents[6] and 32.6% of college students in North America[7] reporting cannabis use in the past 30 days. High usage rates of cannabis by youth could partially reflect difficulty obtaining alcohol in this age group.[8] The changing legal landscape for this drug has been associated with increased usage, availability, and potency of cannabis products, as well as with a reduced perception of harm of cannabis use.[9]

In the past decade, there has been a dramatic increase in the availability of cannabis products. Since the 1996 enactment of the first state law allowing the medical use of cannabis, 33 US states and the District of Columbia have legalized medical marijuana. More than 17 states allow products that are high in CBD and low in THC[10] and 11 states allow essentially unregulated cannabis for recreational use.[11] Of note, there are no standardized definitions of medical marijuana, high-CBD products, or low-THC products.[12] It is difficult to identify the amount of THC in commercial products in the United States now, because products vary from batch to batch, often lack standardized testing, and have been reported to be inaccurately labeled.[13]

Concomitant with increased general availability, the authors have seen both increased THC potency of standard cannabis products as well as increased availability of novel high-potency products. Percentage THC content in illicit (street) and commercial flower marijuana markets increased from 3.96% ($\pm$1.82%) THC content in 1995 to 11.84% ($\pm$6.6%) THC content in 2014,[14] with no change in CBD levels.[15] Synthetic cannabinoids (eg, spice/K2), highly potent, full CD1 (cluster of differentiation 1) receptor agonists, as well as skunk or resin products have recently become popular; these products produce more intense effects than whole-plant cannabis.[16] There has been an enormous increase in the availability of CBD products (eg, CBD oil, gummies, edibles, vapes, or bath products), which are generally considered safe, helpful, and homeopathic by a large segment of users who do not elect to use products containing THC. Despite minimal, generally low-quality evidence for medical benefits, they are touted to cause relief from pain, anxiety, depression, insomnia, and even psychosis.[2,17] (An exception is CBD for certain forms of pediatric epilepsy, including Lennox-Gastaut syndrome[18] and Dravet syndrome.[19]) Of note, US Food and Drug Administration tests have shown that some CBD products sold in the United States contain little to no CBD, and contain high levels of THC.[20,21] This finding suggests that individuals may be unaware that they are consuming THC and its itinerant potential negative effects on mental health, highlighting the need for additional regulation of CBD and commercial cannabis products to protect consumers.[19]

Clinicians should be aware of novel methods of consumption; for example, so-called vaping or dabbing, and ingestion of edibles, which may increase the appeal of using cannabis products and be more difficult for observers to detect than smoked cannabis. Vape pens for cannabis can be indistinguishable from electronic cigarettes, and there are Web sites that instruct youth how to be stealthy, including using an electronic cigarette to vape cannabis products. Dabbing is accomplished by extracting concentrated doses of cannabis into a sticky oil, which is heated on a hot surface (typically a nail) and inhaled through a device that can resemble a bong. Because of different pharmacokinetics of smoking versus ingesting cannabis, edibles delay the timing and increase both the duration and intensity of intoxication. Ingesting cannabis produces a 30-minute to 60-minute delay to peak high and up to a 3 times longer high (2 hours vs 6 hours) than smoking cannabis,[22] which, in an effort to experience intoxication, has resulted in accidental ingestion of too much cannabis and associated adverse effects.[23]

EFFECTS OF CANNABIS USE IN PEOPLE WITH PSYCHOTIC DISORDERS

Cannabis use is common in people with chronic schizophrenia[24] and first-episode psychosis (FEP)[25] and has been associated with a poor prognosis.[26,27] Cannabis use after FEP worsens both psychotic symptoms and psychosocial functioning, controlling for other risk factors.[28–30] In laboratory studies, a single dose of THC causes transient psychotic symptoms in a greater proportion of people with schizophrenia than healthy volunteers.[1] Synthetic cannabinoids (eg, spice/K2) also trigger psychotic symptoms, aggression, and suicidal thoughts[31,32] in those with prior psychosis, suggesting THC use as a risk factor for poor outcomes in those with psychosis.

Persistent cannabis use after the first episode of schizophrenia has been associated with relapse,[33] increasing the risk for relapse 2.2-fold, even after controlling for confounding factors, including medication adherence.[34] Although some research has suggested the association is bidirectional,[35] cross-lagged analyses indicate that cannabis use predicts risk of relapse, rather than relapse predicting cannabis use.[33] Cannabis use in FEP has been associated with increased frequency of hospital admissions,[36] longer duration of first hospital stay, and greater odds of having more than 20 hospitalizations.[37] Critically important, discontinuation of cannabis use after FEP significantly reduces relapse risk to the level of nonusers,[38] improving both symptoms[38] and functioning.[39] Cannabis discontinuation increases the probability of remission in FEP,[40] supporting cannabis abstinence as one of the few modifiable clinical targets to improve psychotic disorder outcomes. Although the negative impact of persistent cannabis use on recovery from a psychotic disorder[37] has long been recognized, new research has begun to support the independent contribution of early initiation, frequent use, and use of high-potency cannabis to the onset and course of new psychotic disorders.[37,41]

DOES CANNABIS CAUSE PSYCHOTIC DISORDERS?

The cause of psychotic disorders is multifactorial, influenced by genes,[42] environment,[43] and their interaction.[44] In recent years, there has been increased attention to the role of cannabis as a potentially preventable environmental risk factor for psychosis.[45] Evidence in support of a causal relationship between cannabis and psychosis includes several factors, such as the plausibility of cannabis use as compromising adolescent brain structure and function, evidence of cannabis use as preceding the onset of a psychotic disorder, and a strong dose-dependent association between cannabis use and psychotic disorder. Alternatively, epidemiologic data have yet to empirically show the expected increased incidence of psychotic disorders associated with increased availability and usage of cannabis. It has also been difficult to disentangle contributions of shared genetic and environmental factors and there is some evidence for a common genetic pathway to both psychotic disorders and cannabis use.

Late adolescence is a particularly vulnerable period, because the brain is undergoing extensive changes, including the development of higher cognitive functions[46] and an increase in white matter volume enabling rapid flow of information throughout the brain.[47] Psychosis usually develops during this vulnerable period in late adolescence,[48] and is also associated with impaired brain function[49] and reduced cognitive performance[50] (See Philip D. Harvey and Elizabeth C. Isner's article, "Cognition, Social Cognition, and Functional Capacity in Early Onset Schizophrenia," in this issue). Cannabis use during development of critical higher-order cognitive functioning may produce long-term changes on the brain, as shown by studies with adult cannabis users showing both immediate and long-term impacts on brain structure, connectivity, and function,[51–53] including cognitive performance,[54,55] motivation,[41] and emotional processing.[56] A recent literature review highlighted the strong connection between early, frequent, and heavy adolescent cannabis exposure and poor cognitive and psychiatric outcomes in adulthood (in both clinical and preclinical studies).[57] US Department of Health and Human Services increased awareness of the effects of cannabis use on cognitive functioning in adolescence and, as a consequence, the link to school absences, dropouts, and even suicide attempts.[58,59]

Motivations for cannabis use in people with severe mental illness have been debated. So-called self-medication has been proposed to suggest cannabis use as a method of relieving mental health symptoms,[60] which suggests the possibility that the manifestations of a psychotic disorder could precede cannabis use and violate the assumption of temporality required to show a causal relationship. However, a fair amount of evidence against the self-medication theory has amassed[61,62]: most importantly, findings of large temporal periods separating the onset of cannabis use and the onset of psychosis or other apparent significant mental health symptoms.[54] Several studies provide compelling evidence that cannabis use precedes the onset of psychotic illness[55] and psychotic symptoms,[63] even in people with no reported lifetime psychotic symptoms.[61] In a 35-year follow-up of a large cohort study of 50,087 conscripts, frequent cannabis users had a 3.7-fold greater incidence of psychotic outcomes compared with nonusers.[64] Moreover, it has been found that 28% to 45% of those initially diagnosed with a substance-induced psychosis convert to schizophrenia or bipolar disorder,[65–67] suggesting that frank psychotic symptoms in the context of cannabis use could herald syndromal illness and warrant intervention.

Importantly, a strong dose effect for both frequency and THC potency on risk of psychotic disorder has been well replicated. Greater frequency of cannabis use is associated with increased risk of psychotic disorder,[68] with studies showing a 50% to 200% increase in risk for participants who used most heavily.[69] Youth who use high-THC-potency cannabis show a 3-fold increase in risk of a psychotic disorder compared with those who never used cannabis.[70] Daily users of high-potency cannabis show the highest risk of developing a psychotic disorder.[70]

Recently, a large study of 901 people with FEP and 1237 controls in Europe and Brazil provided evidence to support a causal relationship between cannabis use and new-onset psychosis. This study collected data on frequency of cannabis use and potency of cannabis used, and amalgamated data on regional incidence of FEP with expected concentration of THC in cannabis for sites (eg, London and Amsterdam were considered high-potency sites and Italy and Spain were considered low-potency sites). Daily cannabis use was associated with an increase in the risk for psychosis nearly 4 times higher compared with never users and, for daily users of high-potency THC cannabis, the risk was nearly 5 times higher (even when controlling for risk factors).[71] Importantly, the investigators estimate that, if high-potency cannabis were no longer available, 12% to 50% of all FEP cases could be prevented across the sites.

This study also highlighted that people who use cannabis and develop schizophrenia do so at a significantly younger age than those who did not use cannabis,[71] replicating a prior report.[72] Men who used high-potency cannabis daily had psychotic illness onset an average of 6 years earlier than non–cannabis users.[73] Earlier age at onset of cannabis use predicted earlier onset of psychotic symptoms,[62] a marker of poor outcome,[74] particularly those who initiated cannabis before age 16 years.[71]

There remains controversy regarding whether the same factors increase risk of psychosis and risk of cannabis use or whether this association is entirely caused by cannabis increasing psychosis risk because studies have failed to take into account the confounding of correlated genetic and environmental factors,[75] including childhood trauma,[76] tobacco,[77] and urbanicity,[43] which may interact synergistically to increase risk of psychosis.[78] In addition, epidemiologic data have not supported the expected increased incidence of schizophrenia with increased cannabis use over 3 decades in Australia, as would be predicted if increased cannabis use was directly related to schizophrenia.[63] Heritable variations in dopamine neurotransmission have been found to moderate individual sensitivity to the psychotogenic effects of cannabis. For example, the AKT1 pathway has been implicated in schizophrenia,[79,80] is linked to dopamine signaling,[81] and is activated by cannabinoids.[82] The interaction between Protein kinase B (AKT1) and cannabis use predicted a 2-fold increase of risk of psychotic disorder with cannabis use,[83,84] supporting a gene-environment interaction. A meta-analysis of a large genome-wide association study of lifetime cannabis use indicated that genetic risk factors for cannabis use and schizophrenia are positively correlated.[85] Moreover, it has been suggested that a large portion of the association between cannabis abuse and schizophrenia derived from monozygotic twin studies is related to familial factors.[86] In contrast, meta-analyses have not supported an interaction between the genes (COMT [catechol-O-methyltransferase] genotype) and a cannabis-psychosis link,[87,88] suggesting that, despite early, positive reports, the genetic risk for schizophrenia at this particular locus predicts only a small amount of the risk for using cannabis.[41,89] Although a possible link with genetic variations does not disregard a link between cannabis and psychosis, it does suggest that the association is far more nuanced than was previously thought.[75]

Although cannabis use has been associated with symptoms of psychosis and people with a psychotic disorder are more likely to use cannabis than those without a psychotic disorder, the question remains whether these associations represent a causal relationship between cannabis use and psychosis in individuals without an underlying risk. The relationship between cannabis and psychosis seems to fulfill many of the standard criteria for causality, including temporality, biological gradient, plausibility, evidence, consistency, and coherence.[90] However, assessing the effect of dose and exposure (biological gradient) has been challenging because THC content varies considerably and, because of ethical and feasibility issues, assessing the impact of long-term cannabis use has been difficult.

CLINICAL RECOMMENDATIONS

Given the changing landscape, continued research and attention to the relationship between psychosis and cannabis is critical for identifying risk factors and informing intervention. Risk factors for developing psychosis with cannabis use may include genetic risk (eg, having a first-degree family member with schizophrenia spectrum or bipolar disorder), male gender, frequent (daily) cannabis use (particularly of high-potency cannabis), and younger age of initiation of cannabis use. Pediatricians and other child and adolescent care providers can have an impact by monitoring cannabis use, assessing for psychotic symptoms and changes in behavior, expressly advising siblings of individuals with a history of psychosis against cannabis use, and educating young people on the risks of cannabis use (eg, addiction, psychotic symptoms, and negative effects on learning and memory[91,92]). For individuals with FEP and using cannabis, coordinated specialty care programs can be beneficial because they include an integrated substance use component.[93] However, there is currently a lack of evidence-based practice for addressing cannabis use in this population.[94–96] The Recovery After an Initial Schizophrenia Episode (RAISE)-Early Treatment Program (ETP) study randomized 404 individuals with FEP[97] (See Abigail Wright and colleagues' article, "Evidence-Based Psychosocial Treatment for Individuals with Early Psychosis," in this issue) to receive usual care or coordinated specialty care, a multicomponent intervention that included educational, motivational, and cognitive-behavior strategies for clients and their families to address substance use disorders. Although half the participants enrolled met criteria for a substance use disorder (35% for a cannabis use disorder), there were no changes in substance use after the program, highlighting the need for future enhancements to this component of the intervention as well as clinician training.[98]

Studies with general-population adolescents have shown positive outcomes using voucher-based contingency management to incentivize cannabis abstinence,[99] applicable to serious mental illness.[100] Schuster and colleagues[101] showed that 90% of youth in such a program achieved biochemically validated sobriety from cannabis for 30 days. A later study supported the effectiveness of contingency management for achieving abstinence and showed improvements in memory with abstinence[102]; however, 94% of individuals who stopped using cannabis resumed regular cannabis use within 2 weeks.[101] Abstaining from using cannabis for a prolonged time can be difficult for youth who have become accustomed to using and may use cannabis for several reasons, including facilitation of social activities, pleasure, stress reduction, sleep, or as a way of feeling more independent. In such cases, recommending a reduction in the frequency of cannabis use, a brief trial period of abstinence (as a method to allow for evaluating the pros and cons of abstinence), or a switch to low-potency cannabis could reduce harm, strengthen the treatment alliance, and potentially lay a foundation for future abstinence from cannabis.

SUMMARY

If the current course of broadening commercialization of increasingly potent cannabis products is maintained, clinicians are likely to begin to see effects that were rare in the past, when cannabis use was not as widespread. Vulnerable populations, particularly young people and individuals with genetic risk for psychosis, seem to be at increased risk of psychosis, especially with exposure to products with higher THC potency. New routes of administration, including vaped and edible products, and a culture of rapidly changing norms and reduced perceptions of risk make it possible that the current, limited knowledge of the effect of cannabis exposure on risk for psychotic illness may no longer be accurate. Clinicians should routinely monitor for cannabis use, changes in behavior or functioning, and presence of attenuated or frank psychotic symptoms. There is a pressing and growing need to identify interventions with long-term effectiveness for cannabis reduction and abstinence. The time is right for the United States to follow Canada's lead and invest in public health education and messaging regarding cannabis as legal, but not safe, for younger users, particularly of high-potency products.[103] There is a need for science-based campaigns and prevention programs to inform vulnerable groups of the risks, and these risks should be reinforced by organizations at the local, state, and national level.[59] Prevention efforts, such as a reduction in the availability of high-potency cannabis and early identification of risk factors (eg, younger age of initiation, daily use, and use of high-potency cannabis) have the potential to delay or even prevent the onset of a psychotic disorder.

REFERENCES

1. D'Souza DC, Perry E, MacDougall L, et al. The psychotomimetic effects of intravenous delta-9-tetrahydrocannabinol in healthy individuals: implications for psychosis. Neuropsychopharmacology 2004;29(8):1558–72.

2. Zuardi AW, Hallak JEC, Dursun SM, et al. Cannabidiol monotherapy for treatment-resistant schizophrenia. J Psychopharmacol 2006;20(5):683–6.
3. Zuardi A, Crippa Z, Hallack J, et al. A critical review of the antipsychotic effects of cannabidiol: 30 years of a translational investigation. Curr Pharm Des 2012; 18(32):5131–40.
4. SAMHSA. Results from the 2010 national survey on drug use and health: summary of national findings. Rockville (MD): Substance Abuse and Mental Health Services Administration; 2011.
5. Hasin DS, Saha TD, Kerridge BT, et al. Prevalence of marijuana use disorders in the United States between 2001-2002 and 2012-2013. JAMA Psychiatry 2015; 72(12):1235–42.
6. Simons-Morton B, Pickett W, Boyce W, et al. Cross-national comparison of adolescent drinking and cannabis use in the United States, Canada, and The Netherlands. Int J Drug Policy 2010;21(1):64–9.
7. Allen J, Holder MD. Marijuana use and well-being in University students. J Happiness Stud 2014;15(2):301–21.
8. Crost B, Guerrero S. The effect of alcohol availability on marijuana use: evidence from the minimum legal drinking age. J Health Econ 2012;31(1):112–21.
9. Pacek LR, Mauro PM, Martins SS. Perceived risk of regular cannabis use in the United States from 2002 to 2012: differences by sex, age, and race/ethnicity. Drug Alcohol Depend 2015;149:232–44.
10. Maxwell JC, Mendelson B. What do we know about the impact of the laws related to marijuana? Journal of Addiction Medicine 2016;25(3):289–313.
11. DISA Global Solutions. Map of marijuana legality by state. Available at: https://disa.com/map-of-marijuana-legality-by-state. Accessed June 13, 2019.
12. Mead A. The legal status of cannabis (marijuana) and cannabidiol (CBD) under U.S. law. Epilepsy Behav 2017;70:288–91.
13. Vandrey R, Raber JC, Raber ME, et al. Cannabinoid dose and label accuracy in edible medical cannabis products. JAMA 2015;313(24):2491–3.
14. ElSohly MA, Mehmedic Z, Foster S, et al. Changes in cannabis potency over the last 2 decades (1995-2014): analysis of current data in the United States. Biol Psychiatry 2016;79(7):613–9.
15. ElSohly MA, Ross SA, Mehmedic Z, et al. Potency trends of delta9-THC and other cannabinoids in confiscated marijuana from 1980-1997. J Forensic Sci 2000; 45(1):24–30. Available at: http://www.ncbi.nlm.nih.gov/pubmed/10641915.
16. Every-Palmer S. Synthetic cannabinoid JWH-018 and psychosis: an explorative study. Drug Alcohol Depend 2011;117(2–3):152–7.
17. Abrams D. Integrating cannabis into clinical cancer care. Curr Oncol 2016; 23(2):8–14.
18. Lattanzi S, Brigo F, Cagnetti C, et al. Efficacy and safety of adjunctive cannabidiol in patients with Lennox–Gastaut syndrome: a systematic review and meta-analysis. CNS Drugs 2018;32(10):905–16.
19. Devinsky O, Patel AD, Thiele EA, et al. Randomized, dose-ranging safety trial of cannabidiol in Dravet syndrome. Neurology 2018;90(14):e1204–11.
20. U.S. Food and Drug Administration. Warning letters and test results 2015. Available at: https://www.fda.gov/news-events/public-health-focus/warning-letters-and-test-results-cannabidiol-related-products. Accessed May 8, 2019.
21. U.S. Food and Drug Administration. Warning letters and test results 2016. Available at: https://www.fda.gov/news-events/public-health-focus/warning-letters-and-test-results-cannabidiol-related-products. Accessed May 8, 2019.

22. Lemberger L, Weiss J, Watanabe A, et al. Delta-9-tetrahydrocannabinol. Temporal correlation of the psychologic effects and blood levels after various routes of administration. N Engl J Med 1972;316(23):1430–5.
23. Wang GS, Le Lait MC, Deakyne SJ, et al. Unintentional pediatric exposures to marijuana in Colorado, 2009-2015. JAMA Pediatr 2016;170(9):e160971.
24. Toftdahl NG, Nordentoft M, Hjorthøj C. Prevalence of substance use disorders in psychiatric patients: a nationwide Danish population-based study. Soc Psychiatry Psychiatr Epidemiol 2016;51(1):129–40.
25. Barnett JH, Werners U, Secher SM, et al. Substance use in a population-based clinic sample of people with first-episode psychosis. Br J Psychiatry 2007;190:515–20.
26. Van Os J, Bak M, Hanssen M, et al. Cannabis use and psychosis: a longitudinal population-based study. Am J Epidemiol 2002;156(4):319–27.
27. Arseneault L, Cannon M, Poulton R, et al. Cannabis use in adolescence and risk for adult psychosis: longitudinal prospective study. BMJ 2002;325(7374):1212–3.
28. Foti DJ, Kotov R, Guey LT, et al. Cannabis use and the course of schizophrenia: 10-year follow- up after first hospitalization. Am J Psychiatry 2010;167(8):987–93.
29. Stone JM, Fisher HL, Major B, et al. Cannabis use and first-episode psychosis: relationship with manic and psychotic symptoms, and with age at presentation. Psychol Med 2014;44(3):499–506.
30. Seddon JL, Birchwood M, Copello A, et al. Cannabis use is associated with increased psychotic symptoms and poorer psychosocial functioning in first-episode psychosis: a report from the UK National EDEN study. Schizophr Bull 2016;42(3):619–25.
31. Hurst D, Loeffler G, McLay R. Psychosis associated with synthetic cannabinoid agonists: a case series. Am J Psychiatry 2011;168(10):1119.
32. Roberto AJ, Lorenzo A, Li KJ, et al. First-episode of synthetic cannabinoid-induced psychosis in a young adult, successfully managed with hospitalization and risperidone. Case Rep Psychiatry 2016;2016:1–4.
33. Schoeler T, Petros N, Di Forti M, et al. Association between continued cannabis use and risk of relapse in first-episode psychosis a quasi-experimental investigation within an observational study. JAMA Psychiatry 2016;73(11):1173–9.
34. Alvarez-Jimenez M, Priede A, Hetrick SE, et al. Risk factors for relapse following treatment for first episode psychosis: a systematic review and meta-analysis of longitudinal studies. Schizophr Res 2012;139(1–3):116–28.
35. Ferdinand RF, Sondeijker F, Van Der Ende J, et al. Cannabis use predicts future psychotic symptoms, and vice versa. Addiction 2005;100(5):612–8.
36. Patel R, Wilson R, Jackson R, et al. Association of cannabis use with hospital admission and antipsychotic treatment failure in first episode psychosis: an observational study. BMJ Open 2016;6(3):1–9.
37. Manrique-Garcia E, Zammit S, Dalman C, et al. Prognosis of schizophrenia in persons with and without a history of cannabis use. Psychol Med 2014;44(12):2513–21.
38. Schoeler T, Monk A, Sami MB, et al. Continued versus discontinued cannabis use in patients with psychosis: a systematic review and meta-analysis. Lancet Psychiatry 2016;3(3):215–25.
39. González-Pinto A, Alberich S, Barbeito S, et al. Cannabis and first-episode psychosis: different long-term outcomes depending on continued or discontinued use. Schizophr Bull 2011;37(3):631–9.

40. Lambert M, Conus P, Lubman DI, et al. The impact of substance use disorders on clinical outcome in 643 patients with first-episode psychosis. Acta Psychiatr Scand 2005;112(2):141–8.
41. Volkow ND, Swanson JM, Evins AE, et al. Effects of cannabis use on human behavior, including cognition, motivation, and psychosis: a review. JAMA Psychiatry 2016;73(3):292–7.
42. Cannon TD, Cadenhead K, Cornblatt B, et al. Prediction of psychosis in youth at high clinical risk: a multisite longitudinal study in North America. Arch Gen Psychiatry 2011;65(1):28–37.
43. Krabbendam L, Van Os J. Schizophrenia and urbanicity: a major environmental influence - conditional on genetic risk. Schizophr Bull 2005;31(4):795–9.
44. Rutten BPF, Mill J. Epigenetic mediation of environmental influences in major psychotic disorders. Schizophr Bull 2009;35(6):1045–56.
45. Henquet C, Di Forti M, Morrison P, et al. Gene-environment interplay between cannabis and psychosis. Schizophr Bull 2008;34(6):1111–21.
46. Paus TT, Keshavan M, Giedd JN. Why do many psychiatric disorders emerge during adolescence? Nat Rev Neurosci 2008;9(12):947–57.
47. Paus T. Mapping brain maturation and cognitive development during adolescence. Trends Cogn Sci 2005;9(2):60–8.
48. Kessler RC, Amminger GP, Aguilar-Gaxiola S, et al. Age of onset of mental disorders: a review of recent literature. Curr Opin Psychiatry 2007;20(4):359–64.
49. Wu C-H, Hwang T-J, Chen Y-J, et al. Primary and secondary alterations of white matter connectivity in schizophrenia: a study on first-episode and chronic patients using whole-brain tractography-based analysis. Schizophr Res 2015; 169(1–3):54–61.
50. Schaeffer DJ, Rodrigue a L, Burton CR, et al. White matter structural integrity differs between people with schizophrenia and healthy groups as a function of cognitive control. Schizophr Res 2015;169(1–3):62–8.
51. Bloomfield MAP, Hindocha C, Green SF, et al. The neuropsychopharmacology of cannabis: a review of human imaging studies. Pharmacol Ther 2018;195: 132–61.
52. Crane NA, Schuster RM. Effects of cannabis on neurocognitive functioning: recent advances, neurodevelopmental influences, and sex differences. Neuropsychol Rev 2013;23(2):117–37.
53. Englund A, Morrison PD, Nottage J, et al. Cannabidiol inhibits THC-elicited paranoid symptoms and hippocampal-dependent memory impairment. J Psychopharmacol 2013;27(1):19–27.
54. Di Forti M, Morrison PD, Butt A, et al. Cannabis use and psychiatric and cognitive disorders: the chicken or the egg? Curr Opin Psychiatry 2007;20(3): 228–34. Available at: http://ovidsp.ovid.com/ovidweb.cgi?T=JS&PAGE= reference&D=emed8&NEWS=N&AN=2007183226.
55. Schimmelmann BG, Conus P, Cotton SM, et al. Cannabis use disorder and age at onset of psychosis - a study in first-episode patients. Schizophr Res 2011; 129(1):52–6.
56. Bhattacharyya S, Morrison PD, Fusar-Poli P, et al. Opposite effects of δ-9-tetrahydrocannabinol and cannabidiol on human brain function and psychopathology. Neuropsychopharmacology 2010;35(3):764–74.
57. Levine A, Clemenza K, Rynn M, et al. Evidence for the risks and consequences of adolescent cannabis exposure. J Am Acad Child Adolesc Psychiatry 2017; 56(3):214–25.

58. Silins E, Horwood LJ, Patton GC, et al. Young adult sequelae of adolescent cannabis use: an integrative analysis. Lancet Psychiatry 2014;1(4):286–93.

59. U.S. Department of Health & Human Services. U.S. Surgeon general's advisory: marijuana use and the developing brain. 2019.

60. Khantzian EJ. The self-medication hypothesis of substance use disorders: a reconsideration and recent applications. Harv Rev Psychiatry 1997;4(5): 231–44. Available at: http://www.tandfonline.com/doi/abs/10.3109/10673229709030550.

61. Kuepper R, Van Os J, Lieb R, et al. Continued cannabis use and risk of incidence and persistence of psychotic symptoms: 10 year follow-up cohort study. BMJ 2011;342(7796):537.

62. Dragt S, Nieman DH, Schultze-Lutter F, et al. Cannabis use and age at onset of symptoms in subjects at clinical high risk for psychosis. Acta Psychiatr Scand 2012;125(1):45–53.

63. Degenhardt L, Hall W, Lynskey M. Testing hypotheses about the relationship between cannabis use and psychosis. Drug Alcohol Depend 2003;71(1):37–48.

64. Manrique-Garcia E, Zammit S, Dalman C, et al. Cannabis, schizophrenia and other non-affective psychoses: 35 years of follow-up of a population-based cohort. Psychol Med 2012;42(6):1321–8.

65. Starzer MSK, Nordentoft M, Hjorthøj C. Rates and predictors of conversion to schizophrenia or bipolar disorder following substance-induced psychosis. Am J Psychiatry 2018;175(4):343–50.

66. Arendt M, Rosenberg R, Foldager L, et al. Cannabis-induced psychosis and subsequent schizophrenia-spectrum disorders: follow-up study of 535 incident cases. Br J Psychiatry 2005;187:510–5.

67. Crebbin K, Mitford E, Paxton R, et al. First-episode drug-induced psychosis: a medium term follow up study reveals a high-risk group. Soc Psychiatry Psychiatr Epidemiol 2009;44(9):710–5.

68. Marconi A, Di Forti M, Lewis CM, et al. Meta-analysis of the association between the level of cannabis use and risk of psychosis. Schizophr Bull 2016;42(5): 1262–9.

69. Moore TH, Zammit S, Lingford-Hughes A, et al. Cannabis use and risk of psychotic or affective mental health outcomes: a systematic review. Lancet 2007; 370(9584):319–28.

70. Di Forti M, Marconi A, Carra E, et al. Proportion of patients in south London with first-episode psychosis attributable to use of high potency cannabis: a case-control study. Lancet Psychiatry 2015;2(3):233–8.

71. Di Forti M, Quattrone D, Freeman TP, et al. The contribution of cannabis use to variation in the incidence of psychotic disorder across Europe (EU-GEI): a multi-centre case-control study. Lancet Psychiatry 2019;6(5):427–36.

72. Veen ND, Selten J-P, van der Tweel I, et al. Cannabis use and age at onset of schizophrenia ingeborg van der Tweel. Am J Psychiatry 2004;161:501–6. Available at: http://ajp.psychiatryonline.org.

73. Di Forti M, Sallis H, Allegri F, et al. Daily use, especially of high-potency cannabis, drives the earlier onset of psychosis in cannabis users. Schizophr Bull 2014;40(6):1509–17.

74. Immonen J, Jääskeläinen E, Korpela H, et al. Age at onset and the outcomes of schizophrenia: a systematic review and meta-analysis. Early Interv Psychiatry 2017;11(6):453–60.

75. Gillespie NA, Pasman JA, Treur JL, et al. High-potency cannabis and incident psychosis: correcting the causal assumption. Lancet Psychiatry 2019;6(6):e14.

76. Harley M, Kelleher I, Clarke M, et al. Cannabis use and childhood trauma interact additively to increase the risk of psychotic symptoms in adolescence. Psychol Med 2010;40(10):1627–34.

77. Myles N, Newall H, Compton MT, et al. The age at onset of psychosis and tobacco use: a systematic meta-analysis. Soc Psychiatry Psychiatr Epidemiol 2012;47(8):1243–50.

78. Gilman J, Sobolewski SM, Evins AE. Cannabis use as an independent risk factor for, or component cause of, schizophrenia and related psychotic disorders. In: Compton M, Manseau M, editors. The complex connection between cannabis and schizophrenia. London: Academic Press; 2018. p. 221–46.

79. Thiselton DL, Vladimirov VI, Kuo PH, et al. AKT1 is associated with schizophrenia across multiple symptom dimensions in the Irish study of high density schizophrenia families. Biol Psychiatry 2008;63(5):449–57.

80. Norton N, Williams HJ, Dwyer S, et al. Association analysis of AKT1 and schizophrenia in a UK case control sample. Schizophr Res 2007;93(1–3):58–65.

81. Tan HY, Nicodemus KK, Chen Q, et al. Genetic variation in AKT1 is linked to dopamine-associated prefrontal cortical structure and function in humans. J Clin Invest 2008;118(6):2200–8.

82. Ozaita A, Puighermanal E, Maldonado R. Regulation of PI3K/Akt/GSK-3 pathway by cannabinoids in the brain. J Neurochem 2007;102(4):1105–14.

83. Van Winkel R, Kahn RS, Linszen DH, et al. Family-based analysis of genetic variation underlying psychosis-inducing effects of cannabis: sibling analysis and proband follow-up. Arch Gen Psychiatry 2011;68(2):148–57.

84. Di Forti M, Iyegbe C, Sallis H, et al. Confirmation that the AKT1 (rs2494732) genotype influences the risk of psychosis in cannabis users. Biol Psychiatry 2012;72(10):811–6.

85. Pasman J, Verweij K, Gerring Z, et al. GWAS of lifetime cannabis use reveals new risk loci, genetic overlap with psychiatric traits, and a causal influence of schizophrenia. Nature neuroscience 2016;118(24):6072–8.

86. Giordano GN, Ohlsson H, Sundquist K, et al. The association between cannabis abuse and subsequent schizophrenia: a Swedish national co-relative control study. Psychol Med 2015;45(2):407–14.

87. Vaessen TSJ, De Jong L, Schäfer AT, et al. The interaction between cannabis use and the Val158Met polymorphism of the COMT gene in psychosis: a trans-diagnostic meta ± analysis. PLoS One 2018;13(2):1–22.

88. Zammit S, Owen MJ, Evans J, et al. Cannabis, COMT and psychotic experiences. Br J Psychiatry 2011;199(5):380–5.

89. Power RA, Verweij KJH, Zuhair M, et al. Genetic predisposition to schizophrenia associated with increased use of cannabis. Mol Psychiatry 2014;19(11):1201–4.

90. Radhakrishnan R, Wilkinson ST, D'Souza DC. Gone to pot-a review of the association between cannabis and psychosis. Front Psychiatry 2014;5:1–24.

91. Schuster RM, Hoeppner SS, Evins AE, et al. Early onset marijuana use is associated with learning inefficiencies. Neuropsychology 2016;30(4):405–15.

92. Crane NA, Schuster RM, Gonzalez R. Preliminary evidence for a sex-specific relationship between amount of cannabis use and neurocognitive performance in young adult cannabis users. J Int Neuropsychol Soc 2013;19(9):1009–15.

93. Mueser KT, Penn DL, Addington J, et al. The NAVIGATE program for first-episode psychosis: rationale, overview, and description of psychosocial components. Psychiatr Serv 2015;66(7):680–90.

94. Barrowclough C, Marshall M, Gregg L, et al. A phase-specific psychological therapy for people with problematic cannabis use following a first episode of psychosis: a randomized controlled trial. Psychol Med 2014;44(13):2749–61.

95. Edwards J, Elkins K, Hinton M, et al. Randomized controlled trial of a cannabis-focused intervention for young people with first-episode psychosis. Acta Psychiatr Scand 2006;114(2):109–17.

96. Madigan K, Brennan D, Lawlor E, et al. A multi-center, Randomized controlled trial of a group psychological intervention for psychosis with comorbid cannabis dependence over the early course of illness. Schizophr Res 2013;143(1): 138–42.

97. Kane JM, Robinson DG, Schooler NR, et al. Comprehensive versus usual community care for first episode psychosis: two-year outcomes from the NIMH RAISE early treatment program. Am J Geriatr Psychiatry 2016;173(4):362–72.

98. Cather C, Brunette MF, Mueser KT, et al. Impact of comprehensive treatment for first episode psychosis on substance use outcomes: a randomized controlled trial. Psychiatry Res 2018;268:303–11.

99. Stanger C, Budney AJ. Contingency management approaches for adolescent substance use disorders. Child Adolesc Psychiatr Clin N Am 2010;19(3): 547–62.

100. Sigmon SC, Higgins ST. Voucher-based contingent reinforcement of marijuana abstinence among individuals with serious mental illness. J Subst Abuse Treat 2006;30(4):291–5.

101. Schuster R, Hanly A, Gilman J, et al. A contingency management method for 30-days abstinence in non-treatment seeking young adult cannabis users. Drug and Alcohol Dependence 2016;5(6):1–8.

102. Schuster RM, Gilman J, Schoenfeld D, et al. One month of cannabis abstinence in adolescents and young adults is associated with improved memory. J Clin Psychiatry 2018;79(6) [pii:17m11977].

103. New Brunswick Medical Society. Legal, not safe. Available at: https://www.legalnotsafe.ca/. Accessed June 13, 2019.

Neurobiology of Psychosis in Youth

Genetics of Childhood-onset Schizophrenia 2019 Update

Jennifer K. Forsyth, PhD[a],*, Robert F. Asarnow, PhD[a,b,c],*

KEYWORDS

- Childhood-onset schizophrenia • Genetics • Common variants • GWAS
- Copy number variants • Rare variants • De novo mutations
- Autism spectrum disorder

KEY POINTS

- Childhood-onset schizophrenia (COS) shares considerable genetic overlap with adult-onset schizophrenia.
- The risk architecture of COS involves common and rare variants, including copy number variants.
- COS shares genetic overlap with earlier-onset neurodevelopmental disorders, such as autism spectrum disorder.
- The utility of genetic screening for diagnosis and individualized treatment is currently limited; however, genetic testing may be useful in some cases and identifying common neural pathways on which risk variants act offers promise toward developing novel interventions.

INTRODUCTION

Childhood-onset schizophrenia (COS) is defined as schizophrenia with onset before age 13 years and is a rare and early-onset variant of the much more common adult onset-schizophrenia (AOS). The prevalence of true COS is fewer than 1 in 10,000.[1] In contrast, the lifetime prevalence of AOS is 4.0 in 1,000.[2] Note that before Diagnostic and Statistical Manual of Mental Disorders, Third Edition (DSM-III), there were no uniform diagnostic criteria for COS. Early studies of COS therefore included children who

Disclosures and funding sources: R. Asarnow, Della Martin Foundation, NIMH grant MH72697; J.K. Forsyth, NIMH K08MH118577, NARSAD Young Investigator Award. The authors have no conflicts of interest to disclose.
[a] Department of Psychiatry & Biobehavioral Sciences, University of California, Los Angeles, 760 Westwood Plaza, Los Angeles, CA 90095, USA; [b] Department of Psychology, University of California, Los Angeles, 502 Portola Plaza Los Angeles, CA 90095, USA; [c] Brain Research Institute, University of California, Los Angeles, 695 Charles E Young Dr S, Los Angeles, CA 90095, USA
* Corresponding authors. 760 Westwood Plaza, Los Angeles, CA 90095.
E-mail addresses: jforsyth@mednet.ucla.edu (J.K.F.); rasarnow@mednet.ucla.edu (R.F.A.)

now would receive DSM-V[3] diagnoses of autism spectrum disorder, unspecified neu-rodevelopmental disorder, or schizophrenia, and there were significant variations between clinicians in how COS was diagnosed.

Epidemiologic and family studies in the twentieth century clearly established that genetic factors play a major role in the cause of AOS. In the past decade, modern genome-wide association studies (GWASs) have begun to identify many specific genetic factors that are associated with AOS. Because of the low prevalence of COS, less is known about the individual genetic factors that increase risk for COS. Nevertheless, genetic studies of COS have generally paralleled studies of the much more common AOS, and initial findings suggest that many genetic factors that confer risk for AOS also confer risk for COS.

To highlight the historical evolution of genetic studies of COS, this article first discusses familial aggregation studies of AOS and COS. It then provides a brief overview of modern understandings of the human genome and classes of genetic variation as they relate to the genetic architecture of schizophrenia. The article subsequently provides an overview of major genetic findings for AOS, including reviewing studies of common, rare, and copy number variants (CNVs) in AOS. Finally, it reviews genetic studies of COS, more specifically. Of note, many modern, large-scale GWASs of schizophrenia involve minimal patient characterization aside from establishing schizophrenia case status. As such, age of onset is often not reported. Because most patients with schizophrenia have their first psychotic episode in adulthood, this article refers to studies of patients with broadly ascertained schizophrenia as AOS studies. In addition, in the discussion of familial aggregation studies, the focus is on studies that examined risk in parents of schizophrenia probands rather than risk in siblings, because the siblings of COS probands typically have not entered the classic age of risk for schizophrenia.

FAMILIAL AGGREGATION OF SCHIZOPHRENIA

Initial genetic studies of AOS and COS examined family members of patients with AOS or COS to test the hypotheses that schizophrenia and/or schizophrenia spectrum disorders show familial aggregation. Every modern study that used narrow, operationalized criteria for schizophrenia found that schizophrenia strongly aggregated in families of patients with AOS relative to families of community controls. Modern family studies found a 3-fold increase in the relative risk (RR) for schizophrenia among parents of AOS probands compared with the parents of controls.[4] Similarly, the morbid schizophrenia risk for parents and siblings of AOS probands was 6% and 9%, respectively, compared with 1% in the general population.[5] Adoption and twin studies further suggested that the increased risk of schizophrenia among family members of AOS probands was largely due to shared genetic factors, rather than shared environmental factors.[4]

In studies of COS, an early twin study found a concordance for COS diagnosis for monozygotic twins of 88.2% compared with a concordance of 22.3% in dizygotic twins.[6] This concordance yielded a heritability estimate of 84.5%, suggesting that COS is highly heritable. Two modern studies that used DSM-III-R criteria and collected data through both personal interview and interviews of family members similarly suggested that schizophrenia aggregates in the families of COS probands. Thus, the University of California, Los Angeles (UCLA) study found an RR of 17 for schizophrenia in the parents of COS probands compared with those of controls.[7] The NIMH Child Psychiatry Branch study of 95 patients with COS found 1 case of schizophrenia in parents of COS probands and none in parents of community control probands.[8] Together, these family aggregation studies suggested that genes may play a role in the etiology of schizophrenia.

FAMILIAL AGGREGATION OF SCHIZOPHRENIA SPECTRUM DISORDERS

Family studies also found that, in addition to schizophrenia, several other psychiatric disorders tend to aggregate in families of AOS probands. These disorders are termed schizophrenia spectrum disorders, and include schizoaffective disorder (depressed type), schizotypal personality disorder, schizophreniform and atypical psychosis, and paranoid personality disorder. The only 2 studies that determined the RR of schizophrenia spectrum disorders separately for parents (ie, not combined with siblings) of AOS probands found RRs of schizotypal personality and/or paranoid personality disorders of 6.6[9] and 3.0[10] in parents of AOS probands.

In the 2 modern family studies of COS, the RRs for schizotypal personality and/or paranoid personality disorders in parents of COS probands were 10.5[7] and 15.2.[8] When schizophrenia was included as a schizophrenia spectrum disorder, the RR for schizophrenia spectrum disorders was 16.9[7] and 15.9[8] in parents of COS probands. The RR for just schizophrenia, schizotypal, or paranoid personality disorders was 15.1 in parents of COS probands.[7] Compared with the RR of 5.8 for schizophrenia, schizotypal, or paranoid personality disorder found in a large family study of AOS probands that used similar diagnostic approaches as the UCLA study,[9] the RR risk of schizophrenia and schizophrenia spectrum disorders appears to be greater in parents of COS probands than in parents of AOS probands. This increased rate of schizophrenia spectrum disorders in relatives of COS probands suggests that schizophrenia spectrum disorders may aggregate more strongly in the families of COS probands compared with AOS probands.

FAMILIAL AGGREGATION OF NEUROBIOLOGICAL ABNORMALITIES

Several neurobiological abnormalities present in patients with AOS and COS are also present in a substantial number of their nonpsychotic first-degree relatives. These abnormalities are sometimes referred to as endophenotypes. Endophenotypes are thought to reflect the effects of genetic risk for schizophrenia and are considered intermediate phenotypes that may be closer to the biological effects of risk genes than DSM-V symptoms of schizophrenia.[11] Some investigators have argued that identifying endophenotypes may help elucidate causal pathways between putative risk genes and "their expression as a clinically identifiable phenotype."[12]

Abnormalities found in the nonpsychotic relatives of patients with AOS include impairments in neurocognitive functioning and smooth-pursuit eye movements, and abnormalities in brain structure and electrical activity.[13,14] Many similar abnormalities are found in the nonpsychotic relatives of COS probands. For example, a combination of scores on 3 tests that detect neurocognitive deficits in nonpsychotic relatives of AOS probands identified 20% of mothers and fathers of COS probands compared with 0% of the mothers or fathers of community control probands. Scores on these neurocognitive tests also showed some diagnostic specificity, with a cutoff that identified 12% of mothers of COS probands identifying 0% of mothers with attention-deficit/hyperactivity disorder.[15] Nonpsychotic first-degree relatives of patients with COS also showed impairments in attention/executive function[16] and smooth-pursuit eye tracking.[17] Nonpsychotic siblings of COS probands showed deficits on a procedural skill learning task supported by a cortical-striatal network,[18] widespread reductions in white matter microstructural integrity,[19] and reduced gray matter volume in several cortical and subcortical regions, but increased gray matter volume in the lingual gyrus and cerebellum.[20] A longitudinal study also found that, before adolescence, the nonpsychotic siblings of COS probands showed reduced cortical gray matter in superior temporal and prefrontal areas[21]; however, these reductions normalized during adolescence. In general, the first-degree relatives of patients with COS show subtle impairments on some tasks identified as potential endophenotypes in studies of relatives of patients with AOS, suggesting that these deficits do not merely reflect the effects of psychosis, and instead are likely to reflect genetic factors.

Interestingly, a family study of first-degree and second-degree relatives of community controls with and without family histories of schizophrenia found that impairment in neurocognitive functioning and incidence of schizophrenia spectrum disorders were relatively independent expressions of familial liability to schizophrenia.[22] Given that schizophrenia is a complex, polygenic disorder, the genes associated with neurobiological endophenotypes may not be the same set of genes that are associated with psychotic symptoms. In addition, a recent family study of COS, AOS, and community control probands examined familial transmission of neurocognitive function. In families with AOS, this study found shared familial effects on attention and working memory, but not on verbal learning and memory for faces. By contrast, in families with COS, there were significant shared familial effects on verbal learning and memory for faces, but not on attention and working memory.[23] Thus, the familial architecture of neurocognitive functions may differ between nuclear families with COS and AOS.

It is important to recognize that paralleling the heterogeneity of findings in studies of patients with COS and AOS patients, many first-degree relatives of patients with schizophrenia do not have neurobiological abnormalities. However, although there is considerable heterogeneity among relatives in what abnormalities they do have, type of neurocognitive impairment does tend to run in families. The neurobiological abnormalities identified in nonpsychotic relatives of patients with COS seem to tap diverse neural networks. Heterogeneity of neurobiological abnormalities may indicate that impairments in specific neural networks are associated with different sets of susceptibility genes. If this is the case, endophenotypes may help identify biologically meaningful subtypes of schizophrenia linked to specific genotypes, thereby providing a clearer link between genetic and phenotypic variation.[24]

BRIEF INTRODUCTION TO THE HUMAN GENOME AND CLASSES OF SPECIFIC GENETIC VARIANTS

Recent genetic studies of AOS and COS have focused on identifying specific genetic factors that increase risk for schizophrenia. The ability to rigorously pursue such questions has accelerated rapidly since 2003, when the human genome was first sequenced and established as a reference genome to enable subsequent scientific discovery.[25] Understanding of the range of classes of genetic variants observed in the human population, the frequency at which different classes of variants exist in the average person's genome, and the overall genetic architecture of complex traits such as schizophrenia have improved dramatically since this landmark achievement. It is now known that there are ~3 billion nucleotide base pairs (bp) in the human genome, comprising the 4 nucleotide bases, adenine (A), cytosine (C), guanine (G), and thymine (G). Approximately 1.5% of this DNA sequence encodes proteins,[26] which form the building blocks of every cell and organ in the human body. A substantial portion of the remaining DNA sequence encodes non–protein-coding RNA transcripts or regulatory sequences that are critical for temporally and spatially regulating the expression of the ~20,000 protein-coding genes in the human genome.

However, estimates of the exact proportion of non–protein-coding DNA having a functional role vary widely (eg, <10% to up to 80%[27–29]), and a significant portion of noncoding DNA likely has no functional role.[29]

The vast majority of DNA sequence is identical between 2 individual humans (>99.8%).[30] Nevertheless, given the total length of the human genome, the average individual differs from the reference human genome at approximately 4 to 5 million locations in the genome,[30] yielding a huge pool of variants to examine for potential association with psychiatric traits such as schizophrenia. Broadly, each variation in sequence can be categorized based on the frequency at which it is observed in the population, the size and type of variant (eg, number of affected nucleotides), and the functional consequence of the variant. Thus, common variants (ie, traditionally defined as variants found in >5% of the population) are observed more frequently than rare variants (ie, <0.5%–1% of the population). Relatedly, single nucleotide variants, which are called single nucleotide polymorphisms (SNPs) when they are common in a population, affect only 1 bp and are generally smaller or affect shorter DNA sequence than short insertions or deletions (ie, indels; 1–49 bp in length). Short indels, in turn, are smaller than structural variants, which include inversions, translocations, deletions, and duplications of larger sequences of DNA (ie, >50 bp) that affect chromosomal structure.[31] Owing to the effect of natural selection, in which deleterious mutations affect the ability of individuals to mate and/or have viable offspring, or are lethal altogether, common variants are less likely to have damaging effects compared with rare or de novo variants. However, new mutations, known as de novo mutations (DNMs), occur in every offspring (ie, are not observed in either parent) and are thereby continuously introduced into the population. Thus, all individuals carry rare variants and DNMs. Although most variants observed in a single individual's genome are common and small (>99.9% of variants), the average human genome also contains more than 2000 structural variants, and 40,000 to 200,000 rare variants (ie, 1%–4% of variants per genome).[7,30] Regardless of variant class or the frequency at which a variant is observed in a population, the ultimate importance of a given variant rests on whether it exerts a molecular or phenotypic consequence, such as by qualitatively altering the structure of a protein and/or altering its level of expression.[31] Most variants are currently thought to have benign or minimal phenotypic consequences; however, annotating the functional consequences of a variant remains a complex task, particularly for non–protein-coding regions of the genome.

These advances in the understanding of the range and scale of genetic variation present in the human genome have ushered in a new era of psychiatric genetics, focused largely on using genome-wide approaches to identify variants associated with disease, as well as understanding how disease-associated variants disrupt biological processes to cause disease. Given the frequency with which variants of all classes are observed in the average individual genome, finding robust associations between individual variants and complex traits is a major challenge. However, as new tools and standards for genetic studies have been developed and refined, psychiatric genetics has begun to yield major insights into the genetic architecture and specific variants associated with complex psychiatric traits such as AOS and COS.

THE NEW ERA OF PSYCHIATRIC GENOMICS

Psychiatric genetics in the 1990s and 2000s was dominated by small to moderate-sized studies of candidate genes and linkage studies that frequently failed to replicate.[32–34] In contrast, over the last decade, large-scale collaborative studies, often genotyping thousands to tens of thousands of minimally phenotyped patients and controls, have begun to identify many specific variants that are robustly associated with disease. The advent and eventual success of these large-scale studies was facilitated by technological improvements that dramatically reduced the cost of genome-wide genotyping and sequencing, as well as the realization that critical confounds such as SNPs occurring at varying rates in populations with different ancestries (ie, that can lead to spurious associations if patient and control groups are not carefully matched in genetic ancestry), needed to be carefully accounted for in genetic studies.[35]

Thus far, most GWASs of schizophrenia have investigated different classes of genetic variants through independent studies (ie, studying common, rare, or de novo variants separately). In addition, given that COS is a rare condition, existing studies largely involved patients with AOS. Therefore, results from well-powered, seminal studies of the most typical AOS are reviewed here first, for each broad class of genetic variants. Evidence for the multifactorial/polygenic threshold model of risk for schizophrenia across variant classes is also discussed. Finally, studies that are specific to COS are reviewed, as well as studies that explore genetic associations in relation to age of psychosis onset. Across this review of studies, the focus is on findings based on genome-wide approaches, given the now well-established problems with replicability in candidate gene studies.

OVERVIEW OF GENETIC STUDIES OF ADULT-ONSET SCHIZOPHRENIA

It is now clear that the genetic architecture of AOS is complex and high polygenic, involving hundreds to thousands of genes, with risk variants spanning the range of possible allelic frequencies and variant classes. Thus, in a seminal GWAS of common variants in 36,989 schizophrenia cases and 113,075 controls, 108 independent loci were found to be significantly associated with schizophrenia status.[36] Although each significantly associated loci conferred only a small increase in risk (ie, median odds ratio [OR] per associated SNP = 1.08), when the effects of all nominally associated ($P<.05$) loci were considered together as a single polygenic risk score (PRS), schizophrenia PRS was able to explain 18.4% of the variance in case versus control status.[36] Although 40% of the 108 significantly associated loci were located within the sequence boundaries of a single protein-coding gene, the remaining associated SNPs were located in non–protein-coding regions of the genome, and only 10 loci were credibly associated with nonsynonymous polymorphisms predicted to directly alter the amino-acid sequence of a protein. This finding suggests that many common variants associated with AOS are likely to contribute to disease risk by altering the level of expression of specific proteins, rather than more directly altering protein structure. Notable genes implicated by associated loci included DRD2, which encodes the dopamine D2 receptor, which is the primary target of almost all antipsychotic drugs; numerous genes involved in glutamatergic signaling and plasticity, including GRIA1, GRIN2A, and SRR; and genes encoding voltage-gated calcium channels, such as CACNA1C and CACNB2, thus providing genetic evidence for existing etiologic hypotheses of schizophrenia involving dopaminergic and glutamatergic signaling. These schizophrenia-associated variants were also found to map to genes that are expressed specifically in pyramidal neurons (ie, the primary glutamatergic/excitatory neurons of the cortex), medium spiny neurons of the striatum (ie, primary dopaminergic neurons), and cortical interneurons (ie, primary GABAergic/inhibitory neurons).[37] A more recent meta-analytic GWAS of common variants in schizophrenia included an additional 5220 schizophrenia cases and 18,823 controls, and identified 145 independent loci significantly associated with schizophrenia.[38] The identified schizophrenia-associated SNPs were enriched for genes that are intolerant to mutation (ie, found to be very rarely mutated in humans, suggesting that mutation in these genes is under strong selective pressure), genes involved in synaptic transmission, and genes that are targets of the fragile X mental retardation protein (FMRP), which is known to regulate the protein-level expression of genes involved in brain development and synaptic plasticity. Together, these seminal studies provided compelling evidence that common risk variants for schizophrenia converge onto neuronal and synaptic gene sets. As sample sizes continue to increase, the number of common variants significantly associated with AOS will continue to increase, along with the understanding of the convergent biological processes affected by risk variants for AOS.

Studies of rare variants have also yielded insights into the genetic etiology of AOS, although, given the inherent low frequency of individual rare variants, disease associations are generally tested after aggregating variants to summary levels such as the gene or gene-set level. Thus, patients with schizophrenia have been found to carry an increased burden of rare[39] and ultrarare[40] deleterious mutations, overall, compared with controls, although the effect size of this overall increased burden is small (eg, $OR = 1.07$ for damaging and disruptive ultrarare variants[40]). Nevertheless, aggregated at the gene-set level, rare deleterious mutations in patients with schizophrenia were found to be enriched for genes that are intolerant to mutation, genes that are expressed specifically in neurons, gene targets of FMRP,[41] and genes that are components of synaptic gene sets, such as the N-methyl-D-aspartate receptor (NMDAR) and activity-regulated cytoskeleton-associated protein (Arc) complexes,[39,40,42] which are critically involved in modulating synaptic plasticity. Protein-altering DNMs in patients with schizophrenia have been found to be similarly increased in genes involved in neuronal and synaptic function, including genes that are components of the postsynaptic density, the NMDAR and Arc complexes, and targets of FMRP,[43] as well as among genes involved in regulating the expression of other genes.[44] Thus, compelling evidence indicates that damaging rare variants and DNMs in AOS also converge on genes involved in neuronal and synaptic function.

CNVs are a particular class of structural variants in which large segments of DNA are deleted or duplicated, resulting in genomic imbalances in the normal number of copies of DNA in the region. CNVs frequently arise in genomic hotspot regions that contain repeats of DNA sequence, known as segmental duplications, because these repeat DNA sequences make them prone to unequal crossing over during meiotic recombination (ie, nonallelic homologous recombination). As an overall class, large (eg, >100 kb), rare CNVs (ie, observed in <1% of the population) have been consistently associated with schizophrenia (eg, $OR = 1.15$[45,46]) and have yielded important insights into the genetic causes of schizophrenia.[45–50] The overall increased burden of CNVs associated with schizophrenia is concentrated in CNVs that overlap genes[48] and several recurrent CNV loci have been associated with schizophrenia, including deletions at the 22q11.2, 2p16.3 (NRXN1), 3q29, 15q11.2, and 15q13.3 loci, duplications at the 16p11.2 and 7q11.23 loci, and deletions or duplications at the 1q21.1 and 7p36.3 (VIPR2) loci. About 2.5% of patients with schizophrenia are estimated to carry CNVs at 1 or more schizophrenia-associated loci.[49] Note that CNVs at many of these specific loci have pleiotropic effects, because they are also associated with broader neurodevelopmental disorders such as autism spectrum disorder (ASD) and intellectual disability (ID).[47,51,52] Similar to common variants associated with schizophrenia, as well as other rare and de novo variants, schizophrenia-associated CNVs disproportionately affect neuronal and synaptic gene sets,[53] including components of the postsynaptic density, NMDAR and Arc complexes,[47,54] and sets of genes that are involved in excitatory and inhibitory neurotransmission.[55]

Notably, although common variants are expected to account for the largest proportion of overall genetic liability for schizophrenia at the clinical population level (30%–50%), each individual common variant confers only a small increase in risk.[36] In contrast, deleterious rare variants, de novo variants, and CNVs may account for a smaller proportion of schizophrenia liability at the clinical population level; however, when present in a given individual, deleterious rare variants can increase risk substantially (eg, ORs up to ~20–68 for the most highly penetrant CNVs[48]).

Growing evidence also indicates that common and rare variants interact to increase risk. Thus, the total burden of common schizophrenia-associated risk alleles that given individuals carry can be summarized by their schizophrenia PRSs, which are calculated as their weighted sum of schizophrenia risk-associated SNP alleles based on recent GWAS (eg, Ref.[36]). Although patients with schizophrenia have higher PRSs than controls, regardless of CNV carrier status, patients who carry risk CNVs that have previously been associated with schizophrenia have lower PRSs compared with patients without risk CNVs.[56,57] Furthermore, the increased burden of common schizophrenia risk alleles in patients who also carry risk CNVs was found to be inversely proportional to the effect size of the risk CNV.[57] Similarly, patients with schizophrenia with damaging de novo variants in genes that are intolerant to mutation, or are associated with neurodevelopmental disorders more broadly, were found to have lower transmission of schizophrenia PRSs from parents compared with patients without de novo variants in these genes.[58]

Together, these findings suggest that there is significant heterogeneity in the specific risk variants carried by each individual patient with AOS, and that risk variants converge across variants classes and the allelic frequency spectrum to increase risk in an additive manner. Overall, this is consistent with long-standing multifactorial/polygenic threshold models of schizophrenia, which postulate that schizophrenia results when an accumulation of risk factors crosses a threshold of liability.[59]

GENETIC STUDIES OF CHILDHOOD-ONSET SCHIZOPHRENIA

Given that COS is rare, there are few genetic studies of COS, and most of these have focused on establishing the extent to which risk for COS is conferred through similar genetic mechanisms as AOS. Preliminary evidence suggests that, in addition to sharing genetic risk factors with AOS, the genetic architecture of COS may include greater loading from variants that also confer risk for other neurodevelopmental disorders, such as ASD, ID, and epilepsy. Thus, in a study of 130 COS probands and 103 of their healthy siblings, COS probands had significantly higher schizophrenia PRSs than their siblings, as well as higher polygenic risk for ASD.[60] Increased rates of large CNVs have also been found in COS,[50] including in CNVs associated with schizophrenia and other neurodevelopmental disorders. Of note, rates of large, rare CNVs seem to be higher in patients with COS compared not only to controls but also to patients with AOS. Thus, 11.9% of COS probands were estimated to have a neurodevelopmental disease–associated CNV compared with 1.5% of their healthy siblings and 1.4% to 4.9% of patients with AOS.[61–63] In particular, many COS probands have been found to carry CNVs at the well-known 22q11.2 locus, which is known to increase risk for multiple psychiatric and developmental disorders, including schizophrenia, ASD, ID, and attention-deficit/hyperactivity disorder.[61–63]

Studies of DNMs using exome sequencing in COS have been small; however, one study of 17 COS proband-parent trios found an overall protein-coding DNM rate of 1.17 per COS exome, which was similar to rates found in other psychiatric diseases.[64] DNMs in patients with COS were enriched in loss-of-function intolerant genes, similar to AOS and other neurodevelopmental disorders.[64] Numerous DNMs were found in these small COS samples that affect genes implicated in broader neurodevelopmental disorders, including ATP1A3, which encodes a subunit of the neuron-specific ATP-dependent transmembrane sodium-potassium pump[65,66]; UPF3B, which is involved in regulating nonsense-mediated decay of messenger RNAs[67]; SRCAP, which is a component of the chromatin-remodeling SRCAP complex and can function as a transcriptional activator in Notch-mediated and CREB-mediated transcription; and PNKP, which is involved in DNA-strand repair (Sanders, personal communication, 2014). Together, these initial studies suggest that DNMs in COS are enriched for neurodevelopmental disorder–associated genes; however, further research is needed to systematically test this specific hypothesis.

Interestingly, two moderately sized, independent studies (ie, 2762 cases and 3187 controls,[68] and 1067 patients and 1169 controls[69]) that largely involved patients with AOS found that earlier age of psychosis onset was *not* associated with higher schizophrenia PRS. In contrast, in one of these studies which also assessed environmental risk factors, a high loading of environmental risk from perinatal insult, head injury, and/or cannabis use was associated with earlier psychosis onset.[69] Given that so-called earlier onset in these studies seemed to generally involve patients with adolescent or early-adult onset, this raises the intriguing possibility that the risk architecture of psychosis onset within an intermediate, adolescent range may include a greater accumulation of risk from environmental factors compared with later psychosis onset in early adulthood to mid-adulthood. In contrast, as noted earlier, the genetic architecture of COS may be characterized by a joint loading of variants that confer risk for AOS, as well as variants that are strongly associated with early-onset neurodevelopmental disorders such as ASD and ID. This possibility is consistent with the increased rates of autism spectrum or pervasive developmental disorder diagnoses found among patients with COS.[70–72] Together, this raises the possibility that different genetic and environmental risk architectures may underlie childhood, versus adolescent, versus adult onset of schizophrenia. However, this is largely speculative. Large-scale studies that concurrently assess various environmental risk factors and a comprehensive range of genetic variants associated with AOS and early neurodevelopmental disorders in large samples of patients with schizophrenia whose ages of onset span the full range possible are needed to elucidate the risk architecture and specific genetic variants underlying variation in age of psychosis onset.

SUMMARY AND IMPLICATIONS FOR CLINICAL PRACTICE

Overall, the extant literature suggests that the risk architecture of COS involves contributions from common variants that are associated with AOS, common variants that are associated with ASD, and a potentially higher contribution from large, rare CNVs that are associated with multiple neurodevelopmental disorders, including schizophrenia, ASD, and ID, relative to AOS.

As the cost of genotyping and sequencing continues to decrease, and knowledge of the genetic causes of COS, specifically, as well as schizophrenia, more broadly, and other neurodevelopmental disorders continues to improve, the promise of using genetic information to refine the diagnostic categories and develop individualized treatments for COS is increasingly salient.[73] Indeed, harnessing the power of next-generation sequencing to accelerate biomedical discovery and develop better targeted treatments that leverage genetic and molecular information at the individual patient level is a driving force behind the 2015 NIH Precision Medicine Initiative.[74] Precision medicine approaches have already been incorporated into drug discovery trials and patient care in other areas of medicine. This progress is most notable for cancer, in which screening for known highly penetrant genetic mutations and molecular profiling of tumors is beginning to affect clinical decision making and guide the development and use of targeted therapies for specific tumor subtypes.[75–77]

The path to precision medicine in psychiatry has a considerable way to go before gene discovery successes are translated into individualized treatments. Nevertheless, one early target for genomic screening might be for patients with COS with notable developmental characteristics, such as facial dysmorphology, ID, language delay, or health problems such as congenital heart defects that are linked to CNV-related syndromes (eg, 22q11.2, 3q29, or 15q11.2 deletion syndrome). Even in the absence of current, direct treatment implications, genetic testing to assess for the presence of potential pathogenic CNVs may be useful for improving patient and caregiver knowledge of disease causes, as well as improving access to medical benefits and social services.[78,79] As major advances in gene discovery continue in the coming years, identifying convergent pathways through which multiple genes associated with COS adversely affect brain development and function offers great promise for developing novel therapeutic targets for this debilitating condition.

REFERENCES

1. Burd L, Kerbeshian J. A North Dakota prevalence study of schizophrenia presenting in childhood. J Am Acad Child Adolesc Psychiatry 1987;26(3):347–50.
2. McGrath J, Saha S, Chant D, et al. Schizophrenia: a concise overview of incidence, prevalence, and mortality. Epidemiol Rev 2008;30:67–76.
3. American Psychiatric Association. (2013). Diagnostic and statistical manual of mental disorders (5th ed.). Arlington, VA: Author. Available at: https://dsm.psychiatryonline.org/doi/pdf/10.1176/appi.books.9780890420249.dsm-iv-tr Accessed September 26, 2019.
4. Kendler KS, Diehl SR. The genetics of schizophrenia: a current, genetic-epidemiologic perspective. Schizophr Bull 1993;19(2):261–85.
5. Tsuang M. Schizophrenia: genes and environment. Biol Psychiatry 2000;47(3):210–20. Available at: https://www.ncbi.nlm.nih.gov/pubmed/10682218.
6. Kallmann FJ, Roth B. Genetic aspects of preadolescent schizophrenia. Am J Psychiatry 1956;112(8):599–606.
7. Asarnow RF, Nuechterlein KH, Fogelson D, et al. Schizophrenia and schizophrenia-spectrum personality disorders in the first-degree relatives of children with schizophrenia: the UCLA family study. Arch Gen Psychiatry 2001;58(6):581–8. Available at: https://www.ncbi.nlm.nih.gov/pubmed/11386988.
8. Nicolson R, Brookner FB, Lenane M, et al. Parental schizophrenia spectrum disorders in childhood-onset and adult-onset schizophrenia. Am J Psychiatry 2003;160(3):490–5.
9. Kendler KS, McGuire M, Gruenberg AM, et al. The roscommon family study. I. Methods, diagnosis of probands, and risk of schizophrenia in relatives. Arch Gen Psychiatry 1993;50(7):527–40. Available at: https://www.ncbi.nlm.nih.gov/pubmed/8317947.
10. Baron M, Gruen R, Asnis L, et al. Familial transmission of schizotypal and borderline personality disorders. Am J Psychiatry 1985;142(8):927–34.
11. Gottesman II, Shields J. Genetic theorizing and schizophrenia. Br J Psychiatry 1973;122(566):15–30. Available at: https://www.ncbi.nlm.nih.gov/pubmed/4683020.

12. Nenadic I, Gaser C, Sauer H. Heterogeneity of brain structural variation and the structural imaging endophenotypes in schizophrenia. Neuropsychobiology 2012; 66(1):44–9.

13. Cannon TD. The inheritance of intermediate phenotypes for schizophrenia. Curr Opin Psychiatry 2005;18(2):135–40. Available at: https://www.ncbi.nlm.nih.gov/pubmed/16639165.

14. Allen AJ, Griss ME, Folley BS, et al. Endophenotypes in schizophrenia: a selective review. Schizophr Res 2009;109(1–3):24–37.

15. Asarnow RF, Nuechterlein KH, Subotnik KL, et al. Neurocognitive impairments in nonpsychotic parents of children with schizophrenia and attention-deficit/hyperactivity disorder: the University of California, Los Angeles Family Study. Arch Gen Psychiatry 2002;59(11):1053–60. Available at: https://jamanetwork.com/journals/jamapsychiatry/article-abstract/206880.

16. Gochman PA, Greenstein D, Sporn A, et al. Childhood onset schizophrenia: familial neurocognitive measures. Schizophr Res 2004;71(1):43–7.

17. Sporn A, Greenstein D, Gogtay N, et al. Childhood-onset schizophrenia: smooth pursuit eye-tracking dysfunction in family members. Schizophr Res 2005;73(2–3): 243–52.

18. Wagshal D, Knowlton BJ, Cohen JR, et al. Deficits in probabilistic classification learning and liability for schizophrenia. Psychiatry Res 2012;200(2–3):167–72.

19. Waltzman D, Knowlton BJ, Cohen JR, et al. DTI microstructural abnormalities in adolescent siblings of patients with childhood-onset schizophrenia. Psychiatry Res Neuroimaging 2016;258:23–9.

20. Wagshal D, Knowlton BJ, Cohen JR, et al. Cognitive correlates of gray matter abnormalities in adolescent siblings of patients with childhood-onset schizophrenia. Schizophr Res 2015;161(2–3):345–50.

21. Mattai AA, Weisinger B, Greenstein D, et al. Normalization of cortical gray matter deficits in nonpsychotic siblings of patients with childhood-onset schizophrenia. J Am Acad Child Adolesc Psychiatry 2011;50(7):697–704.

22. Asarnow RF, Nuechterlein KH, Asamen J, et al. Neurocognitive functioning and schizophrenia spectrum disorders can be independent expressions of familial liability for schizophrenia in community control children: the UCLA family study. Schizophr Res 2002;54(1–2):111–20. Available at: https://www.ncbi.nlm.nih.gov/pubmed/11853985.

23. Bigdeli TB, Nuechterlein KH, Sugar CA, et al. Evidence of shared familial factors influencing neurocognitive endophenotypes in adult- and childhood-onset schizophrenia. Psychol Med 2019. [Epub ahead of print].

24. Greenwood TA, Lazzeroni LC, Murray SS, et al. Analysis of 94 candidate genes and 12 endophenotypes for schizophrenia from the Consortium on the Genetics of Schizophrenia. Am J Psychiatry 2011;168(9):930–46. Available at: https://ajp.psychiatryonline.org/doi/abs/10.1176/appi.ajp.2011.10050723.

25. Collins FS, Morgan M, Patrinos A. The human genome project: lessons from large-scale biology. Science 2003;300(5617):286–90.

26. Lander ES, Linton LM, Birren B, et al. Initial sequencing and analysis of the human genome. Nature 2001;409(6822):860–921.

27. ENCODE Project Consortium. An integrated encyclopedia of DNA elements in the human genome. Nature 2012;489(7414):57–74.

28. Rands CM, Meader S, Ponting CP, et al. 8.2% of the Human genome is constrained: variation in rates of turnover across functional element classes in the human lineage. PLoS Genet 2014;10(7):e1004525.

29. Kellis M, Wold B, Snyder MP, et al. Defining functional DNA elements in the human genome. Proc Natl Acad Sci U S A 2014;111(17):6131–8.

30. 1000 Genomes Project Consortium, Auton A, Brooks LD, Durbin RM, et al. A global reference for human genetic variation. Nature 2015;526(7571):68–74.

31. Lappalainen T, Scott AJ, Brandt M, et al. Genomic analysis in the age of human genome sequencing. Cell 2019;177(1):70–84.

32. Owen MJ, Cardno AG. Psychiatric genetics: progress, problems, and potential. Lancet 1999;354(Suppl 1):SI11–4.

33. NCI-NHGRI Working Group on Replication in Association Studies, Chanock SJ, Manolio T, Boehnke M, et al. Replicating genotype-phenotype associations. Nature 2007;447(7145):655–60.

34. Arango C. Candidate gene associations studies in psychiatry: time to move forward. Eur Arch Psychiatry Clin Neurosci 2017;267(1):1–2.

35. Hellwege JN, Keaton JM, Giri A, et al. Population stratification in genetic association studies. Curr Protoc Hum Genet 2017;95:1.22.1–1.22.23.

36. Schizophrenia Working Group of the Psychiatric Genomics Consortium. Biological insights from 108 schizophrenia-associated genetic loci. Nature 2014; 511(7510):421–7.

37. Skene NG, Bryois J, Bakken TE, et al. Genetic identification of brain cell types underlying schizophrenia. Nat Genet 2018. https://doi.org/10.1038/s41588-018-0129-5.

38. Pardiñas AF, Holmans P, Pocklington AJ, et al. Common schizophrenia alleles are enriched in mutation-intolerant genes and in regions under strong background selection. Nat Genet 2018. https://doi.org/10.1038/s41588-018-0059-2.

39. Loohuis LMO, Vorstman JAS, Ori AP, et al. Genome-wide burden of deleterious coding variants increased in schizophrenia. Nat Commun 2015;6:7501.

40. Genovese G, Fromer M, Stahl EA, et al. Increased burden of ultra-rare protein-altering variants among 4,877 individuals with schizophrenia. Nat Neurosci 2016;19(11):1433–41.

41. Richards AL, Leonenko G, Walters JT, et al. Exome arrays capture polygenic rare variant contributions to schizophrenia. Hum Mol Genet 2016;25(5):1001–7.

42. Purcell SM, Moran JL, Fromer M, et al. A polygenic burden of rare disruptive mutations in schizophrenia. Nature 2014;506(7487):185–90.

43. Fromer M, Pocklington AJ, Kavanagh DH, et al. De novo mutations in schizophrenia implicate synaptic networks. Nature 2014;506(7487):179–84.

44. McCarthy SE, Gillis J, Kramer M, et al. De novo mutations in schizophrenia implicate chromatin remodeling and support a genetic overlap with autism and intellectual disability. Mol Psychiatry 2014;19(6):652–8.

45. International Schizophrenia Consortium. Rare chromosomal deletions and duplications increase risk of schizophrenia. Nature 2008;455(7210):237–41.

46. Kirov G, Grozeva D, Norton N, et al. Support for the involvement of large copy number variants in the pathogenesis of schizophrenia. Hum Mol Genet 2009; 18(8):1497–503.

47. Kirov G, Rees E, Walters JTR, et al. The penetrance of copy number variations for schizophrenia and developmental delay. Biol Psychiatry 2014;75(5):378–85.

48. Marshall CR, Howrigan DP, Merico D, et al. Contribution of copy number variants to schizophrenia from a genome-wide study of 41,321 subjects. Nat Genet 2017; 49(1):27–35.

49. Rees E, Walters JTR, Georgieva L, et al. Analysis of copy number variations at 15 schizophrenia-associated loci. Br J Psychiatry 2014;204(2):108–14.

50. Walsh T, McClellan JM, McCarthy SE, et al. Rare structural variants disrupt multiple genes in neurodevelopmental pathways in schizophrenia. Science 2008; 320(5875):539–43.
51. Sanders SJ, He X, Willsey AJ, et al. Insights into autism spectrum disorder genomic architecture and biology from 71 risk loci. Neuron 2015;87(6):1215–33.
52. Rees E, Kendall K, Pardiñas AF, et al. Analysis of intellectual disability copy number variants for association with schizophrenia. JAMA Psychiatry 2016;73(9): 963–9.
53. Forsyth JK, Nachun D, Gandal MJ, et al. Synaptic and gene regulatory mechanisms in schizophrenia, autism, and 22q11.2 CNV mediated risk for neuropsychiatric disorders. bioRxiv 2019;555490. https://doi.org/10.1101/555490.
54. Kirov G, Pocklington AJ, Holmans P, et al. De novo CNV analysis implicates specific abnormalities of postsynaptic signalling complexes in the pathogenesis of schizophrenia. Mol Psychiatry 2012;17(2):142–53.
55. Pocklington AJ, Rees E, Walters JTR, et al. Novel findings from CNVs implicate inhibitory and excitatory signaling complexes in schizophrenia. Neuron 2015; 86(5):1203–14.
56. Tansey KE, Rees E, Linden DE, et al. Common alleles contribute to schizophrenia in CNV carriers. Mol Psychiatry 2016;21(8):1085–9.
57. Bergen SE, Ploner A, Howrigan D, et al. Joint contributions of rare copy number variants and common SNPs to risk for schizophrenia. Am J Psychiatry 2018. https://doi.org/10.1176/appi.ajp.2018.17040467.
58. Rees E, Han J, Morgan J, et al. Analyses of rare and common alleles in parent-proband trios implicate rare missense variants in SLC6A1 in schizophrenia and confirm the involvement of loss of function intolerant and neurodevelopmental disorder genes. bioRxiv 2019;607549. https://doi.org/10.1101/607549.
59. McGue M, Gottesman II, Rao DC. The transmission of schizophrenia under a multifactorial threshold model. Am J Hum Genet 1983;35(6):1161–78. Available at: https://www.ncbi.nlm.nih.gov/pubmed/6650500.
60. Ahn K, An SS, Shugart YY, et al. Common polygenic variation and risk for childhood-onset schizophrenia. Mol Psychiatry 2014;21:94.
61. Ahn K, Gotay N, Andersen TM, et al. High rate of disease-related copy number variations in childhood onset schizophrenia. Mol Psychiatry 2014;19(5):568–72.
62. Sagar A, Bishop JR, Tessman DC, et al. Co-occurrence of autism, childhood psychosis, and intellectual disability associated with a de novo 3q29 microdeletion. Am J Med Genet A 2013;161(4):845–9. Available at: https://onlinelibrary.wiley.com/doi/abs/10.1002/ajmg.a.35754.
63. Vorstman JAS, Morcus MEJ, Duijff SN, et al. The 22q11.2 deletion in children: high rate of autistic disorders and early onset of psychotic symptoms. J Am Acad Child Adolesc Psychiatry 2006;45(9):1104–13.
64. Ambalavanan A, Girard SL, Ahn K, et al. De novo variants in sporadic cases of childhood onset schizophrenia. Eur J Hum Genet 2016;24(6):944–8.
65. Chaumette B, Ferrafiat V, Ambalavanan A, et al. Missense variants in ATP1A3 and FXYD gene family are associated with childhood-onset schizophrenia. Mol Psychiatry 2018. https://doi.org/10.1038/s41380-018-0103-8.
66. Smedemark-Margulies N, Brownstein CA, Vargas S, et al. A novel de novo mutation in ATP1A3 and childhood-onset schizophrenia. Cold Spring Harb Mol Case Stud 2016;2(5):a001008.
67. Jolly LA, Homan CC, Jacob R, et al. The UPF3B gene, implicated in intellectual disability, autism, ADHD and childhood onset schizophrenia regulates neural

progenitor cell behaviour and neuronal outgrowth. Hum Mol Genet 2013;22(23): 4673–87.

68. Bergen SE, O'Dushlaine CT, Lee PH, et al. Genetic modifiers and subtypes in schizophrenia: investigations of age at onset, severity, sex and family history. Schizophr Res 2014;154(1–3):48–53.

69. Stepniak B, Papiol S, Hammer C, et al. Accumulated environmental risk determining age at schizophrenia onset: a deep phenotyping-based study. Lancet Psychiatry 2014;1(6):444–53.

70. Rapoport J, Chavez A, Greenstein D, et al. Autism spectrum disorders and childhood-onset schizophrenia: clinical and biological contributions to a relation revisited. J Am Acad Child Adolesc Psychiatry 2009;48(1):10–8.

71. Hollis C. Child and adolescent (juvenile onset) schizophrenia. A case control study of premorbid developmental impairments. Br J Psychiatry 1995;166(4): 489–95.

72. Sporn AL, Addington AM, Gogtay N, et al. Pervasive developmental disorder and childhood-onset schizophrenia: comorbid disorder or a phenotypic variant of a very early onset illness? Biol Psychiatry 2004;55(10):989–94.

73. Gandal MJ, Leppa V, Won H, et al. The road to precision psychiatry: translating genetics into disease mechanisms. Nat Neurosci 2016;19(11):1397–407.

74. Khoury MJ, Iademarco MF, Riley WT. Precision public health for the era of precision medicine. Am J Prev Med 2016;50(3):398–401.

75. Bettaieb A, Paul C, Plenchette S, et al. Precision medicine in breast cancer: reality or utopia? J Transl Med 2017;15(1):139.

76. Dienstmann R, Vermeulen L, Guinney J, et al. Consensus molecular subtypes and the evolution of precision medicine in colorectal cancer. Nat Rev Cancer 2017;17(2):79–92.

77. Cardon LR, Harris T. Precision medicine, genomics and drug discovery. Hum Mol Genet 2016;25(R2):R166–72.

78. Bouwkamp CG, Kievit AJA, Markx S, et al. Copy number variation in syndromic forms of psychiatric illness: the emerging value of clinical genetic testing in psychiatry. Am J Psychiatry 2017;174(11):1036–50.

79. Costain G, Chow EWC, Ray PN, et al. Caregiver and adult patient perspectives on the importance of a diagnosis of 22q11.2 deletion syndrome. J Intellect Disabil Res 2012;56(6):641–51.

Cognition, Social Cognition, and Functional Capacity in Early-Onset Schizophrenia

Philip D. Harvey, PhD[a],*, Elizabeth C. Isner, BS[b]

KEYWORDS

- Schizophrenia • Social cognition • Functional capacity
- Attenuated psychosis syndrome • Neurocognition

KEY POINTS

- Cognitive impairment in early-onset schizophrenia (EOS) has the same general profile as that seen in adult-onset cases and in individuals with attenuated psychosis syndrome (APS) who convert to psychosis.
- Social cognitive performance is related to real-world social outcomes. Early-onset cases with schizophrenia also have deficits in social cognition, as do cases with APS.
- Impairments in the ability to perform everyday functional skills, referred to as functional capacity, are also impaired in APS, and EOS cases, with these impairments nearly as substantial as those seen in more chronic patients.
- Early-onset cases require immediate intervention to reduce morbidity.

Schizophrenia is well known for its positive and negative symptoms that form the definitional core of the disorder. However, the cognitive deficits also present have emerged as an area of increasing research over time. Deficits begin to manifest in the premorbid phase,[1] worsening in some cases in the prodromal phase,[2] and have been shown to be fully developed at the time of the first diagnosable episode of

Disclosure Statement: In the past year, Dr P.D. Harvey has received consulting fees or travel reimbursements from Alkermes, Boehringer Ingelheim, Intra-Cellular Therapies, Lundbeck Pharma, Minerva Pharma, Otsuka America (Otsuka Digital Health), Roche Pharma, Sanofi Pharma, Sunovion Pharma, Takeda Pharma, and Teva. He receives royalties from the Brief Assessment of Cognition in Schizophrenia and the MATRICS Consensus Battery. He is chief scientific officer of i-Function, Inc. He has a research grant from Takeda and from the Stanley Medical Research Foundation. These activities are not directly related to the content of this article. Ms E.C. Isner has nothing to disclose.

[a] Department of Psychiatry and Behavioral Sciences, University of Miami Miller School of Medicine, Research Service, Bruce W. Carter VA Medical Center, 1120 Northwest 14th Street, Suite 1450, Miami, FL 33136, USA; [b] University of Miami Miller School of Medicine, 1120 Northwest 14th Street, Suite 1450, Miami, FL 33136, USA
* Corresponding author.
E-mail address: philipdharvey1@cs.com

psychosis.[3] These deficits predict the well-known functional deficits in schizophrenia better than the level of psychotic symptoms, and clinical remission is typically not accompanied by functional recovery. Multiple domains of cognition are affected, ranging from processing speed to working memory to social cognition. A variety of performance-based assessments have been developed to measure impairment across domains at various stages of illness. Further, an additional critical development has been the development of performance-based assessments of the ability to perform everyday functional, vocational, and social skills. These competence-based measures are globally referred to as indices of "functional capacity,"[4] and have been determined to be an intermediate influence on everyday functioning; shown on one hand to be affected by cognitive and social cognitive deficits, and on the other, influencing everyday functioning across domains.[5,6]

ONSET OF SCHIZOPHRENIA AND COGNITIVE FUNCTIONING

The typical age of diagnosis of schizophrenia is very early adulthood, with the age of onset approximately 7 to 10 years later in women. Thus, there are some cases with onset in childhood, including very early childhood, and more cases in which there are pre-illness changes detected in the years before age 18. As childhood schizophrenia is much rarer and because the illness may not develop as insidiously as it does in older individuals, our discussion of premorbid and prodromal signs of impairment in schizophrenia may not apply as fully to childhood-onset as later-onset. However, there are clear cognitive changes before adulthood in many individuals who are diagnosed in adulthood but cognitively impaired in childhood.

REVIEW OF THE MOST RELEVANT COGNITIVE DOMAINS IN SCHIZOPHRENIA

Neurocognitive domains in general have been separated into attention, episodic and working memory, executive functions, language skills, processing speed, and crystallized knowledge, among others.[7] The authors briefly describe the relevant domains and comment on any differences between childhood-onset and adult-onset schizophrenia. They also add in a detailed discussion of social cognition and functional capacity, which are important outcome-related features of cognition and its correlates. **Table 1** shows the level of impairment in various cognitive domains, several of which are discussed herein. This table is based on the results of several review articles, including Harvey and Bowie[8] and Dickinson and colleagues.[9]

Attention has been long understood to be a building block for other functional domains of cognition, as it is fundamental in establishing memory as well as the ability to function socially, aiding in tasks such as carrying out work and conversation. Earlier reviews[7] considered attention to be one of the least affected domains, but this ability shows the most consistent decline after the first-episode psychosis resolved when compared with healthy children.

In contrast, memory for the early-onset schizophrenia (EOS) population is consistently affected before onset of psychosis and after clinical stabilization. Working memory, verbal memory, and learning have been found to be severely affected domains in several studies. Working memory was found to remain stable over time, whereas learning declined when compared with healthy children. The ability to acquire new memories is the primary domain of impairment, not consolidation and recall. In adults, working memory is also a severely affected domain, and only part of the deficits can be accounted for by issues with attention. Further, visual memory data were inconsistent with a study showing severe impairment and a study showing minimal impairment. Like with attention, memory has been shown to be one of the primary

Table 1
Level of impairment in cognitive abilities in schizophrenia

	Adult			Child
	Mild	Moderate	Severe	Similarity
Crystallized knowledge	X			More impaired
Perceptual skills		X		Similar
Manual dexterity		X		More impaired
Attention				
Sustained attention			X	Less impaired
Selective attention		X		Less impaired
Working memory				
Spatial working memory		X		More impaired
Verbal working memory			X	Similar
Episodic memory				
Verbal learning			X	Similar
Nonverbal memory (spatial memory)		X		Mixed
Delayed recall		X		Similar
Delayed recognition	X			Similar
Procedural memory		X		Similar
Executive functions		X		Similar
Processing speed			X	Similar
Verbal skills				
Naming	X			Unknown
Verbal fluency		X		Unknown

contributors to functional impairment, as it prevents patients from remaining employed and being able to carry out everyday tasks required of them. Research has shown that adult schizophrenic patients use similar strategies to learn as healthy patients, but they are not as efficient as their counterparts.

Executive functioning is the ability to solve problems, use abstract thinking, and to coordinate other cognitive skills, commonly also referred to as "reasoning and problem solving." In EOS patients, executive functioning deficits are one of the areas in which impairment does not seem as substantial during prodromal periods, but impairments are seen at the time of the first episode and tend to be persistent. In adults, it is found to be moderately impaired; however, it is difficult to tell if these deficits are specific to this domain or if they are connected to other frequently affected domains. Adult impairment in executive functioning has been shown to be connected to a worse course of disease.

Processing speed appears as well to be one of the most impaired domains across onset age, whereas language skills seem to be one of the least impaired. In reference to processing speed, EOS patients fail to improve with age as healthy individuals do. In adults, processing speed is one of the severely affected domains, and it has been shown to be related to higher-level functions, as it plays a role in what can be processed into memory.[10] Language skills have been less well investigated, with less information about verbal fluency than later-onset cases. Crystallized knowledge and global IQ appear to be more impaired in EOS cases than in adult-onset cases, although there is limited decline after illness onset. The reduced time available to acquire a knowledge base before the onset of psychosis is likely the cause of these greater intellectual limitations compared with later-onset cases. For EOS patients, using IQ as a measure of general intellectual ability, there is little change over time and patients generally do not show significant declines in their IQ, even after disease onset. However, the early disadvantage may well be the origin of the greater functional impairments seen in EOS cases.

WHAT IS THE INTERFACE BETWEEN PRODROMAL STATES AND EARLY-ONSET PSYCHOSIS?

Prodromal features of schizophrenia have been described for many decades and have typically included deterioration in social, everyday activities, and academic/productive functioning before the onset of psychotic symptoms. Furthermore, cognitive functioning appears to change over the time course of psychotic symptom development. These states are variably defined as attenuated psychosis syndrome (APS), clinical high risk (CHR), and with other terms. Seidman and colleagues[11] noted that, "there is ample evidence of significant but milder impairments during the premorbid phase, greater deficits during the prodromal or clinical high-risk (CHR) period [of psychosis], culminating in relatively severe deficits in the first episode and chronic phases."

Several large-scale studies addressed cognition in APS, including the North American Prodrome Longitudinal Study Phase 1 (NAPLS-1)[12] and 2 (NAPLS-2),[11] the Longitudinal Youth at-Risk Study (LYRIKS) in Singapore,[13] and several other studies conducted in Europe and Australia.[14,15] Data from NAPLS-2 revealed that among 609 patients at CHR, 74 (12%) converted to psychosis, 242 (40%) did not convert, and 293 (48%) went on to develop other outcomes.[16] As of 2018, 10% of patients in the LYRIKS study were converters; of those who did not convert, 54% were found to remit and the other 46% remained impaired during the rest of the study.[13] Longer-term studies up to 10 years suggest that those who are stably impaired after 2 years do not show increased risk for conversion to psychosis or remission of symptoms.[17]

COGNITIVE IMPAIRMENT IN ATTENUATED PSYCHOSIS SYNDROME

Numerous studies have examined the cognitive-impairment profile of APS,[3,11–13,16] but we focus only on the baseline profile and subsequent course. Cognitive deficits diminish when patients remit from APS; however, for non-remitters, cognition remains poor and appears to be associated with sustained poor functional outcome.[13] NAPLS-1 found that the cognitive deficits present in APS appeared similar to those seen in first-episode psychosis (FEP),[3] with this finding replicated in NAPLS-2.[11] Cognitive deficits were present across the whole NAPLS APS population; however, those who converted to psychosis demonstrated the most substantial levels of cognitive impairment, particularly regarding attention/working memory and declarative memory. Interestingly, these cognitive impairments were present at the time of detection of APS (ie, baseline) in those patients who converted to psychosis.[3,11,13,18] There was no evidence of cognitive decline in the longitudinal follow-up study from detection of the prodrome to development of psychosis in cases who convert.[19]

FUNCTIONAL CAPACITY

These measures are designed to examine the critical skills that are required to function socially and in the community. These indices demonstrate a close association to cognitive test data, as well as real-world functioning, and may be better ways to measure functional abilities compared with older methods because they reduce the bias that occurs when the patient or an informant provides ratings. Performance-based measures of functional capacity actually measure what the patient can do, in functional and social domains. Several performance-based measures have recently been investigated, in domains of both social and everyday functional skills. Two of these, The Maryland Assessment of Social Competence (MASC) and the Social Skills Performance Assessment, measure functional capacity through a rater's observation and scoring of patient social competence during role playing.[20,21] Another frequently used measure of functional capacity is the University of California, San Diego Performance-Based Skills Assessment (UPSA).[22] The UPSA takes approximately 30 minutes and measures performance in several domains of everyday living, such as counting money, planning an outing, and designating times to take certain medications. An abbreviated version of the UPSA, the UPSA-B,[23] has been very widely used across different conditions and has generally similar psychometric properties compared with the longer versions.

There have been relatively few studies of functional capacity in early-onset psychosis, but there is some potentially important data on performance-based, everyday activities measures. The Map test, developed by the NAPLS group to assess functional capacity in adolescent and young-adult high-risk populations, has been applied to approximately 80% (n = 609) of the NAPLS CHR study sample (n = 764).[16] The task requires participants to complete a set of errands as part of a simulated errand-running and shopping trip, emphasizing the ability to process multiple instructions simultaneously, and thus measuring the specific skill-set required to perform a particular real-world function as efficiently as possible. Map task performance, and therefore functional capacity and efficiency, was able to significantly predict conversion to psychosis, independent of intellectual deficits, clinical symptoms, and real-world role achievement. In specific, Map test performance was 0.7 SD worse in the CHR group in general compared with healthy controls. Further, those cases who converted to psychosis performed 1.4 SD worse than healthy controls, whereas the impairment seen in nonconverters was 0.6 SD worse than healthy controls and, as a result, 0.8 SD better than those who converted.

A study of patients with first-episode psychosis[24] found substantial baseline impairments in patients on the UPSA-B, with every cognitive domain assessed correlated with performance. There was a substantial practice effect on the test, with many patients achieving ceiling after being retested, with a single form, 3 times in a year. However, baseline performance was still quite impaired compared with older healthy controls: 77 for first episode patients (perfect score = 100), 88 for healthy control (d = 0.8), with scores that were somewhat better than those seen in much older (mean age: 50), much more chronic patients on whom the UPSA-B was standardized: mean = 64. Thus, functional capacity limitations were present and had correlates in first-episode patients that were similar to those seen in much more chronic patients.

SOCIAL COGNITION

An important domain not discussed in Frangou's[7] review that has been rapidly gaining research interest is social cognition, defined by the National Institute of Mental Health as the "mental operations that underlie social interactions, including perceiving, interpreting, and generating responses to the intentions, dispositions, and behaviors of others."[25] Social cognitive deficits have a unique role in that they have been shown to be particularly important for success in social interactions and these different skills have substantial age-relevant implications. For example, many neurocognitive skills are particularly important for a patient to finish school, seek and obtain employment, and live independently as an adult. However, childhood-onset has different implications, because it is not expected at this time for children to have the skills to be self-supporting, either in terms of financially supporting themselves or living independently. Consequently, social interactions are a critical functional skill area, relevant to both functioning at school and at home, and play a central role in relating to others in childhood and adolescence. Thus, social cognitive abilities would appear to be particularly relevant to childhood-onset psychotic disorders and they have not been nearly as well studied.

DOMAINS OF SOCIAL COGNITION

Only recently have experts systematically attempted to reach an agreement on the core domains of social cognition. The Social Cognition Psychometric Evaluation (SCOPE) study was a multiphase project designed to improve measurement of social cognition in schizophrenia.[26–28] Through review of literature and expert panels, it helped identify 4 core social cognitive domains: emotion processing, social perception, theory of mind/mental state attribution, and attributional style/bias.

Emotion Processing

This domain is broadly defined as perceiving and using emotion.[25] It subsumes 3 subdomains that represent both lower-level and higher-level processes. At a lower perceptual level is the first subdomain, emotion perception/recognition (identifying and recognizing emotional displays from facial expressions and/or nonface cues, such as voice). At a higher level are the 2 subdomains of understanding emotions (ie, comprehending others' emotional displays) and managing emotions (ie, correctly reacting to emotional displays).

Social Perception

Social perception refers to decoding and interpreting social cues in others.[29–31] It includes social context processing and social knowledge, which can be defined as knowing social rules, roles, and goals (RRGs), using those RRGs, and understanding how such RRGs may influence others' behaviors.[32,33]

Theory of Mind/Mental State Attribution

This domain is defined as the ability to comprehend and represent the mental states of others, including the inference of intentions, dispositions, and/or beliefs.[34,35] Theory of mind is also referred to as mentalizing, mental state attribution, or cognitive empathy.[36]

Attributional Style/Bias

Attributional style describes the way in which individuals explain or make sense of the cause of social events or interactions.[25,35]

The SCOPE study deemed 3 tasks from the domains of emotion processing and mental state attribution suitable for immediate use in clinical trials: The Bell Lysaker Emotion Recognition Task (BLERT),[36] the Hinting task,[37] and the Penn Emotion Recognition Task (ER-40).[38] Three other measures showed adequate psychometric properties but with limitations: Reading the Mind in the Eyes (Eyes),[39] The Awareness of Social Inferences Task (TASIT),[40] and Intentionally Bias Task (IBT).[41] All of the acceptable social cognitive indices showed significant correlations with at least one outcome measure, which included indices of real-world functioning, cognitive performance, and functional capacity.

A component of the SCOPE study was a study of patients with first-episode psychosis with the SCOPE measures to look at this specific population.[42] Across the measures there was general sensitivity to diagnostic effects. The largest effect size was for the TASIT (d = 1.0) with effect sizes in the moderate or larger range for the ER-40, Eyes, and Hinting tasks. The Eyes Test was the only test correlated with clinician/informant ratings of everyday outcomes. This is potentially a limitation of the social cognition measures because the Eyes Test is known to be highly correlated with intelligence and social class variables.

Studies of social cognition in both first-episode psychosis and in prodromal states have been conducted. In a meta-analysis of studies on emotion recognition in early-onset and first-episode psychosis, a large effect size for differences between psychotic patients and healthy controls was detected (d = 0.88).[43] Specific negative emotions posed more recognition and intensity assessment challenges. In a study comparing CHR and first-episode psychosis groups,[44] the CHR group was less impaired than first-episode patients, but more impaired than healthy controls. In another small study (total n = 49, 13 converters) it was reported that performance on theory of mind tasks and neurocognitive measures both predicted conversion.[45] In this study, only baseline performance was used to predict conversion, leaving open the question regarding decline in social cognition during the prodrome. A larger-scale study[46] with a total of 147 prodromal individuals reported that theory of mind deficits did account for more variance in conversion to EOS than IQ.

Another critical finding relevant to social cognition and social competence is the finding from the NAPLS study[47] that declining social functioning, measured by clinical ratings of social competence over the course of the follow-up, was a much more relevant predictor of conversion from a prodromal state to psychosis than changes in role functioning. Role functioning did not have the same overall predictive potential and did not worsen over time to the same extent. It is of high interest, given that neurocognitive and social cognitive abilities have differential predictive power for social and nonsocial (ie, role) functioning, that neurocognitive abilities were also not found to decline over time during the prodrome in several different studies. Thus, the finding that social, but not role, functioning declines are predictive of conversion is due to differences in progression of impairment over time. The predictors of role functioning (cognitive abilities) are themselves stable after detection of the prodrome and not declining.

Although it is not clear if additional large-scale CHR studies will be performed, it is a very viable hypothesis that declining social cognitive ability during critical prodromal periods may underlie the social functioning deterioration that precedes conversion to psychosis. As neurocognitive impairment is most severe in patients who convert, in-line with their greater impairment in functional capacity, it seems possible that from a cognitive perspective, a significant neurocognitive impairment combined with declining social cognitive abilities is the risk signature for predicting the transition from prodromal states to early-onset psychosis. The studies that have used social cognitive measures have either had very small samples or have not presented longitudinal social cognition data.

There are a few caveats to consider when exploring social cognition in child and adolescent minds. First, we must consider the level of education achieved by the patients versus the healthy controls. Second, we also should consider gender as a factor in social cognition, given that a healthy male individual and healthy female individual will show differences in ability, likely due to the way that each sex processes perceived emotions, and these differences could vary in psychotic individuals. For example, Erol and colleagues[48] compared healthy and schizophrenic women versus healthy and schizophrenic men on their performance on a facial emotion recognition test. The differences between the genders were similar in both the healthy and the schizophrenic groups, with women outperforming men. But, when patients with first-episode psychosis were compared with healthy controls who matched their age group in their ability to recognize facial emotions and with theory of mind,[49] there were no differences between men and woman in their performance on social cognitive performance.

TREATMENTS
Computerized Cognitive Training

Computerized cognitive training (CCT) is commonly used with demonstrated efficacy for the treatment of cognitive deficits in schizophrenia[50] and may have benefits for patients with APS and EOS. A pilot study assessing the effect of CCT on cognition (40 hours for 8 weeks) revealed significant improvements in processing speed in a pre-CCT to post-CCT CHR population.[51] The study found that most of the benefit came in the first 20 to 25 hours of CCT, with only minimal subsequent improvements. A later randomized controlled trial comparing CCT (40 hours for 8 weeks) with a computer game control revealed verbal memory to be significantly improved following CCT in a CHR population.[52] In addition, CCT (up to 40 hours) induced significant gains in global cognition, verbal memory, and problem solving in patients with recent-onset schizophrenia, versus a computer game control group.[53]

Social Cognition Training

Social cognitive and interaction training (SCIT) and various forms of computerized social cognitive training (CSCT) have also been developed in recent years following the success of CCT in the treatment of cognitive impairment and resultant functional deficits in severe mental illness. Combs and colleagues[54] developed SCIT, which is a group intervention based on a manualized strategy. It combines psychoeducation, skill practice, and homework assignments in which participants are encouraged to practice outside of the group. The results suggested modest benefits in improving social functioning and negative symptoms, but not in the realm of social cognition. Later, larger scale studies have confirmed the efficacy of the training and again suggested that dose effects are important.[55]

Considering that the SCIT program requires a trained clinician team, long treatment durations, and organized patient groups, there are limits to the practicality of these treatments. To address this, Nahum and colleagues[56] evaluated the feasibility of SocialVille, an online program designed to treat social cognition deficits in patients with schizophrenia by affect perception, social cue perception, theory of mind, and self-referential processing with 19 computerized exercises. Finally, Lindenmayer and colleagues[57] tested a computerized intervention originally developed for autism spectrum patients, Mind Reading: an Interactive Guide to Emotions, in a sample of patients with chronic schizophrenia, finding benefits of combined CCT and CSCT.

In a study of prodromal cases, Alvarez-Jimenez and colleagues[58] developed and delivered a socially based intervention aimed at mindfulness and motivation, delivered through a social media platform. The investigators reported very positive preliminary results in increasing social engagement. As this is the feature that worsens during the transition to EOS in many cases, as described previously, this may have positive preventive benefits. In another small-scale study, SCIT training was used to treat social cognitive deficits in patients with first-episode psychosis.[59] Although the sample size was quite small, the investigators reported that the intervention was feasible.

SUMMARY

Early-onset psychosis has a number of important features, including cognitive and social cognitive performance, that seem quite similar to that seen in patients with a later-onset age. Social cognition is not as well studied, particularly in prodromal cases, as neurocognition, but the importance of social deterioration for prediction of the development of first-episode psychosis suggests an important role. Finally, functional capacity, although studied in patients with later-onset ages, has been minimally addressed in prodromal and early-onset cases. The data that are available suggest considerable impairment and considerable importance for the prediction of conversion to a diagnosis of psychosis.

Treatment will remain a critical goal and computerized training interventions have shown promise in prodromal and first-episode samples. The feasibility of these interventions with older, much more chronic patients suggests feasibility for these interventions in targeting cognitive and social cognitive impairments, which would have the potential to limit the considerable morbidity of schizophrenia, particularly in cases with early onset or those with prodromal features.

REFERENCES

1. Woodberry KA, Giuliano AJ, Seidman LJ. Premorbid IQ in schizophrenia: a meta-analytic review. Am J Psychiatry 2008;165:579–87.
2. Mesholam-Gately RI, Giuliano AJ, Goff KP, et al. Neurocognition in first-episode schizophrenia: a meta-analytic review. Neuropsychology 2009;23:315–36.
3. Seidman LJ, Giuliano AJ, Meyer EC, et al. Neuropsychology of the prodrome to psychosis in the NAPLS consortium: relationship to family history and conversion to psychosis. Arch Gen Psychiatry 2010;67:578–88.
4. Harvey PD, Velligan DI, Bellack AS. Performance-based measures of functional skills: usefulness in clinical treatment studies. Schizophr Bull 2007;33(5):1138–48.
5. Strassnig MT, Raykov T, O'Gorman C, et al. Determinants of different aspects of everyday outcome in schizophrenia: the roles of negative symptoms, cognition, and functional capacity. Schizophr Res 2015;165(1):76–82.
6. Kalin M, Kaplan S, Gould F, et al. Social cognition, social competence, negative symptoms and social outcomes: inter-relationships in people with schizophrenia. J Psychiatr Res 2015;68:254–60.
7. Frangou S. Neurocognition in early onset schizophrenia. Child Adolesc Psychiatr Clin N Am 2013;22(4):715–26.
8. Harvey PD, Bowie CR. Cognition in severe mental illness: schizophrenia, bipolar disorder, and depression. In: Husain M, Schott JM, editors. Oxford handbook of cognitive neurology and dementia. Oxford (UK): OUP; 2016. p. 463–70.
9. Dickinson D, Schaefer J, Weinberger DR. The multifacted "global" cognitive impairment profiles in schizophrenia. In: Harvey PD, editor. Cognitive impairment in schizophrenia. New York: Cambridge University press; 2013. p. 24–49.
10. Dickinson D, Harvey PD. Systemic hypotheses for generalized cognitive deficits in schizophrenia: a new take on an old problem. Schizophr Bull 2009;35:403–14.
11. Seidman LJ, Shapiro DI, Stone WS, et al. Association of neurocognition with transition to psychosis: baseline functioning in the second phase of the North American prodrome longitudinal study. JAMA Psychiatry 2016;73(12):1239–48.
12. Cannon TD, Cadenhead KS, Cornblatt B, et al. Prediction of psychosis in youth at high clinical risk: a multi-site longitudinal study in North America. Arch Gen Psychiatry 2008;65:28–37.

13. Lam M, Lee J, Rapisarda A, et al. Longitudinal cognitive changes in young individuals at ultrahigh risk for psychosis. JAMA Psychiatry 2018;75(9):929–39.

14. Mollon J, David AS, Zammit S, et al. Course of cognitive development from infancy to early adulthood in the psychosis spectrum. JAMA Psychiatry 2018;75:270–9.

15. Nelson B, Yuen HP, Wood SJ, et al. Long-term follow-up of a group at ultra high risk ("prodromal") for psychosis: the PACE 400 study. JAMA Psychiatry 2013;70:793–802.

16. McLaughkin D, Carrion RE, Auther AM, et al. Functional capacity assessed by the map task in individuals at clinical high-risk for psychosis. Schizophr Bull 2016;42:1234–42.

17. Klosterkotter RJ, Hellmich M, Steinmeyer EM, et al. Diagnosing schizophrenia in the initial prodromal phase. Arch Gen Psychiatry 2001;58:158–64.

18. Harvey PD. The course of cognition and functioning in patients at ultrahigh risk of developing psychosis: the roles of remission and persistent nonconverting symptoms. JAMA Psychiatry 2018;75:882–3.

19. Carrion RE, Walder DJ, Auther AM, et al. From the psychosis prodrome to the first-episode of psychosis: no evidence of a cognitive decline. J Psychiatr Res 2018;96:231–8.

20. Bellack AS, Sayers M, Mueser KT, et al. An evaluation of social problem solving in schizophrenia. J Abnorm Psychol 1994;103:371–8.

21. Patterson TL, Moscona S, McKibbin CL, et al. Social skills performance assessment among older patients with schizophrenia. Schizophr Res 2001;482-3:351–60.

22. Patterson TL, Goldman S, McKibbin CL, et al. UCSD performance-based skills assessment: development of a new measure of everyday functioning for severely mentally ill adults. Schizophr Bull 2001;27:235–45.

23. Mausbach BT, Harvey PD, Pulver AE, et al. Relationship of the Brief UCSD Performance-based Skills Assessment (UPSA-B) to multiple indicators of functioning in people with schizophrenia and bipolar disorder. Bipolar Disord 2010;12:45–55.

24. Vesterager L, Christensen TO, Olsen BB, et al. Cognitive and clinical predictors of functional capacity in patients with first episode schizophrenia. Schizophr Res 2012;141:251–6.

25. Green MF, Penn DL, Bentall R, et al. Social cognition in schizophrenia: an NIMH workshop on definitions, assessment, and research opportunities. Schizophr Bull 2008;34(6):1211–20.

26. Pinkham AE, Penn DL, Green MF, et al. The social cognition psychometric evaluation study: results of the expert survey and RAND panel. Schizophr Bull 2014;40(4):813–23.

27. Pinkham AE, Penn DL, Green MF, et al. Social cognition psychometric evaluation: results of the initial psychometric study. Schizophr Bull 2016;42(2):494–504.

28. Pinkham AE, Harvey PD, Penn DL. Social cognition psychometric evaluation: results of the final validation study. Schizophr Bull 2018;44(4):737–48.

29. Penn DL, Ritchie M, Francis J, et al. Social perception in schizophrenia: the role of context. Psychiatry Res 2002;109(2):149–59.

30. Sergi MJ, Green MF. Social perception and early visual processing in schizophrenia. Schizophr Res 2003;59(2–3):233–41.

31. Toomey R, Schuldberg D, Corrigan P, et al. Nonverbal social perception and symptomatology in schizophrenia. Schizophr Res 2002;53(1–2):83–91.

32. Addington J, Saeedi H, Addington D. Influence of social perception and social knowledge on cognitive and social functioning in early psychosis. Br J Psychiatry 2006;189:373–8.

33. Corrigan PW, Green MF. Schizophrenic patients' sensitivity to social cues: the role of abstraction. Am J Psychiatry 1993;150(4):589–94.

34. Frith C. The cognitive neuropsychology of schizophrenia east. Sussex (UK): Psychology Press; 1992.

35. Penn D, Addington J, Pinkham A. Social cognitive impairments. In: Stroup TS, Lieberman JA, Perkins DO, editors. The American Psychiatric Publishing textbook of schizophrenia. Arlington (VA): American Psychiatric Publishing, Inc.; 2006. p. 261–74.

36. Bryson G, Bell M, Lysaker P. Affect recognition in schizophrenia: a function of global impairment or a specific cognitive deficit. Psychiatry Res 1997;71(2): 105–13.

37. Corcoran R, Mercer G, Frith CD. Schizophrenia, symptomatology and social inference: investigating "theory of mind" in people with schizophrenia. Schizophr Res 1995;17(1):5–13.

38. Kohler CG, Turner TH, Bilker WB, et al. Facial emotion recognition in schizophrenia: intensity effects and error pattern. Am J Psychiatry 2003;160(10): 1768–74.

39. Baron-Cohen S, Wheelwright S, Hill J, et al. The 'Reading the mind in the eyes' Test revised version: a study with normal adults, and adults with Asperger syndrome or high-functioning autism. J Child Psychol Psychiatry 2001;42(2):241–51.

40. Shamay-Tsoory SG. The neural bases for empathy. Neuroscientist 2011;17(1): 18–24.

41. Rosset E. It's no accident: our bias for intentional explanations. Cognition 2008; 108(3):771–80.

42. Ludwig KA, Pinkham AE, Harvey PD, et al. Social cognition psychometric evaluation (SCOPE) in people with early psychosis: a preliminary study. Schizophr Res 2017;190:136–43.

43. Barkl SJ, Lah S, Harris AWF. Facial emotion identification in early onset and first-episode psychosis: a systematic review with meta-analysis. Schizophr Res 2014; 159:62–9.

44. Thompsopn A, Papas A, Bartholomeusz C, et al. Social cognition in clinical "at risk" for psychosis and first episode psychosis populations. Schizophr Res 2012;141:204–9.

45. Kim HS, Shin AY, Jang JH, et al. Social cognition and neurocognition as predictors of conversion to psychosis in individuals at ultra-high risk. Schizophr Res 2011;130:170–5.

46. Healey KM, Penn DL, Perkins D, et al. Theory of mind and social judgments in people at clinical high risk of psychosis. Schizophr Res 2013;150(2–3):498–504.

47. Carrión RE, Auther AM, McLaughlin D, et al. The global functioning: social and role scales—further validation in a large sample of adolescents and young adults at clinical high risk for psychosis. Schizophr Bull 2019;45(4):763–72.

48. Erol A, Putgul G, Kosger F, et al. Facial emotion recognition in schizophrenia: the impact of gender. Psychiatry Investig 2013;10(1):69–74.

49. Danaher H, Allott K, Killackey E, et al. An examination of sex differences in neurocognition and social cognition in first-episode psychosis. Psychiatry Res 2018; 259:36–43.

50. Wykes T, Huddy V, Cellard C, et al. A meta-analysis of cognitive remediation for schizophrenia: methodology and effect sizes. Am J Psychiatry 2011;168:472–85.

51. Hooker CI, Carol EE, Eisenstein TJ, et al. A pilot study of cognitive training in clinical high risk for psychosis: initial evidence of cognitive benefit. Schizophr Res 2014;157:314–6.
52. Loewy R, Fisher M, Schlosser DA, et al. Intensive auditory cognitive training improves verbal memory in adolescents and young adults at clinical high risk for psychosis. Schizophr Bull 2016;42(Suppl 1):S118–26.
53. Fisher M, Loewy R, Carter C, et al. Neuroplasticity-based auditory training via laptop computer improves cognition in young individuals with recent onset schizophrenia. Schizophr Bull 2015;41:250–8.
54. Combs DR, Adams SD, Penn DL, et al. Social Cognition and Interaction Training (SCIT) for inpatients with schizophrenia spectrum disorders: preliminary findings. Schizophr Res 2007;91(1–3):112–6.
55. Roberts DL, Combs DR, Willoughby M, et al. A randomized, controlled trial of Social Cognition and Interaction Training (SCIT) for outpatients with schizophrenia spectrum disorders. Br J Clin Psychol 2014;53(3):281–98.
56. Nahum M, Fisher M, Loewy R, et al. A novel, online social cognitive training program for young adults with schizophrenia: a pilot study. Schizophr Res Cogn 2014;1(1):e11–9.
57. Lindenmayer JP, Khan A, McGurk SR, et al. Does social cognition training augment response to computer-assisted cognitive remediation for schizophrenia? Schizophr Res 2018;201:180–6.
58. Alvarez-Jimenez M, Gleeson JF, Bendall S, et al. Enhancing social functioning in young people at Ultra High Risk (UHR) for psychosis: a pilot study of a novel strengths and mindfulness-based online social therapy. Schizophr Res 2018; 202:369–77.
59. Bartholomeusz CF, Allott K, Killackey E, et al. Social cognition training as an intervention for improving functional outcome in first-episode psychosis: a feasibility study. Early Interv Psychiatry 2013;7(4):421–6.

Management and Interventions
for Psychosis in Youth

Psychopharmacologic Treatment of Schizophrenia in Adolescents and Children

Esther S. Lee, MD*, Hal Kronsberg, MD, Robert L. Findling, MD, MBA

KEYWORDS

- Adolescents • Antipsychotic medication • Antipsychotic side effects • Children
- Psychopharmacology • Psychosis • Schizophrenia

KEY POINTS

- Several antipsychotic medications have demonstrated efficacy in the treatment of children and adolescents with schizophrenia.
- As with adults, clozapine demonstrated superior efficacy in treating adolescent schizophrenia in treatment-resistant patients.
- In large head-to-head studies, several of which included first-generation agents, symptom improvement was often comparable among different medications.
- Side-effect profiles vary considerably across medications and can often be more severe in youths than adults.

INTRODUCTION

The development of antipsychotic agents has revolutionized the treatment of schizophrenia. Beginning with the development of chlorpromazine in 1950, originally intended as an anesthetic potentiate, there were more than 40 antipsychotic medications introduced by 1990. Despite the significant effect, there were clinical concerns for the acute extrapyramidal symptoms (EPS) that became associated with antipsychotic use. These considerations eventually led to the development and use of clozapine, which was particularly useful for the treatment-resistant population. A wave of "atypical" antipsychotics soon followed that demonstrated efficacy for both positive and negative symptoms as well as a more favorable EPS profile.[1] Although there are currently 11 second-generation antipsychotic agents approved by the Food and Drug Administration (FDA), clinical trials for antipsychotic medications to date have

Division of Child and Adolescent Psychiatry, Department of Psychiatry and Behavioral Sciences, Johns Hopkins University School of Medicine, 1800 Orleans Street, Bloomberg Children's Center, Suite 12344, Baltimore, MD 21287, USA
* Corresponding author.
E-mail address: elee121@jhmi.edu

Child Adolesc Psychiatric Clin N Am 29 (2020) 183–210
https://doi.org/10.1016/j.chc.2019.08.009
1056-4993/20/© 2019 Elsevier Inc. All rights reserved.

predominantly focused on treatment in adults, and there is a relative dearth of comparable data in children and adolescents.[2]

Schizophrenia is recognized for its significant pediatric disease burden, one of the highest among high-income countries, with an estimated loss of 479,009 disability-adjusted life-years in children between 0 and 17 years. Despite this, only 4.6% of schizophrenia trials between 2006 and 2011 included pediatric subjects (20/430).[3] Although the diagnostic criteria for schizophrenia remain consistent throughout the life cycle, the disease presentation can differ greatly between youths and adults, and the existing evidence suggests that the efficacy, tolerability, and safety of antipsychotic agents can also differ between the different age groups. Although knowledge regarding antipsychotic medications in this younger population has increased exponentially in the last decade, additional studies are still needed to translate knowledge of these medications into safe clinical practice. Although a multimodal approach is recommended when developing a treatment plan, the intention of this article is to review some of the seminal pharmacologic studies that helped inform antipsychotic treatment practices for schizophrenia in children and adolescents, in addition to clinical considerations for commonly used agents (**Table 1**).

DISCUSSION
First-Generation Antipsychotics

The first-generation antipsychotics act on the dopaminergic system, blocking D_2 receptors in mesolimbic, nigrostriatal, and tuberoinfundibular areas.[4] One of the largest randomized controlled trials (RCT) examining the role of these medications in youth with schizophrenia was conducted by Pool and colleagues[5] in 1974. Upon comparing haloperidol (mean dose 9.8 mg/d), loxapine (mean dose 87.5 mg/d), and placebo over 4 weeks, both active treatments were found to have similar and significant symptom improvement but also higher rates of EPS. In another study, Realmuto and colleagues[6] compared the efficacy of thiothixene and thioridazine in a 4- to 6-week single-blinded study. There were no differences in outcome measures or overall occurrence of side effects. Despite statistically significant symptomatic improvement, participants continued to have elevated Brief Psychiatric Rating Scale (BPRS) scores, and 42.9% of participants were rated "slightly improved," "not improved," or "worse" according to Clinical Global Impression (CGI) scores.

Second-Generation Antipsychotics

Clozapine
Introduced in 1990, clozapine has demonstrated significantly greater efficacy compared with other antipsychotics in treating schizophrenia in children and adults who have not responded to multiple antipsychotic medication trials (**Table 2**).[7] Clozapine has binding affinity to $5\text{-}HT_{2A}$ and D_2 receptors, among others,[8] and comes with an increased risk of seizures and agranulocytosis compared with other agents. Ninety-five percent of cases for the latter occur within the first 6 months of treatment, and there are mandatory monitoring systems requiring absolute neutrophil counts.[9] In addition, blocking muscarinic receptors can cause constipation in more than half of users.[10] Although not FDA approved for treatment in children and adolescents, clozapine has been investigated in multiple head-to-head trials.[11–13]

In the earliest double-blind (DB) trial, Kumra and colleagues[11] compared clozapine against haloperidol with concurrent benztropine administration in adolescents with schizophrenia who had not previously responded to neuroleptics. Clozapine (mean

Table 1
Summary of prescribing information for second-generation antipsychotic agents

Medication	FDA Approval for Adolescent Schizophrenia	Recommended Dosages	Available Strengths	Treatment Considerations for FDA-Approved Agents
Clozapine	No			General warnings/precautions
Risperidone	Yes (13–17 y)	Initial: 0.5 mg Target: 3 mg Effective range: 1–6 mg Maximum: 6 mg/d	Tablets: 0.25, 0.5, 1, 2, 3, 4 mg Oral solution: 1 mg/mL Orally disintegrating tablets: 0.5, 1, 2, 3, 4 mg	• Neuroleptic malignant syndrome • Tardive dyskinesia • Hyperglycemia and diabetes mellitus • Hyperprolactinemia (higher risk with risperidone)
Olanzapine	Yes (13–17 y)	Initial: 2.5–5 mg Target: 10 mg/d Maximum: 20 mg/d	Tablets (not scored): 2.5, 5, 7.5, 10, 15, 20 mg Orally disintegrating tablets: 5, 10, 15, 20 mg Intramuscular injection: 10 mg vial	• Orthostatic hypotension • Leukopenia, neutropenia, and agranulocytosis (elevated risk with clozapine) • Suicidality • Hyperlipidemia (higher risk with clozapine, olanzapine in adult studies)
Quetiapine	Yes (13–17 y)	Initial: 25 mg bid Target: 400–800 mg/d Max: 800 mg/d	Tablets: 25, 50, 100, 200, 300, 400 mg	• Weight gain (higher risk with clozapine, olanzapine in adult studies) • Cardiovascular changes (higher risk of QTc prolongation with ziprasidone, higher risk of myocarditis with clozapine)
Aripiprazole	Yes (13–17 y)	Initial: 2 mg Target: 10 mg/d Maximum: 30 mg/d	Tablets: 2, 5, 10, 15, 20, 30 mg Orally disintegrating tablets: 10, 15 mg Oral solution: 1 mg/mL Intramuscular injection: 9.75 mg/1.3 mL single-dose vial	• Seizure (clozapine associated with greatest risk increase) • Potential for cognitive and motor impairment • Hypothyroidism (observed with quetiapine) • Cataracts (observed with long-term quetiapine use)
Paliperidone	Yes (12–17 y)	Initial: 3 mg Target: 3–6 mg/d (<51 kg), 3–12 mg/d (≥51 kg) Maximum: 6 mg/d (<51 kg), 12 mg/d (≥51 kg) * Tablet must be swallowed whole	Tablets: 1.5, 3, 6, 9 mg	General monitoring recommendations Baseline • Detailed personal, family, and lifestyle history (to be updated regularly) • Parkinsonism, akathisia • Tardive dyskinesia • Height, weight (every visit) • Blood pressure, pulse

(continued on next page)

Table 1
(continued)

Medication	FDA Approval for Adolescent Schizophrenia	Recommended Dosages	Available Strengths	Treatment Considerations for FDA-Approved Agents
Lurasidone	Yes (13–17 y)	Initial: 40 mg Target: 40–80 mg/d Maximum: 80 mg/d * Tablet should be taken with food (at least 350 calories)	Tablets: 20, 40, 60, 80, 120 mg	• Electrolytes, complete blood count, renal, and liver function • Fasting blood glucose and lipids • Liver function tests At 3 mo • Parkinsonism, akathisia • Tardive dyskinesia • Blood pressure, pulse • Fasting blood glucose and lipids • Liver function tests annually • Parkinsonism, akathisia • Tardive dyskinesia • Blood pressure, pulse • Electrolytes, complete blood count, renal and liver function (monitor more frequently with clozapine) • Fasting blood glucose and lipids (every 6 mo) • Liver function tests Other • Prolactin: obtain if symptomatic • Electrocardiogram: obtain at baseline for ziprasidone (also during titration and at maximum dose) and clozapine • Thyrotropin and free T4: baseline and follow-up measures recommended with quetiapine • Eye examination: recommended at baseline and 6-mo intervals with quetiapine
Ziprasidone	No			
Asenapine	No			
Iloperidone	No			
Cariprazine	No			

* Denotes important med administration considerations.
Data from Refs. [110–116]

Table 2
Summarization of selected second-generation antipsychotic studies

Medication	Publication	Study Design, Duration	N	Age (y)	Target Dose (mg/d)	Primary Efficacy Measure/Purpose	Effectiveness/ Findings	Noteworthy AEs
Clozapine	Kumra et al,[11] 1996	Randomized, DB trial against haloperidol & benztropine, 6 wk	21	6–17	Flexible dosing: clozapine up to 525 mg/d (mean 176 mg/d), haloperidol up to 27 mg/d (mean 16 mg/d)	Mean reduction in BPRS, Bunney-Hamburg Psychosis Rating Scale, Children's Global Assessment Scale, Scale for Assessment of Negative Symptoms, Scale for Assessment of Positive Symptoms	Clozapine had statistically significant improvement over haloperidol on all measures of psychosis	Drowsiness and salivation higher in clozapine, no changes in AIMS for either group. For the clozapine group, 2/10 dropped out from neutropenia (even after stopping and restarting medication), 2/10 had significant seizure activity
Clozapine	Shaw et al,[13] 2006	Randomized, DB, head-to-head trial against olanzapine, 6 wk	25	7–16	Flexible dosing: clozapine up to 900 mg/d (mean 327 mg/d), olanzapine up to 20 mg/d (mean 18.1 mg/d)	Mean reduction in CGI-S, Scale for the Assessment of Negative Symptoms, Scale for the Assessment of Positive Symptoms, BPRS, Bunney-Hamburg Psychosis Rating Scale	Moderate to large treatment effects in favor of clozapine, but given sample size only statistically significant improvement in negative symptoms	Clozapine group had more AEs, especially nocturnal enuresis, tachycardia, and hypertension. Similar weight gain in both groups
Clozapine	Kumra et al,[12] 2008	Randomized, DB, head-to-head trial against high-dose olanzapine, 6 wk	39	10–18	Flexible dosing: clozapine up to 900 mg/d (mean 403.1 mg/d), olanzapine up to 30 mg/d (mean 26.2 mg/d)	Response defined as a decrease of ≥30% in BPRS and a CGI improvement rating of 1 or 2	66% taking clozapine met responder criteria compared with 33% taking olanzapine	AE profiles were similar between groups with substantial metabolic effects and higher levels of sweating and salivation in the clozapine group

(continued on next page)

Table 2
(continued)

Medication	Publication	Study Design, Duration	N	Age (y)	Target Dose (mg/d)	Primary Efficacy Measure/Purpose	Effectiveness/Findings	Noteworthy AEs
Risperidone	Haas et al,[20] 2009	Randomized double-blind controlled trial vs lowdose risperidone, 8 wk	257	13–17	Flexible dosing: standard dose between 1.5 and 6 mg/d (mean 4 mg/d), low-dose between 0.15 and 0.6 mg/d (mean 0.4 mg/d)	Mean improvement in PANSS scores	Statistically significant improvement over low dose and an average reduction of 23.6 in PANSS scores, effect size of 0.49	74.4% in standard-dose group had an AE, most dose adjustments were for somnolence (19%). 33% of this group had EPS-related AEs, and 56% were prescribed an antiparkinsonian agent. 70% of the standard-dose group had prolactin elevations beyond the upper limit of normal
Risperidone	Haas et al,[21] 2009	RDBPCT, 6 wk	160	13–17	Flexible dosing: 4- 6 mg/d (mode 6 mg) vs 1-3 mg/d (mode 3 mg/d) vs placebo	Mean improvement in PANSS scores and response defined as reduction in PANSS of greater or equal to 20%	Statistically significant improvement over placebo by both active groups, high dose by 12.8 and low dose by 12.0. Overall improvement by high-dose group was 23.7 and 23.0 in low-dose group	AEs in 75% low-dose and 76% high-dose groups, most often somnolence, and changes in AIMS were minimal in both arms. No glucose-related AEs, weight gain was 1.3 kg in low-dose and 1.5 kg in high-dose groups

Drug	Study	Design	N	Age	Dosing	Outcome measure	Results	Serious AEs
Risperidone	Pandina et al,[22] 2012	OLE of the above trials, 6 or 12 mo	390	13–17	Flexible dosing between 2 and 6 mg/d (median mode dose 3.8 mg/d for 6-mo group and 3.0 mg/d for 12-mo group)	Mean improvement in PANSS scores and response defined as ≥20% reduction in PANSS total score	PANSS scores decreased 13.6 from baseline at 6 mo, 61.8% response at 6 mo	Serious AEs experienced by 16%, with 86% experiencing any AE. Weight gain was reported as a treatment AE in 15% with a mean gain of 4.0 kg. Prolactin-related AE in 9%. 32.3% of participants dropped out of the study, 31% experienced an EPS-related AE, and 27% reported somnolence
Olanzapine	Kryzhanovskaya et al,[29] 2009	RDBPCT, 6 wk	107	13–17	Flexible dosing between 2.5 and 20 mg/d (mean 11.1 mg/d)	Mean change in BPRS-C total score	Significant improvement with olanzapine over placebo (−19.4 vs −9.3) starting at week 2	Significant increases with olanzapine in terms of weight, prolactin levels, fasting triglycerides, uric acid, and alanine aminotransferase
Olanzapine	Kemp et al,[30] 2013	RDBPCT, 6 wk, post hoc analysis of study by Kryzhanovskaya et al,[29] 2009	107	13–17	Flexible dosing between 2.5 and 20 mg/d	Study possible association between weight gain and treatment outcome	Significant weight gain appeared to indicate greater treatment efficacy, but effect cancels out once duration is included as a covariate	

(continued on next page)

Table 2
(continued)

Medication	Publication	Study Design, Duration	N	Age (y)	Target Dose (mg/d)	Primary Efficacy Measure/Purpose	Effectiveness/ Findings	Noteworthy AEs
Quetiapine	Findling et al,[34] 2012	RDBPCT, 6 wk	222	13–17	400 mg/d or 800 mg/d in divided doses	Mean change in PANSS total score	Both 400-mg/d and 800-mg/d groups demonstrated significant mean improvement compared with placebo, with LS mean changes from baseline to endpoint being −27.3 and −28.44 vs placebo (−19.15)	Most common TEAEs included somnolence, headache, and dizziness. Active groups also had increased weight (2.2 kg for 400 mg/ d, 1.8 mg for 800 mg/d, −0.4 kg for placebo), and increases in total cholesterol, LDL cholesterol, and triglycerides. Quetiapine showed a decrease in mean total thyroxine levels (with mean increase in thyroid stimulating hormone in the 400-mg/d group) and greater mean changes in pulse rate

Aripiprazole	Findling et al,[38] 2008	RDBPCT, phase 3, 6 wk	302	13–17	10 mg/d or 30 mg/d	Mean change in PANSS total score	Aripiprazole statistically superior to placebo at both 10 mg/d (−26.7) and 30 mg/d (−28.6) vs placebo (−21.2)	Extrapyramidal disorder, somnolence, and tremor were most common, with higher incidence in the 30-mg/d group. Both active groups had worsening in Simpson-Angus Scale scores (+0.5 for 10 mg/d, +0.3 with 30 mg/d, −0.3 for placebo). There were reductions in serum prolactin in all groups and minimal weight changes (−0.8 kg for placebo, 0.0 in 10 mg/d, and +0.2 kg for 30 mg/d).
Aripiprazole	Correll et al,[39] 2017	RDBPCT, 52 wk	146	13–17	10–30 mg/d	Time from randomization to exacerbation of psychotic symptoms/impending relapse	Significantly longer time to exacerbation for treatment group (hazard ratio = 0.46) and fewer meeting criteria for exacerbation (19.4% vs 37.5%)	TEAEs reported in a similar proportion in both groups with none being related to neuroleptic malignant syndrome, seizures, orthostasis, glucose levels, or prolactin levels. There was a comparable incidence of weight gain and somnolence

(continued on next page)

Table 2
(continued)

Medication	Publication	Study Design, Duration	N	Age (y)	Target Dose (mg/d)	Primary Efficacy Measure/Purpose	Effectiveness/ Findings	Noteworthy AEs
Paliperidone	Singh et al,[44] 2011	RDBPCT, 6 wk	201	12–17	Weight-based, fixed doses ranging from low (1.5 mg/d), medium (3 or 6 mg/d), and high (6 or 12 mg/d)	Mean change in PANSS total score	Significant for the medium-treatment group (−17.3, $P = .006$) vs the high- (−13.8, $P = .09$) and low-treatment (−9.8, $P = .51$) groups as well as placebo (−7.9)	Most common TEAEs included somnolence, akathisia, tremor, insomnia, and headache, many of which were dose related
Paliperidone	Savitz et al,[40] 2015	OLE trial (Singh et al,[44] 2011), 2 y (36 patients involved in a 6-mo study)	220	12–17	Flexible dosing between 1.5 and 12 mg/d (6 mg/d most common dose)	Primary objective was to evaluate long-term safety parameters; secondary objective was efficacy per PANSS, CGI-S, and Children's Global Assessment Scale scales	Improvement in PANSS total score observed within 3 mo of treatment initiation and continued to endpoint, with the mean change in score being −19.1%, and 41.7% of patients achieving remission. Safety profile consistent with that of paliperidone in adults, and risperidone in adolescents	TEAEs experienced by 85.3% of patients, with somnolence and weight gain being most common (18.3% each). 4.3% participants showed a shift to high glucose levels, 9.3% suicidality-related TEAEs, and 9.3% a potentially prolactin-related event (18.5% in girls, 3.3% in boys). EPS-related events were most commonly related to Parkinsonism (15.5%) and hyperkinesia (13.8%)

| Lurasidone | Goldman et al,[47] 2017 | RDBPCT, 6 wk | 326 | 13–17 | 40 mg/d or 80 mg/d | Mean change in PANSS total score | LS mean change significant for both 40-mg/d and 80-mg/d groups (−18.6, −18.3) vs placebo (−10.5), with separation apparent starting at week 1. A greater proportion of 40-mg/d and 80-mg/d participants also met criteria for response (63.9% and 65.1% vs 42.0% placebo) | Lower overall incidence of serious AEs with treatment (3.6% at 40 mg/d, 1.9% at 80 mg/d) vs placebo (8.0%), and no clinically significant differences for body weight, lipid parameters, glycemic indices, and prolactin levels. Higher incidence of akathisia (9.1% for 40 mg/d, 8.7% for 80 mg/d, and 1.8% for placebo) and other EPS-related AE (6.4% at 40 mg/d, 3.8% in 80 mg/d, 1.8% with placebo) |

(continued on next page)

Table 2
(continued)

Medication	Publication	Study Design, Duration	N	Age (y)	Target Dose (mg/d)	Primary Efficacy Measure/Purpose	Effectiveness/ Findings	Noteworthy AEs
Ziprasidone	Findling et al,[50] 2013	RDBPCT, 6 wk followed by 26-wk open extension	283	13–17	Flexible dosing 40–160 mg/d (mean modal dose 129.3 mg/d)	Mean change in BPRS-A, PANSS, CGI-S scores	In the RCT, no significant separation in BPRS-A or other measures, statistically significant improvement in PANSS-positive subscale	In the RCT, somnolence (19.7%) and EPS (11.4%) were the most common AEs. No difference in AIMS and small increase in QT interval corrected by Fridericia's formula (3.9 ms to 10.8 ms) ziprasidone was generally well tolerated with minimal associated changes in body mass index and no differences in metabolic AEs
Asenapine	Findling et al,[53] 2015	RDBPCT, 8 wk followed by 26-wk open extension	306	12–17	Fixed doses, either 5 mg/d or 10 mg/d	Mean change in PANSS scores	In the RCT, PANSS scores did not separate from placebo despite numerical improvement. In OLE, 48% had a 30% decrease in PANSS total	In the RCT, somnolence, sedation, hypersomnia, and gastrointestinal disorders were most common AEs. In the RCT, 10% had >7% weight gain, and in the OLE, 14.3% had >7% gain

dose 176 mg/d) showed statistically significant improvement over haloperidol (mean dose 16 mg/d) in all outcome measures. Two subsequent DB RCTs compared clozapine with olanzapine at different dosages in youth with schizophrenia who were previously antipsychotic nonresponders.[12,13] Shaw and colleagues[13] enrolled children as young as 7 years and used a standard dose of olanzapine (mean dose 18.1 mg/d) over 8 weeks. Multiple treatment measures favored clozapine but, because of sample size, the only statistically significant improvements from baseline were for negative symptoms. Kumra and colleagues[12] conducted a similar trial with "high-dose" olanzapine (mean dose 26.2 mg/d) and clozapine. After 12 weeks, 66% in the clozapine group met criteria for response versus 33% in the olanzapine group.

Overall, all 3 RCTs support the use of clozapine for treatment-refractory youth with schizophrenia. However, caution was recommended given clozapine's greater incidence of adverse events (AEs) during clinical trials.

Risperidone

Risperidone was first approved for the treatment of adult schizophrenia in 1993 and has since gained approval for adolescents (13–17 years).[14] Risperidone has high antagonistic affinity for 5-HT$_{2A}$ receptors and a moderately high affinity for D$_2$, $\alpha 1$, $\alpha 2$, and H$_1$ receptors.[15] Owing to its D$_2$ blockage, risperidone may be more likely to induce hyperprolactinemia compared with other atypical agents and is also associated with other metabolic and extrapyramidal side effects.[16] Some of risperidone's side effects may be mitigated by slower titration to find the lowest optimal dose.[17,18] A review of long-acting injectable antipsychotics in youth suggests that side effects are similar with both preparations.[19]

There are several RCTs demonstrating risperidone's efficacy in treating children and adolescents with schizophrenia.[20–22] Haas and colleagues[20] determined that standard-dose risperidone (median of 4 mg/d) shows significant improvement in Positive and Negative Syndrome Scale (PANSS) scores compared with low-dose risperidone (median of 0.4 mg/d) in adolescents with an acute exacerbation. In a similarly blinded RCT, Haas and colleagues[21] found that low-dose (1-3 mg/d) and high-dose risperidone (4-6 mg/d) showed similar improvements in PANSS scores over placebo. The investigators concluded that the risk-benefit profile favored a lower dose for adolescents. In an open-label extension (OLE) of both the above-mentioned studies, Pandina and colleagues[22] found that improvements from the blinded RCTs were generally maintained over the course of the 6- or 12-month trials.

Risperidone has been investigated as a possible early intervention for high-risk youth, but clinical trials against supportive psychotherapy and placebo do not yet support a role in preventing the transition to psychosis.[23]

Olanzapine

Introduced in 1996, olanzapine currently has FDA approval in children for the treatment of schizophrenia (13–17 years).[14] In addition to working as an antagonist of D$_2$ and 5-HT$_{2A}$ receptors, it has been hypothesized that its antagonistic effects at 5-HT$_{2C}$, 5-HT$_3$, 5-HT$_6$, D$_{1-4}$, histamine H$_1$, $\alpha 1$-adrenoreceptors, γ-aminobutyric acid$_a$, β-adrenoreceptors, and muscarinic M$_{1-5}$ receptors are responsible for its adverse effects.[24] Olanzapine demonstrates a similar pharmacokinetic profile between pediatric and adult patients, and it is not necessary to adjust dosage for age, weight, or gender.[25] Olanzapine is found in lower concentrations in smokers compared with nonsmokers, suggesting an increased clearance rate.[26–28]

The efficacy of olanzapine in the acute management of adolescent schizophrenia was established by Kryzhanovskaya and colleagues[29] in a 6-week randomized, double-blind, placebo-controlled trial (RDBPCT). With flexible dosing between 2.5 and 20.0 mg/d (mean daily dose 11.1 mg/d, mean modal dose 12.5 mg/d), the olanzapine group demonstrated significant improvement over placebo in Brief Psychiatric Rating Scale for Children (BPRS-C) scores starting at week 2. A post hoc analysis of these data conducted by Kemp and colleagues[30] tested a possible association between obesity, acute weight gain, and treatment response. Although significant weight gain during the trial appeared to indicate greater treatment efficacy, the effect was canceled out once duration was included as a covariate.

Quetiapine

Quetiapine has FDA approval for the treatment of schizophrenia in teenagers (13–17 years).[14] Its pharmacologic mechanism involves weaker antagonism at D_2 and 5-HT_2 receptors, stronger antagonism at $\alpha 1$ receptors, and modest histaminergic effects compared with other atypical agents.[31] Quetiapine has a similar pharmacokinetic profile in children, adolescents, and adults,[32] indicating that dosage adjustments may not be necessary for age.[33]

Findling and colleagues[34] demonstrated the efficacy and safety of quetiapine in the acute management of adolescent schizophrenia in an RDBPC, parallel-group study. Quetiapine treatment groups were titrated to a target dose of 400 mg/d or 800 mg/d. By day 42, both treatment groups demonstrated significant mean improvements in PANSS total score compared with placebo. The efficacy and AE profiles were found to be consistent with earlier quetiapine studies in adolescents and adults with schizophrenia, with quetiapine being generally well tolerated.

Aripiprazole

Aripiprazole has FDA approval for the treatment of schizophrenia in adolescents aged 13 to 17.[14] This atypical antipsychotic works as a partial agonist at D_2 and 5-HT_{1A} receptors and as an antagonist at 5-HT_{2A} receptors.[35] Pharmacokinetic studies have shown a higher C_{max} at steady state for children and adolescents compared with adults.[36] Findling and colleagues[37] demonstrated that steady state is achieved after 14 days of once-daily dosing, and that C_{max} and area-under-the-curve values have a linear relationship to dosage.

Aripiprazole's efficacy in acute management of schizophrenic symptoms was established by Findling and colleagues[38] in a phase 3 RDBPC study with target doses of either 10 mg/d or 30 mg/d By the 6-week endpoint, the mean change in PANSS total score was significant at both dosages over placebo, with active treatment groups showing significantly higher rates of remission. The investigators concluded that aripiprazole was more efficacious than placebo at these fixed doses and generally well tolerated. Longer-term efficacy and safety were demonstrated by Correll and colleagues[39] in a 52-week RDBPC with participants dosed between 10 and 30 mg/d The time to exacerbation of psychotic symptoms/impending relapse, the primary efficacy measure, was significantly longer in the aripiprazole group. The proportion meeting criteria for exacerbation of symptoms was also smaller for the active treatment group. Safety and tolerability measures were thought to be consistent with those described in previous studies, and acceptable overall.

Paliperidone

Paliperidone is the major active metabolite of risperidone and is a full antagonist of D_2 receptors. Its extended-release (ER) formulation is currently FDA approved for use in adolescents (12–17 years) diagnosed with schizophrenia.[40] The FDA has recommended a starting dose of 3 mg/d with subsequent dosing between 3 and 6 mg/d in adolescents weighing less than 51 kg, and 3 to 12 mg/d for those weighing $\geq$51 kg.[41]

The ER preparation allows for gradual plasma concentration increases over a 24-hour period and once-daily dosing.[42] Unlike risperidone, paliperidone is largely eliminated renally.[43]

Paliperidone ER was found to be effective in the acute care of adolescent schizophrenia symptoms by Singh and colleagues,[44] who conducted a 6-week, parallel-group, RDBPC study with treatment patients assigned to 1 of 3 weight-based, fixed doses ranging from 1.5 to 12 mg/d The investigators found that the mean change in PANSS scores was significant for the medium-treatment group (3 or 6 mg/d) versus the high- (6 or 12 mg/d) and low-treatment (1.5 mg/d) groups as well as placebo. PANSS scores were also significant for "actual dose strengths" of 3 mg, 6 mg, and 12 mg compared with placebo. This study was extended into a 2-year (including 36 participants in a 6-month study) open-label trial conducted by Savitz and colleagues[40] that helped to establish longer-term safety and efficacy. Participants were dosed between 1.5 and 12 mg/d with the most common dose being 6 mg/d. Improvement in PANSS total score was generally observed within 3 months of treatment initiation and continued to the endpoint, with 41.7% of patients achieving remission. The investigators concluded that the medication's safety profile for adolescents resembled that of adults as well as risperidone in adolescents.

Lurasidone

Introduced in 2010, lurasidone currently has FDA approval for the treatment of schizophrenia in adolescents 13 to 17 years.[14] Its therapeutic effect is mediated through its high-affinity antagonism for D_2, 5-HT_{2A}, and $5HT_7$ receptors, and moderate-affinity partial agonism at $5HT_{1A}$ receptors.[45] The pharmacokinetic profile of lurasidone is similar in the pediatric and adult populations at a dose range of 20 to 160 mg/d, with lower doses (<120 mg/d) having a more favorable AE profile compared with higher ones.[46]

Lurasidone's efficacy and safety for acute management of adolescent schizophrenic symptoms were established by Goldman and colleagues[47] in a 6-week RDBPC study that randomized participants to fixed-dose lurasidone 40 mg/d, 80 mg/d, or placebo. At the endpoint, the least-squares (LS) mean change in PANSS total score was significant for both active treatment groups versus placebo, with separation apparent starting at week 1. A greater proportion of lurasidone participants also met criteria for response. The study concluded that lurasidone is an effective treatment option with an adolescent safety profile consistent with that of adults with schizophrenia.

Other

Ziprasidone is an antagonist of both the 5-HT_{2A} and the D_2 receptors, with an 8-fold greater affinity for 5-HT_{2A} compared with D_2 receptors.[48] Because of its short half-life, ziprasidone should be administered twice daily, and absorption is increased 2-fold when taken with food.[49] Although FDA approved for the treatment of adults with schizophrenia, it does not have approval for children or adolescents.[14] Findling and colleagues[50] conducted a 6-week RDBPCT followed by a 26-week OLE. At the end of the RDBPC and OLE trials, participants taking ziprasidone did not demonstrate significant improvement in the BPRS-anchored or other measures over placebo, with the exception of a reduction in the PANSS positive symptom subscale. Because of its lack of separation from placebo, it is not recommended as a first-line treatment of schizophrenia in youths.

Derived from a tetracyclic antidepressant, asenapine has a high affinity for and antagonism of serotonergic receptors, as well as potent dopamine, α-adrenergic, and histamine antagonism with low cholinergic activity.[51] Dosed twice daily, asenapine is administered sublingually, and patients should not take water within 5 minutes of administration, because this reduces absorption and bioavailability.[52] In 2015, asenapine became FDA approved to treat children between 10 and 17 years with acute manic or mixed episodes of bipolar I disorder.[14] Findling and colleagues[53] examined the efficacy of 2 different doses (2.5 mg and 5 mg twice daily) in an 8-week RDBPCT followed by a 26-week OLE study. After 8 weeks, reductions in PANSS scores were greater for both dosage groups compared with placebo but did not achieve statistical significance. To the authors' knowledge, no other large-scale, placebo-controlled RCTs for early-onset schizophrenia have been completed at this time.

Iloperidone acts through a combination of D_2 and 5-HT_2 antagonism.[54] It is FDA approved for the treatment of adult schizophrenia, but there are no prospective adolescent schizophrenia RCTs published at this time.[14]

Cariprazine is another atypical antipsychotic that is FDA approved for adult schizophrenia as well as acute manic or mixed episodes of bipolar I disorder.[55] It exhibits high affinity as a partial agonist for D_2, D_3, and 5-HT_{1A} receptors and has low affinity for 5-HT_{2C} and α-1_A adrenergic receptors.[56] There are no adolescent schizophrenia RCTs for cariprazine published at this time.

Although there is some anecdotal evidence indicating that youth with psychosis respond well to long-acting injectable formulations of antipsychotic medications,[57–59] there are no published controlled trials studying the effects on children and adolescents at this time.[19] However, in youth with documented chronic psychotic symptoms and poor treatment compliance, depot antipsychotics may warrant consideration as a treatment option.[60]

Comparison Studies

Several head-to-head trials have been conducted to compare response and side effects between agents (**Table 3**).[61–64] Sikich and colleagues[62] conducted an 8-week DB pilot study in which youth with psychosis (but not necessarily schizophrenia) were randomized to haloperidol (mean dose 5 mg/d), olanzapine (mean dose 12.3 mg/d), or risperidone (mean dose 4.0 mg/d). Overall, 53% of participants taking haloperidol, 74% on risperidone, and 88% on olanzapine met response criteria by BPRS score reductions and CGI improvements; however, overall comparisons failed to show statistically significant differences. Notably, risperidone and olanzapine led to higher rates of AEs than those seen in adults, with more than half of those participants experiencing mild to moderate EPS versus 33% of the haloperidol group withdrawing owing to EPS. All groups experienced significant weight gain. Investigators concluded that although atypical antipsychotics were efficacious, side effects appeared to be more frequent and intense in youth.

Sikich and colleagues[63] followed up the previous study with the largest comparison DBRCT to date. The Treatment of Early Onset Schizophrenia Spectrum Disorders (TEOSS) Study examined the efficacy of molindone (mean dose 59.9 mg/d, administered with benztropine), olanzapine (mean dose 11.4 mg/d), and risperidone (mean dose 2.8 mg/d) in youth with schizophrenia and schizoaffective disorder over 8 weeks. There were no statistically significant differences among the treatment arms, with 50% of those on molindone meeting response criteria compared with 34% with olanzapine and 46% with risperidone. Although 37% of participants experienced at least 1 AE, side effects varied considerably by medication. The molindone group experienced the least weight gain, followed by risperidone and then olanzapine, but experienced more akathisia. The study ultimately stopped randomizing participants to olanzapine because of significant weight gain. Despite the variability of side effects by agent,

---

Table 3
Summarization of selected head-to-head antipsychotic studies

Medications	Publication	Study, Design, Duration	N	Age (y)	Target Dose (mg/d)	Primary Efficacy Measure/Purpose	Effectiveness/Findings	Noteworthy AE
Haloperidol Olanzapine Risperidone	Sikich et al,[62] 2004	Randomized double-blind controlled trial, 8 wk	50	8–19	Flexible dosing: olanzapine 2.5–20 mg/d (mean 12.3 mg/d), haloperidol 1–8 mg/d (mean 5 mg/d), risperidone 1–6 mg/d (mean 4 mg/d)	Mean change in BPRS-C	74% of risperidone, 88% of olanzapine, 53% of haloperidol had significant symptom reduction; between group overall comparisons failed to show statistical improvement differences	Risperidone and olanzapine had higher rates of AEs than in adults and more than half of those on atypicals had mild to moderate EPS; severe EPS was even higher on haloperidol; significant weight gain across all groups
Risperidone Olanzapine Quetiapine	Jensen et al,[61] 2008	Randomized open-label, 12 wk	30	10–18	Flexible dosing: olanzapine 5–20 mg/d (mean 11.4 mg/d), risperidone 0.5–6 mg/d (mean 2.8 mg/d), quetiapine 100–800 mg/d (mean 611 mg/d)	Mean reduction in PANSS	No statistically significant differences between treatment arms, although differences between risperidone > quetiapine approached significance	No significant differences in AIMS. Significant weight gain across all groups
Molindone (with benztropine) Olanzapine Risperidone	Sikich et al,[63] 2008	Randomized double-blind controlled trial, 8 wk	116	8–19	Flexible dosing: olanzapine 2.5–20 mg/d (mean 11.4 mg/d), risperidone 0.5–6 mg/d (mean 2.8 mg/d), molindone 10–140 mg/d (mean 59.9 mg/d)	Response defined as CGI improvement score of 1 or 2 and ≥20% reduction in PANSS	Molindone achieved 50% response, olanzapine achieved 34% response, and risperidone achieved 46% response. No statistically significant differences	Weight gain in olanzapine > risperidone > molindone. Randomization to olanzapine stopped due to weight gain. More changes in lipids and liver function tests in olanzapine group, more akathisia in molindone group

(continued on next page)

199

Table 3
(continued)

Medications	Publication	Study, Design, Duration	N	Age (y)	Target Dose (mg/d)	Primary Efficacy Measure/Purpose	Effectiveness/Findings	Noteworthy AE
Molindone (with benztropine) Olanzapine Risperidone	Findling et al,[64] 2010	DB extension of Sikich et al,[63] 2008 study; up to 44 wk	54	8–19	Flexible dosing (as above): olanzapine mean 9.6 mg/d, risperidone mean 3.9 mg/d, molindone mean 76.5 mg/d	Response defined as CGI improvement score of 1 or 2 and ≥20% reduction in PANSS	PANSS scores varied little during the maintenance period	All groups had statistically significant weight gains but olanzapine > molindone for several weight-related measures. Only 12% of participants completed the study on the same medication they started and only 26% completed the extension trial
Quetiapine Risperidone	Swadi et al,[65] 2010	Open-label, 6 wk	22	<19	Flexible dosing: quetiapine 100–800 mg/d (mean 607 mg/d), risperidone 1.5-5 mg/d (mean 2.9 mg/d)	Response defined as 30% or more reduction in PANSS, BPRS, and CGI-S scores	No significant differences in reduction of symptoms, but risperidone performed better on most outcome measures	Although not statistically significant, greater weight gain was seen with quetiapine and more anticholinergic coadministration for management of EPS with risperidone
Paliperidone Aripiprazole	Savitz et al,[66] 2015	RDBT against aripiprazole, 26 wk	228	12–17	Flexible dosing for paliperidone (3, 6, or 9 mg/d) and aripiprazole (5, 10, or 15 mg/d)	Mean change in PANSS total score	Similar improvement for paliperidone ER and aripiprazole at day 56 (−19.3 vs −19.8) and day 182 (−25.6 vs −26.8). Paliperidone ER and aripiprazole also showed similar rates of response (67.9% and 76.3% at day 56, 76.8% and 81.6% at day 182)	Higher frequency of TEAEs for paliperidone ER compared with aripiprazole (77.0% vs 66.7%); most common TEAEs were akathisia, headache, somnolence, tremor, and weight gain. Incidence of dystonia and hyperkinesia for paliperidone ER was higher (>2%) and also demonstrated more frequent TEAEs related to prolactin (4.4% vs 0.9%)

there were no statistical differences in time to discontinuation, with roughly 40% of participants discontinuing early. Investigators concluded that olanzapine and risperidone did not demonstrate superior efficacy to molindone.

Fifty-four TEOSS participants transitioned to a DB maintenance extension study.[64] During the course of the maintenance period, PANSS scores in all 3 conditions varied little from the beginning of the initial RCT to the end of the maintenance period. However, it is notable that only 12% of participants finished the entire period on the same medication to which they were randomized. Similar to the shorter RCT, all groups experienced statistically significant weight gain, but olanzapine was greatest, particularly in comparison to molindone. Although molindone demonstrated higher levels of akathisia, Abnormal Involuntary Movement Scale (AIMS) scores were not significantly different between arms. The investigators concluded that compared with adult trials, youths with schizophrenia were less likely to maintain the same treatment over 1 year, and minimal improvements were made beyond the initial 8 weeks of treatment.

One additional open-label trial compared risperidone with quetiapine over 6 weeks in youths with psychosis.[65] With response criteria set by changes in PANSS, BPRS, and CGI, there were no statistically significant differences, but risperidone performed better on most outcome measures. In addition, more participants taking quetiapine gained more than 10% of their body weight compared with risperidone, and 4/11 quetiapine participants had to withdraw when their dose exceeded the 800-mg/d threshold. Participants taking risperidone were more likely to take concurrent anticholinergics, but this did not achieve statistical significance.

In another study, Savitz and colleagues[66] compared the efficacy, safety, and tolerability of paliperidone ER against aripiprazole in a DB phase 3 study. Participants were randomized into paliperidone ER (6 mg/d for days 1–7, flexible dosing of 3, 6, or 9 mg/d after day 8) and aripiprazole (10 mg/d by days 5–7, flexible dosing of 5, 10, or 15 mg/d after day 8) treatment groups during an 8-week DB acute treatment period, followed by an 18-week DB maintenance period. Improvements in mean PANSS total scores were similar for both groups at day 56 and day 182, as were the rates of response. Paliperidone ER demonstrated a higher frequency of treatment emergent adverse event (TEAEs) compared with aripiprazole, the most common being akathisia, headache, somnolence, tremor, and weight gain. The incidence of dystonia and hyperkinesia was higher in paliperidone ER, and there were more frequent TEAEs related to prolactin.

Side Effects

With all of the available treatment options that have demonstrated efficacy in adolescent schizophrenia symptoms, the selection of treatment agent often depends on tolerability (see **Table 1**). Although each agent has its unique side-effect profile, there are some possible effects common to the entire class, and monitoring recommendations have been developed to prevent significant AE (see **Table 1**). Some of the more significant treatment risks are briefly discussed.

Metabolic changes

The existing data suggest that weight gain, a well-known side effect of many antipsychotics in adults, may be even more significant in the younger population.[67,68] Adult studies indicate that patients on clozapine and olanzapine are at highest risk of weight gain; quetiapine and risperidone are considered moderate risk, and aripiprazole and ziprasidone are lower risk.[69,70] Along with weight changes, antipsychotic treatment has often been associated with changes in serum lipids in adults, with olanzapine and clozapine conferring the greatest risk of dyslipidemia,[71–73] but the head-to-head comparative data in children and adolescents are relatively limited. Changes in glucose metabolism in treated youth, however, have brought up concerns for the possible development of diabetes mellitus, with 1 prospective study indicating that changes in insulin sensitivity may be apparent within 3 months of medication initiation.[74]

Metabolic syndrome describes the constellation of glucose intolerance, abdominal obesity, dyslipidemia, and hypertension,[75] and there are several ways to mitigate these effects. Multiple metaanalyses have demonstrated the effectiveness of behavioral interventions in alleviating metabolic syndrome in adults,[76,77] and modified versions of these interventions can be effective in children and adolescents.[78] Each antipsychotic agent can present with different metabolic effects,[79] and when weight gain becomes problematic with a particular agent, switching to another with a more favorable profile may be effective.[80] Of the adjunctive medications used to combat significant antipsychotic-induced weight gain, metformin has been most extensively studied in youth with a metaanalysis of 5 studies supporting its potential for reducing weight in this population.[81] In addition, a DB RCT with adults showed topiramate to be effective in reducing weight gain associated with olanzapine treatment,[82] and there is a retrospective chart review indicating possible effectiveness for children and adolescents.[83] Despite some promise, further studies are needed to support the use of these medications for this purpose in a younger population.

Cardiovascular

Cardiovascular changes have been observed during antipsychotic treatment in children, namely QTc prolongation, orthostatic hypotension, tachycardia, and pericarditis.[84] QTc prolongation was particularly relevant for ziprasidone, with a prolongation of 9 to 14 milliseconds longer in adults than risperidone, olanzapine, quetiapine, and haloperidol.[85] Especially in the initial stages of treatment, clozapine has been associated with a higher risk of myocarditis compared with the general population.[86]

Extrapyramidal symptoms

A retrospective review completed by Keepers and colleagues[87] examined 215 adult and child patients receiving neuroleptic medications, 37% of which received prophylactic anticholinergic medications. EPS incidence was observed to decline with age, with peak incidence of dystonia and Parkinsonism in the 10- to 19-years group, and akathisia in the 30- to 39-years group. Divided into age decades, prophylaxis showed statistically significant differences for the 10- to 19-years, 20- to 29-years, and 30- to 39-years groups. Early prophylaxis was particularly valuable for dystonia within first 3 to 4 days of treatment as well as akathisia and Parkinsonism during the first 2 weeks of treatment. The investigators concluded that initial prophylaxis significantly decreased the incidence of dystonia, akathisia, and Parkinsonism and was particularly effective in younger patients between 10 and 30 years.

Neuroleptic malignant syndrome

Characterized by fever, tachycardia, and rigidity, neuroleptic malignant syndrome has been observed in children on both first-generation and second-generation antipsychotics and is a rare but potentially fatal treatment complication.[88]

Prolactin

Several antipsychotics have been associated with increases in prolactin level, with the effect thought to be more pronounced in youths compared with adults.[89,90] Studies indicate that the risk in adults is greatest with risperidone,[90–94] lower with olanzapine and ziprasidone, and minimal with clozapine, quetiapine, and aripiprazole.[95–98]

Although hyperprolactinemia can result in such long-term effects as amenorrhea, erectile dysfunction, decreased libido, hirsutism, and breast symptoms/enlargement,[88] there is some evidence that growth and puberty may not be affected.[99]

Seizures
Although electroencephalogram changes have been reported with this class of medication,[100] clozapine is associated with the greatest increase in seizure risk.[101] Careful administration and monitoring are recommended in at-risk patients.

Agranulocytosis and neutropenia
Although the white blood cell count changes associated with most antipsychotic medications are rarely significant,[102] clozapine has been shown to have an 18-month cumulative incidence of 0.9% for agranulocytosis,[103] with younger age thought to elevate the risk of neutropenia.[104,105] Regular monitoring is essential in avoiding potentially serious complications.

SUMMARY

Although considerable progress has been made in furthering schizophrenia treatment in children and adolescents, there is a clear need for more robust studies to better differentiate between available options.[106] The existing data indicate generally similar efficacy between first- and second-generation antipsychotics with the exception of ziprasidone.[107] Clozapine can also be considered an exception, which has demonstrated clinical superiority in treatment-refractory patients, but is accompanied by a higher risk of major side effects. When selecting an antipsychotic medication in practice, those with FDA approval should generally be considered first. Although major guidelines do not favor any specific agent over another, weight gain with olanzapine may limit its use as a first-line agent.[60,108] As a result, other factors, including side-effect profile, patient and family preference, cost, and availability, may help guide the treatment choice.[109] Despite recent advancements for the younger population, knowledge of this clinical area is still incomplete, and many children and adolescents with schizophrenia may remain symptomatic despite optimal pharmacotherapy.[60] These youth represent one of the most vulnerable pediatric populations within medicine, and additional research and pharmacologic development are required to meet the extraordinary need.

DISCLOSURE

In the past 36 months, Dr. Findling receives or has received research support, acted as a consultant and/or has received honoraria from Acadia, Aevi, Akili, Alcobra, Allergan, Amerex, American Academy of Child & Adolescent Psychiatry, American Psychiatric Press, Arbor, Bracket, Daiichi-Sankyo, Epharma Solutions, Forest, Genentech, Ironshore, KemPharm, Luminopia, Lundbeck, Merck, NIH, Neurim, Noven, Nuvelution, Otsuka, PCORI, Pfizer, Physicians Postgraduate Press, Purinix, Receptor Life Sciences, Roche, Sage, Shire, Sunovion, Supernus Pharmaceuticals, Syneurx, Teva, TouchPoint, Tris, and Validus. Dr Findling discloses the following past or present relationships with the following commercial organizations that could be perceived as a conflict of interest in the past 36 months: Acadia, consultant fees; Aevi, grant research support and consultant fees; Akili, grant research support and consultant fees; Alcobra, grant research support and consultant fees; Allergan, grant research support and consultant fees; Amerex, consultant fees; Am Acad CAP, royalties; American Psychiatric Press, royalties; Arbor, consultant fees; Bracket, honoraria; Daiichi-

Sankyo, royalties; Epharma Solutions, consultant fees; Forest, grant research support; Genentech, consultant fees; Ironshore, consultant fees; KemPharm, consultant fees; Luminopia, consultant fees; Lundbeck, grant research support and consultant fees; Merck, consultant fees; NIH, grant research support and consultant fees; Neurim, grant research support and consultant fees; Noven, consultant fees; Nuvelution, consultant fees; Otsuka, consultant fees; PCORI, grant research support; Pfizer, grant research support; Physicians Postgraduate Press, consultant fees; Purinix, consultant fees; Receptor Life Sciences, consultant fees; Roche, grant research support; Sage, royalties; Shire, grant research support and consultant fees; Sunovion, grant research support and consultant fees; Supernus Pharmaceuticals, grant research support, consultant fees; Syneurx, grant research support; Teva, consultant fees; Touchpoint, consultant; Tris, consultant; Validus, grant research support and consultant fees.

REFERENCES

1. Shen W. A history of antipsychotic drug development. Compr Psychiatry 1999; 40(6):407–14.
2. Whitney Z, Boyda HN, Procyshyn RM, et al. Therapeutic drug levels of second generation antipsychotics in youth: a systematic review. J Child Adolesc Psychopharmacol 2015;25(3):234–45.
3. Bourgeois FT, Murphy S, Pinto C, et al. Pediatric versus adult drug trials for conditions with high pediatric disease burden. Pediatrics 2012;130(2):285–92.
4. Carlsson A. Antipsychotic drugs, neurotransmitters, and schizophrenia. Am J Psychiatry 1978;135(2):164–73.
5. Pool D, Bloom W, Mielke DH, et al. A controlled evaluation of loxitane in seventy-five adolescent schizophrenic patients. Curr Ther Res Clin Exp 1976;19(1):99–104.
6. Realmuto GM, Erickson WD, Yellin AM, et al. Clinical comparison of thiothixene and thioridazine in schizophrenic adolescents. Am J Psychiatry 1984;141(3): 440–2.
7. Olfson M, Gerhard T, Huang C, et al. Comparative effectiveness of second-generation antipsychotic medications in early-onset schizophrenia. Schizophr Bull 2012;38(4):845–53.
8. Meltzer HY. An overview of the mechanism of action of clozapine. J Clin Psychiatry 1994;55(Suppl B):47–52. Available at: http://www.ncbi.nlm.nih.gov/pubmed/7961573.
9. Iqbal MM, Rahman A, Husain Z, et al. Clozapine: a clinical review of adverse effects and management. Ann Clin Psychiatry 2003;15(1):33–48.
10. Chougule A, Praharaj SK, Bhat SM, et al. Prevalence and factors associated with clozapine-related constipation. J Clin Psychopharmacol 2018;38(1):42–6.
11. Kumra S, Frazier JA, Jacobsen LK, et al. Childhood-onset schizophrenia: a double-blind clozapine-haloperidol comparison. Arch Gen Psychiatry 1996; 53(12):1090–7.
12. Kumra S, Kranzler H, Gerbino-Rosen G, et al. Clozapine and "high-dose" olanzapine in refractory early-onset schizophrenia: a 12-week randomized and double-blind comparison. Biol Psychiatry 2008;63(5):524–9.
13. Shaw P, Sporn A, Gogtay N, et al. Childhood-onset schizophrenia. Arch Gen Psychiatry 2006;63(7):721.
14. Lee ES, Vidal C, Findling RL. A focused review on the treatment of pediatric patients with atypical antipsychotics. J Child Adolesc Psychopharmacol 2018; 28(9):582–605.

15. Chopko TC, Lindsley CW. Classics in chemical neuroscience: risperidone. ACS Chem Neurosci 2018;9(7):1520–9.
16. Balijepalli C, Druyts E, Zoratti MJ, et al. Change in prolactin levels in pediatric patients given antipsychotics for schizophrenia and schizophrenia spectrum disorders: a network meta-analysis. Schizophr Res Treatment 2018;2018:1–9.
17. Findling RL, Steiner H, Weller EB. Use of antipsychotics in children and adolescents. J Clin Psychiatry 2005;66(SUPPL. 7):29–40.
18. Keks NA, Culhane C. Risperidone (Risperdal): clinical experience with a new antipsychosis drug. Expert Opin Investig Drugs 2005;8(4):443–52.
19. Lytle S, McVoy M, Sajatovic M. Long-acting injectable antipsychotics in children and adolescents. J Child Adolesc Psychopharmacol 2017;27(1):2–9.
20. Haas M, Eerdekens M, Kushner S, et al. Efficacy, safety and tolerability of two risperidone dosing regimens in adolescent schizophrenia: double-blind study. Br J Psychiatry 2009;194(2):158–64.
21. Haas M, Unis AS, Armenteros J, et al. A 6-week, randomized, double-blind, placebo-controlled study of the efficacy and safety of risperidone in adolescents with schizophrenia. J Child Adolesc Psychopharmacol 2009;19(6):611–21.
22. Pandina G, Kushner S, Karcher K, et al. An open-label, multicenter evaluation of the long-term safety and efficacy of risperidone in adolescents with schizophrenia. Child Adolesc Psychiatry Ment Health 2012;6(1):23.
23. McGorry PD, Nelson B, Phillips LJ, et al. Randomized controlled trial of interventions for young people at ultra-high risk of psychosis. J Clin Psychiatry 2013; 74(04):349–56.
24. Kantrowitz JT, Citrome L. Olanzapine: review of safety 2008. Expert Opin Drug Saf 2008;7:761–9.
25. Lobo ED, Robertson-Plouch C, Quinlan T, et al. Oral olanzapine disposition in adolescents with schizophrenia or bipolar I disorder: a population pharmacokinetic model. Paediatr Drugs 2010;12:201–11.
26. Thiesen FM, Haberhausen M, Schulz E, et al. Serum levels of olanzapine and its n-desmethyl and 2-hydroxymethyl metabolites in child and adolescent psychiatric disorders: effects of dose, diagnosis, age, sex, smoking, and comedication. Ther Drug Monit 2006;28:750–9.
27. Grothe DR, Calis KA, Jacobsen L, et al. Olanzapine pharmacokinetics in pediatric and adolescent inpatients with childhood-onset schizophrenia. J Clin Psychopharmacol 2000;20:220–5.
28. Bigos KL, Pollock BG, Coley KC, et al. Sex, race, and smoking impact olanzapine exposure. J Clin Pharmacol 2008;48:157–65.
29. Kryzhanovskaya L, Schulz SC, McDougle C, et al. Olanzapine versus placebo in adolescents with schizophrenia: a 6-week, randomized, double-blind, placebo-controlled trial. J Am Acad Child Adolesc Psychiatry 2009;48(1):60–70.
30. Kemp DE, Correll CU, Tohen M, et al. Associations among obesity, acute weight gain, and response to treatment with olanzapine in adolescent schizophrenia. J Child Adolesc Psychopharmacol 2013;23(8):522–30.
31. Nasrallah HA. Atypical antipsychotic-induced metabolic side effects: insights from receptor-binding profiles. Mol Psychiatry 2008;13:27–35.
32. Winter HR, Earley WR, Hamer-Maansson JE, et al. Steady-state pharmacokinetic, safety, and tolerability profiles of quetiapine, norquetiapine, and other quetiapine metabolites in pediatric and adult patients with psychotic disorders. J Child Adolesc Psychopharmacol 2008;18:81–98.

33. McConville BJ, Arvanitis LA, Thyrum PT, et al. Pharmacokinetics, tolerability, and clinical effectiveness of quetiapine fumarate: an open-label trial in adolescents with psychotic disorders. J Clin Psychiatry 2000;61:252–60.

34. Findling RL, McKenna K, Earley WR, et al. Efficacy and safety of quetiapine in adolescents with schizophrenia investigated in a 6-week, double-blind, placebo-controlled trial. J Child Adolesc Psychopharmacol 2012;22(5):327–42.

35. Burris KD, Molski TF, Xu C, et al. Aripiprazole, a novel antipsychotic, is a high-affinity partial agonist at human dopamine d2 receptors. J Pharmacol Exp Ther 2002;302:381–9.

36. Mallikaarjun S, Salazar DE, Bramer SL. Pharmacokinetics, tolerability, and safety of aripiprazole following multiple oral dosing in normal healthy volunteers. J Clin Pharmacol 2004;44:179–87.

37. Findling RL, Kauffman R, Sallee FR, et al. An open-label study of aripiprazole: pharmacokinetics, tolerability, and effectiveness in children and adolescents with conduct disorder. J Child Adolesc Psychopharmacol 2009;19:431–9.

38. Findling RL, Robb A, Nyilas M, et al. A multiple-center, randomized, double-blind, placebo-controlled study of oral aripiprazole for treatment of adolescents with schizophrenia. Am J Psychiatry 2008;165(11):1432–41.

39. Correll CU, Kohegyi E, Zhao C, et al. Oral aripiprazole as maintenance treatment in adolescent schizophrenia: results from a 52-week, randomized, placebo-controlled withdrawal study. J Am Acad Child Adolesc Psychiatry 2017;56(9): 784–92.

40. Savitz A, Lane R, Nuamah I, et al. Long-term safety of paliperidone extended release in adolescents with schizophrenia: an open-label, flexible dose study. J Child Adolesc Psychopharmacol 2015;25(7):548–57.

41. Younis IR, Laughren TP, Wang Y, et al. An integrated approach for establishing dosing recommendations: paliperidone for the treatment of adolescent schizophrenia. J Clin Psychopharmacol 2013;33(2):152–6.

42. Boom S, Thyssen A, Crauwels H, et al. The influence of hepatic impairment on the pharmacokinetics of paliperidone. Int J Clin Pharmacol Ther 2009;47: 606–16.

43. Vermeir M, Naessens I, Remmerie B, et al. Absorption, metabolism, and excretion of paliperidone, a new monoaminergic antagonist, in humans. Drug Metab Dispos 2008;36:769–79.

44. Singh J, Robb A, Vijapurkar U, et al. A randomized, double-blind study of paliperidone extended-release in treatment of acute schizophrenia in adolescents. Biol Psychiatry 2011;70(12):1179–87.

45. Ishibashi T, Horisawa T, Tokuda K, et al. Pharmacological profile of lurasidone, a novel antipsychotic agent with potent 5-hydroxytryptramine 7 (5-HT$_7$) and 5-HT$_{1A}$ receptor activity. J Pharmacol Exp Ther 2010;334:171–81.

46. Findling RL, Goldman R, Chiu YY, et al. Pharmacokinetics and tolerability of lurasidone in children and adolescents with psychiatric disorders. Clin Ther 2015; 37:2788–97.

47. Goldman R, Loebel A, Cucchiaro J, et al. Efficacy and safety of lurasidone in adolescents with schizophrenia: a 6-week, randomized placebo-controlled study. J Child Adolesc Psychopharmacol 2017;27(6):516–25.

48. Stimmel GL, Gutierrez MA, Lee V. Ziprasidone: an atypical antipsychotic drug for the treatment of schizophrenia. Clin Ther 2002;24(1):21–37.

49. Elbe D, Carandang CG. Focus on ziprasidone: a review of its use in child and adolescent psychiatry. J Can Acad Child Adolesc Psychiatry 2008;17(4):220–9.

50. Findling RL, Çavuş I, Pappadopulos E, et al. Ziprasidone in adolescents with schizophrenia: results from a placebo-controlled efficacy and long-term open-extension study. J Child Adolesc Psychopharmacol 2013;23(8):531–44.
51. McIntyre R, Wong R. Asenapine: a synthesis of efficacy data in bipolar mania and schizophrenia. Clin Schizophr Relat Psychoses 2012;5(4):217–20.
52. Chwieduk CM, Scott LJ. Asenapine with bipolar I disorder. CNS Drugs 2011; 25(3):251–67.
53. Findling RL, Landbloom RP, Mackle M, et al. Safety and efficacy from an 8 week double-blind trial and a 26 week open-label extension of asenapine in adolescents with schizophrenia. J Child Adolesc Psychopharmacol 2015;25(5): 384–96.
54. Citrome L. Iloperidone: chemistry, pharmacodynamics, pharmacokinetics and metabolism, clinical efficacy, safety and tolerability, regulatory affairs, and an opinion. Expert Opin Drug Metab Toxicol 2010;6(12):1551–64.
55. Citrome L. Cariprazine for acute and maintenance treatment of adults with schizophrenia: an evidence-based review and place in therapy. Neuropsychiatr Dis Treat 2018;14:2563–77.
56. Ágai-Csongor É, Domány G, Nógrádi K, et al. Discovery of cariprazine (RGH-188): a novel antipsychotic acting on dopamine D_3/D_2 receptors. Bioorg Med Chem Lett 2012;22(10):3437–40.
57. Pope S, Zaara S. Efficacy of long-acting injectable antipsychotics in adolescents. J Child Adolesc Psychopharmacol 2016;26:391–4.
58. Fabrega M, Sugranyes G, Baeza I. Two cases of long-acting paliperidone in adolescence. Ther Adv Psychopharmacol 2015;5:304–6.
59. Wisniewski A. New treatment option in resistant schizophrenia in adolescence. Neuropsychiatrie de l'Enfance et de l'adolescence 2012;5:239.
60. McClellan J, Stock S. American Academy of Child and Adolescent Psychiatry Committee on Quality Issues. Practic parameter for the assessment and treatment of children and adolescents with schizophrenia. J Am Acad Child Adolesc Psychiatry 2013;52:976–90.
61. Jensen JB, Kumra S, Leitten W, et al. A comparative pilot study of second-generation antipsychotics in children and adolescents with schizophrenia-spectrum disorders. J Child Adolesc Psychopharmacol 2008;18(4):317–26.
62. Sikich L, Hamer RM, Bashford RA, et al. A pilot study of risperidone, olanzapine, and haloperidol in psychotic youth: a double-blind, randomized, 8-week trial. Neuropsychopharmacology 2004;29(1):133–45.
63. Sikich L, Frazier JA, McClellan J, et al. Double-blind comparison of first- and second-generation antipsychotics in early-onset schizophrenia and schizoaffective disorder: findings from the treatment of early-onset schizophrenia spectrum disorders (TEOSS) study. Am J Psychiatry 2008;165(11):1420–31.
64. Findling RL, Johnson JL, McClellan J, et al. Double-blind maintenance safety and effectiveness findings from the treatment of early-onset schizophrenia spectrum (TEOSS) study. J Am Acad Child Adolesc Psychiatry 2010;49(6): 583–94.
65. Swadi HS, Craig BJ, Pirwani NZ, et al. A trial of quetiapine compared with risperidone in the treatment of first onset psychosis among 15-to 18-year-old adolescents. Int Clin Psychopharmacol 2010;25(1):1–6.
66. Savitz AJ, Lane R, Nuamah I, et al. Efficacy and safety of paliperidone extended release in adolescents with schizophrenia: a randomized, double-blind study. J Am Acad Child Adolesc Psychiatry 2015;54(2):126–37.e1.

67. Safer DJ. A comparison of risperidone-induced weight gain across the age span. J Clin Psychopharmacol 2004;24:429–36.

68. Sport AL, Bobb AJ, Gogtay N, et al. Hormonal correlates of clozapine-induced weight gain in psychotic children: an exploratory study. J Am Acad Child Adolesc Psychiatry 2005;44:925–33.

69. American Diabetes Association, American Psychiatric Association, American Association of Clinical Endocrinologists, North American Association for the Study of Obesity. Consensus development conference on antipsychotic drugs and obesity and diabetes. Diabetes Care 2004;27:596–601.

70. Casey DE, Haupt DW, Newcomer JW, et al. Antipsychotic-induced weight gain and metabolic abnormalities: implications for increased mortality in patients with schizophrenia. J Clin Psychiatry 2004;65(suppl 7):4–18.

71. Wirshing DA, Boyd JA, Meng LR, et al. The effects of novel antipsychotics on glucose and lipid levels. J Clin Psychiatry 2002;63(10):856–65.

72. Koro CE, Fedder DO, L'Italien GJ, et al. An assessment of the independent effects of olanzapine and risperidone exposure on the risk of hyperlipidemia in schizophrenic patients. Arch Gen Psychiatry 2002;59(11):1021–6.

73. Meyer JM. A retrospective comparison of weight, lipid, and glucose changes between risperidone- and olanzapine-treated inpatients: metabolic outcomes after 1 year. J Clin Psychiatry 2002;63(5):425–33.

74. Correll CU, Parikh UH, Mughal T, et al. Development of insulin resistance in antipsychotic-naïve youngsters treated with novel antipsychotics. Biol Psychiatry 2005;57(Suppl 8):36.

75. Maayan L, Correll CU. Weight gain and metabolic risks associated with antipsychotic medications in children and adolescents. J Child Adolesc Psychopharmacol 2011;21(6):517–35.

76. Alvarez-Jiménez M, González-Blanch C, Crespo-Facorro B, et al. Antipsychotic-induced weight gain in chronic and first-episode psychotic disorders: a systematic critical reappraisal. CNS Drugs 2008;22(7):547–62.

77. Gabriele JM, Dubbert PM, Reeves RR. Efficacy of behavioural interventions in managing atypical antipsychotic weight gain. Obes Rev 2009;10(4):442–55.

78. Nicol GE, Kolko R, Lenze EJ, et al. Adiposity, hepatic triglyceride, and carotid intima media thickness during behavioral weight loss treatment in antipsychotic-treated youth: a randomized pilot study. J Child Adolesc Psychopharmacol 2019. https://doi.org/10.1089/cap.2018.0120.

79. Correll CU, Manu P, Olshanskiy V, et al. Cardiometabolic risk of second-generation antipsychotic medications during first-time use in children and adolescents. JAMA 2009;302(16):1765–73.

80. Pramyothin P, Khaodhiar L. Metabolic syndrome with the atypical antipsychotics. Curr Opin Endocrinol Diabetes Obes 2010;17(5):460–6.

81. Ellul P, Delorme R, Cortese S. Metformin for weight gain associated with second-generation antipsychotics in children and adolescents: a systematic review and meta-analysis. CNS Drugs 2018;32(12):1103–12.

82. Narula PK, Rehan HS, Unni KES, et al. Topiramate for prevention of olanzapine associated weight gain and metabolic dysfunction in schizophrenia: a double-blind, placebo-controlled trial. Schizophr Res 2010;118(1–3):218–23.

83. Shapiro M, Reid A, Olsen B, et al. Topiramate, zonisamide and weight loss in children and adolescents prescribed psychiatric medications. Int J Psychiatry Med 2016;51(1):56–68.

84. Findling RL, Drury SS, Jensen PS, et al. Practice parameter for the use of atypical antipsychotic medications in children and adolescents. 2011. Available

at: https://www.aacap.org/App_Themes/AACAP/docs/practice_parameters/ Atypical_Antipsychotic_Medications_Web.pdf. Accessed September 18, 2019.

85. Pfizer Inc., Geodon (ziprasidone) [package insert]. Pfizer Inc, Available at: https:// www.pfizermedicalinformation.com/en-us/geodon, 2015, Accessed September 18, 2019.
86. Wehmeier PM, Heiser P, Remschmidt H. Myocarditis, pericarditis and cardiomyopathy in patients treated with clozapine. J Clin Pharm Ther 2005;30(1):91–6.
87. Keepers GA, Clappison VJ, Casey DE. Initial anticholinergic prophylaxis for neuroleptic-induced extrapyramidal syndromes. Arch Gen Psychiatry 1983;40: 1113–7.
88. Correll CU, Penzner JB, Parikh UH, et al. Recognizing and monitoring adverse events of second-generation antipsychotics in children and adolescents. Child Adolesc Psychiatr Clin N Am 2006;15:177–206.
89. Woods SW, Martin A, Spector SG, et al. Effects of development on olanzapine-associated adverse events. J Am Acad Child Adolesc Psychiatry 2002;41(12): 1439–46.
90. Wudarsky M, Nicolson R, Hamburger SD, et al. Elevated prolactin in pediatric patients on typical and atypical antipsychotics. J Child Adolesc Psychopharmacol 1999;9(4):239–45.
91. Fitzgerald KD, Stewart CM, Tawile V, et al. Risperidone augmentation of serotonin reuptake inhibitor treatment of pediatric obsessive compulsive disorder. J Child Adolesc Psychopharmacol 1999;9:115–23.
92. Findling RL, Kusumakar V, Daneman D, et al. Prolactin levels during long-term risperidone treatment in children and adolescents. J Clin Psychiatry 2003;64: 1362–9.
93. Masi G, Cosenza A, Mucci M. Prolactin levels in young children with pervasive developmental disorders during risperidone treatment. J Child Adolesc Psychopharmacol 2001;11:389–94.
94. Saito E, Correll C, Gallelli K, et al. A prospective study of hyperprolactinemia in children and adolescents treated with atypical antipsychotic agents. J Child Adolesc Psychopharmacol 2004;14:350–68.
95. David SR, Taylor CC, Kinon BJ, et al. The effects of olanzapine, risperidone, and haloperidol on plasma prolactin levels in patients with schizophrenia. Clin Ther 2000;22:1085–96.
96. Haddad PM, Wieck A. Antipsychotic-induced hyperprolactinemia: mechanism, clinical features and management. Drugs 2004;64:2291–314.
97. Meltzer HY, Goode DJ, Schyve PM, et al. Effect of clozapine on human serum prolactin levels. Am J Psychiatry 1979;136:1550–5.
98. Small JG, Hirsch SR, Arvanitis LA, et al. Quetiapine in patients with schizophrenia. A high- and low-dose double-blind comparison with placebo. Seroquel study group. Arch Gen Psychiatry 1997;54:549–57.
99. Dunbar F, Kusumakar V, Daneman D, et al. Growth and sexual maturation during longer-term treatment with risperidone. Am J Psychiatry 2004;161:918–20.
100. Amann BL, Pogarell O, Mergl R, et al. EEG abnormalities associated with antipsychotics: a comparison of quetiapine, olanzapine, haloperidol and healthy subjects. Hum Psychopharmacol 2003;18:641–6.
101. Hedges D, Jeppson K, Whitehead P. Antipsychotic medication and seizures: a review. Drugs Today (Barc) 2003;39(7):551–7.
102. Stubner S, Grohmann R, Engel R, et al. Blood dyscrasias induced by psychotropic drugs. Pharmacopsychiatry 2004;37(Suppl 1):S70–8.

103. Alvir JM, Lieberman JA. Agranulocytosis: incidence and risk factors. J Clin Psychiatry 1994;55(Suppl B):137–8.
104. Alvir JM, Lieberman JA, Safferman AZ, et al. Clozapine-induced agranulocytosis. Incidence and risk factors in the United States. N Engl J Med 1993; 329(3):162–7.
105. Usiskin SI, Nicolson R, Lenane M, et al. Retreatment with clozapine after erythromycin-induced neutropenia. Am J Psychiatry 2000;157(6):1021.
106. Kranzler HN, Cohen SD. Psychopharmacologic treatment of psychosis in children and adolescents. Efficacy and management. Child Adolesc Psychiatr Clin N Am 2013;22(4):727–44.
107. Pagsberg AK, Tarp S, Glintborg D, et al. Acute antipsychotic treatment of children and adolescents with schizophrenia-spectrum disorders: a systematic review and network meta-analysis. J Am Acad Child Adolesc Psychiatry 2017; 56(3):191–202.
108. Kendall T, Hollis C, Stafford M, et al. Recognition and management of psychosis and schizophrenia in children and young people: summary of NICE guidance. BMJ 2013;346:f150.
109. McClellan J. Psychosis in children and adolescents. J Am Acad Child Adolesc Psychiatry 2018;57(5):308–12.
110. Jannsen Pharmaceutical Companies. Risperdal (risperidone) [package insert]. Janssen Pharmaceutical Companies website. 2009. Available at: http://www.janssenlabels.com/package-insert/product-monograph/prescribing-information/RISPERDAL-pi.pdf. Accessed May 29, 2019.
111. Eli Lilly and Company. Zyprexa (olanzapine) [package insert]. Eli Lilly and Company website. 2018. Available at: https://pi.lilly.com/us/zyprexa-pi.pdf. Accessed May 29, 2019.
112. AstraZeneca Pharmaceuticals LP. Seroquel (quetiapine) [package insert]. AstraZeneca Pharmaceuticals LP website. 2018. Available at: https://www.azpicentral.com/seroquel/seroquel.pdf. Accessed May 29, 2019.
113. Otsuka Pharmaceutical Company. Abilify (aripiprazole) [package insert]. Otsuka Pharmaceutical Company website. 2018. Available at: https://www.otsuka-us.com/media/static/Abilify-PI.pdf. Accessed May 29, 2019.
114. Janssen Pharmaceutical Companies. Invega (paliperidone) [package insert]. Janssen Pharmaceutical Companies website. 2019. Available at: http://www.janssenlabels.com/package-insert/product-monograph/prescribing-information/INVEGA-pi.pdf. Accessed May 29, 2019.
115. Sunovion Pharmaceuticals Inc. Latuda (lurasidone) [package insert]. Sunovion Pharmaceuticals Inc. website. Available at: https://www.latuda.com/LatudaPrescribingInformation.pdf. Accessed May 29, 2019.
116. Correll CU. Antipsychotic medications. In: Dulcan MK, editor. Dulcan's textbook of child and adolescent psychiatry. 2nd edition. Arlington (VA): American Psychiatric Association; 2016. p. 795–846.

Evidence-Based Psychosocial Treatment for Individuals with Early Psychosis

Abigail Wright, PhD[a,b],*, Julia Browne, PhD[a,b],
Kim T. Mueser, PhD[c], Corinne Cather, PhD[a,b]

KEYWORDS

- First-episode psychosis • Psychosocial treatment • Family therapy • Psychotherapy

KEY POINTS

- Coordinated specialty care models are an evidence-based practice for first-episode psychosis.
- Individual, group, and family psychological treatments play a key role in recovery from a first episode of psychosis.
- Common elements of these therapies include education, skills training, and a focus on personally meaningful goals.

First-episode psychosis (FEP) usually refers to the initial psychotic episode of a primary psychotic disorder, which often results in fear, confusion, and significant disruption in the individual's life and that of the family. Over the past decade, specialized FEP programs, which combine antipsychotic treatment with psychosocial treatments, have become more widespread in the United States. Individual, group, and family psychotherapy components of comprehensive programs are critical in helping clients and families understand and process the experience of psychosis and learn strategies to promote recovery and well-being.

Coordinated specialty care (CSC) programs (referred to as early intervention services [EISs] in Europe and Australia) provide team-based, comprehensive, evidence-based care, education, and support to engage clients and their families early in the course of illness.[1] The goals of these programs are to reduce the duration of

Disclosure Statement: Drs K.T. Mueser and C. Cather provide training and consultation about implementing NAVIGATE that can include compensation. Drs A. Wright and J. Browne have no disclosures.

[a] Massachusetts General Hospital, Center of Excellence in Psychosocial and Systemic Research, 151 Merrimac Street, 6th Floor, Boston, MA 02114, USA; [b] Harvard Medical School, Boston, MA, USA; [c] Center for Psychiatric Rehabilitation, Boston University, 940 Commonwealth Avenue West, Boston, MA 02215, USA

* Corresponding author. Massachusetts General Hospital, Center of Excellence in Psychosocial and Systemic Research, 151 Merrimac Street, 6th Floor, Boston, MA 02114.

E-mail address: AWRIGHT24@mgh.harvard.edu

untreated psychosis (DUP; ie, the period between onset of symptoms and initiation of antipsychotic medication treatment), prevent further disability, and promote recovery and well-being.

There are differences in the eligibility criteria across programs,[2] but typically CSC programs treat individuals between 15 and 40 years of age (although the United Kingdom has begun offering FEP services to anyone regardless of age)[3] who are within the first few years of the onset of their psychosis. CSC programs are intended for individuals with primary psychosis and are not meant for individuals whose psychotic symptoms are judged to be secondary to substance use (eg, substance-induced psychosis), a mood disorder (eg, bipolar disorder, major depression), a developmental disability (eg, autism), or posttraumatic stress disorder. The most common diagnoses of persons treated in CSC programs are schizophreniform disorder, schizophrenia, and schizoaffective disorder.

RESEARCH SUPPORT

CSC programs have been shown to yield better outcomes than treatment as usual, including fewer symptoms, more school/work participation, less treatment dropout, and reduced use of inpatient services.[4] Studies have consistently highlighted both the importance of well-resourced EISs,[5,6] and of shortening DUP to improve outcomes in persons with FEP.[7–9]

United States

Recovery After an Initial Schizophrenia Episode (RAISE) was a large-scale research initiative, funded by the National Institute of Mental Health (NIMH), which involved 2 studies in the United States, the RAISE-ETP trial[7,10] and the RAISE Connection Program Implementation and Evaluation study.[11] The RAISE-ETP trial enrolled 404 participants in a cluster randomized controlled trial involving 34 community mental health centers in 21 states to deliver 24 months of the NAVIGATE program (a CSC program) or usual care. At 2-year follow-up, participants who received NAVIGATE remained engaged in treatment for a longer period, and demonstrated greater reductions in symptoms, greater improvement in quality of life, better interpersonal relationships, and more involvement in work/school. Outcomes were moderated by DUP, such that those with a shorter DUP (<74 weeks) benefited more from NAVIGATE than those with longer DUP (≥74 weeks).[12] Client and clinician family therapy manuals (and other resources from the NAVIGATE program) are available online: https://navigateconsultants.org/manuals/.

The RAISE Connection Program Implementation and Evaluation study enrolled 65 persons with FEP to receive a CSC program and demonstrated the feasibility of delivering CSC, including high rates of engagement.[11] Another study, the Specialized Treatment Early in Psychosis (STEP) in Connecticut,[13] demonstrated that those engaged in CSC, compared with usual or community care, were less likely to be hospitalized (40.0% in CSC compared with 63.1% in usual care), had significantly fewer inpatient bed days, and showed improvements in vocational engagement.[14]

Across the World

In the United Kingdom, the standard of care requires individuals with FEP be engaged with EISs within 2 weeks of the initial referral, or offered an assessment if considered to have an "At-Risk Mental State," shown to reduce DUP.[15] EISs in the United Kingdom have been linked to reduced hospital admission rates, lower relapse rates and symptom severity, and overall improved access to treatment.[16] Superior effects of CSC programs also have been demonstrated in other countries in Europe, Canada, Australia, and Hong Kong.[17–20]

COMPONENTS AND DELIVERY OF COORDINATED SPECIALTY CARE

CSC is composed of pharmacologic management (once a month), individual psychotherapy (weekly),[21] family psychoeducation,[22] supported employment and education (SEE; weekly),[23,24] case management (weekly), and when available, peer support services.[25] Although there is some variability, CSC programs generally offer time-limited care over a period of 2 to 3 years. However, immediately stopping care at 2 years may be detrimental to an individual's recovery, particularly if the patient has built a good therapeutic relationship.[26] If treatment is required beyond those 2 years, the individual may step down to a lower level of care, with a transition into regular adult services.[27]

CSC involves a multidisciplinary team ,and each team member has a distinct role. For example, the team psychiatrist/prescriber uses a shared decision-making approach in collaboration with the individual with FEP to identify the most effective and tolerable medication(s) at the lowest possible dose.[28] Using an adapted Individual Placement and Support model of supported employment for serious mental illness,[29] the SEE specialist works closely with the client to identify goals related to returning to work and school and provides support across all phases of the employment or education process. Case management focuses on providing resources for basic needs (eg, transportation, insurance) ideally using assertive outreach to promote engagement, respond to crises, or provide services when necessary.[30] Although the peer support role is newer and therefore less well-defined, individuals with lived experience of mental health illness provide valuable support for individuals with FEP,[31] for example, by increasing hopeful attitudes about recovery through sharing their own recovery story, providing support, and facilitating the client's personal goals around community engagement (eg, exercise, going to coffee shops, or becoming more involved in extracurricular school activities). Team meetings are also key to optimal sequencing and coordination of treatment components based on the client's goals. The team typically meets weekly for assessment and treatment planning and communicates closely with outside organizations to provide appropriate community support.

The following section elaborates on the content, goals, and strategies used in individual, group, and family therapies for persons with FEP.

INDIVIDUAL, GROUP, AND FAMILY THERAPIES

The overarching objectives of group, individual, and family therapies in CSC are to

1. Help the client and family understand and cope with the experience of psychosis
2. Promote symptomatic and functional recovery and improve quality of life
3. Support the pursuit of personally meaningful goals of the client[32]

A positive alliance not only helps to engage clients and families in therapy but is also related to improved symptoms and functioning in persons with FEP.[33–36] As such, therapies delivered as part of CSC share several common elements in terms of their primary objectives and focus on promoting engagement and a strong alliance. Psychoeducation about psychosis and its course serves as the backbone for many of these therapies to empower clients and their families to make informed decisions both about treatment and other important aspects of clients' lives (eg, returning to school/work). Further, given that engagement in treatment can be challenging, it is critical for therapists to prioritize developing and maintaining a strong therapeutic alliance with clients and families, which involves agreement on goals and tasks of therapy, as well as the presence of a supportive bond.[37] The use of reflective statements as well as an emphasis on collaboration, shared decision-making, and autonomy can foster a supportive bond as well as improved therapy engagement.[38]

Individual Therapies

Cognitive behavioral therapy for psychosis (CBT-p) aims to help clients understand and cope with symptoms, prevent relapse, and identify and work toward meaningful goals through an improved understanding of how thoughts and beliefs shape emotional reactions and behaviors in response to events.[39–41] CBT-p has garnered substantial support for its use with persons with established schizophrenia and FEP.[16,42,43] Although CBT-p is often delivered as an individual therapy, there is evidence that it also can be effectively delivered as a group psychotherapy.[44,45] Therapists delivering CBT-p often use Socratic questioning techniques to explore clients' understanding of their experiences and to help them identify stressors and vulnerabilities, and the stress-vulnerability model[46] is often used as a framework to discuss precipitants of the initial psychotic episode as well as to identify protective factors to prevent relapse. This therapy includes both psychoeducation about psychosis and collaborative exercises aimed to help clients generate and test out alternative methods for coping with symptoms and appraising current past and present experiences, including the experience of psychosis. CBT-p is typically delivered as 16 weekly sessions over 6 months.[21,47] Persons with FEP are encouraged to complete homework between sessions to promote continued understanding and practice of CBT-p exercises.[43]

Individual Resiliency Training (IRT) served as the individual therapy component of NAVIGATE in the RAISE-ETP study and has been identified as a valuable intervention for persons with FEP.[7,32,48] IRT is rooted in CBT-p, training in illness self-management, and psychiatric rehabilitation. IRT is a manual-based therapy that emphasizes the enhancement of resiliency and strengths to support individuals' pursuit of meaningful goals and to improve their illness management, social functioning, quality of life, and well-being. IRT draws from the structure of the Illness Management and Recovery program[49] and earlier psychotherapeutic approaches for FEP emphasizing positive psychology.[50] IRT contains 7 "standard" modules that are considered foundational for all persons with FEP in CSC as they help to frame the therapy, support the person in setting goals and preventing relapse, provide psychoeducation about psychosis, offer a structure to process the episode of psychosis, and promote resiliency. The standard modules cover the following:

1. Orientation
2. Assessment and goal-setting
3. Education about psychosis
4. Relapse prevention planning
5. Processing the episode
6. Developing resiliency: part one
7. Building a bridge to your goals

IRT also contains 7 "individualized" modules that cover the following:

1. Dealing with negative feelings
2. Coping with symptoms
3. Substance use
4. Having fun and developing good relationships
5. Making choices about smoking

6. Nutrition and exercise
7. Developing resiliency: part two

The decision to offer the content of the individualized modules is made collaboratively between the therapist and client based on the client's personal goals.[48] IRT is typically delivered on a weekly or biweekly basis for as long as needed (eg, delivered for 2 years in the RAISE-ETP trial[7,32,48]).

Group Therapies

Group-based therapies that target social cognition and social skills are effective in promoting functioning[51,52] and negative symptoms[53] among those with established schizophrenia. A few studies have examined their use in FEP populations,[44,54,55] and these studies demonstrate considerable promise given the social cognitive difficulties that persons with FEP experience.[56] Social Skills Training (SST[57]) is an evidence-based intervention that focuses on helping individuals learn and practice skills involved in social interactions (eg, making requests, expressing positive feelings). SST groups often include a discussion of the rationale for a skill, specific steps of the skill, role-play exercises, feedback from the group, and homework assignments. This intervention has been shown to help individuals learn and practice social skills within the group setting and, subsequently, use them effectively in the community. Number of sessions per week and total weeks depend on the needs of the clients and the setting in which it is delivered (eg, mean number of weeks = 19.3 with a range of 2–104 weeks reported in one study).[52]

Cognitive enhancement therapy (CET[58]) has shown benefits in schizophrenia and in early psychosis. CET is composed of computer training (focused on attention, memory, and problem-solving) group therapy (focused on perspective-taking, managing emotions, reading nonverbal cues, and interpreting social situations).[59] CET typically consists of 60 hours of computer training and 45 weekly group sessions. This integrated intervention has been shown to improve social cognition and neurocognition in those with established schizophrenia[60] and in those with FEP.[61]

Stand-alone social cognition training interventions aim to improve individuals' capacity to understand, interpret, and use social information effectively, often targeting one or more of the primary domains of social cognition: theory of mind, emotion perception, social perception, and attributional style.[62] For example, Social Cognition Interaction Training (SCIT), has been examined extensively in established schizophrenia and has been piloted in a sample of persons with FEP.[63] SCIT is delivered as a 20-session to 24-session group psychotherapy typically delivered weekly[64] that includes 3 phases: emotion training (eg, identifying emotions from photos of faces, relationship between emotions and thoughts), figuring out situations (eg, distinguishing between facts and guesses in social situations), and integration (discussion of how information can be applied to salient situations). Individuals learn effective social cognitive strategies, practice them within the groups, and ultimately use them in everyday interactions.

Family Therapies

Historically, family interventions have been underutilized in the treatment of individuals with schizophrenia,[65] despite their clear benefit in reducing relapse and rehospitalization.[66–68] Over recent years, however, family interventions have occupied a more central role in the treatment of FEP.[12] Family intervention, as part of CSC, typically includes education, validation of the impact of psychosis on the family, communication, problem-solving, and goal-setting skills training.

Family education about psychosis and its optimal management serves a number of purposes:

1. Developing a shared language for the treatment team, individual, and the family to talk about psychosis and associated symptoms
2. Providing information so that individuals with psychosis and their families can make informed choices about illness management
3. Orienting the family to how they can support the management of their relative's illness and pursuit of personal goals

Educational topics include information about psychosis and associated symptoms, the stress-vulnerability model of psychosis, diagnosis and prognosis, the role of the family in treatment, early warning signs monitoring, and relapse-prevention planning. Family education provides the opportunity for family members to observe how the clinician talks to the individual with psychosis about symptoms, diagnosis, treatment, and recovery.

Families are often put under tremendous stress due to the disruptions in the family system that result from an episode of psychosis. A key underlying aspect of family interventions is the validation of this stress for the entire family system. Before the onset of the psychosis, the young adult may have been living independently, such that the onset of an illness represents a shifting of roles and worry for the entire family system. Communication, problem-solving, and goal-setting skills training can be important for families during this period of adjustment and heightened stress. Communication skills are aimed at reducing stressful interaction styles characterized by strong displays of negative affect or ambiguous messages and emphasize the use of direct "I statements," reference to specific behaviors, and specific feeling statements taught using the principles skills training (eg, modeling, role playing). Common targets for communication include medication, symptoms, and disclosure of information about the illness with the immediate, as well as the extended, family. In addition, it may be important for family members to reestablish how they will make requests of one another, which dovetails with the question of reasonable expectations of the individual with psychosis during the immediate period following illness onset and beyond.

Fostering problem-solving and goal-setting skills in the family serves the dual purpose of minimizing strife and facilitating recovery through each family member's identification of meaningful goals. Early in treatment, families often work toward the goal of increasing shared pleasant activities, which can increase family connection, shift the focus from illness to enjoyment and fun, and help remediate negative symptoms and demoralization that are commonly associated with the experience of psychosis. Later in treatment, families often take on more challenging goals, such as assisting the young person in returning to school or work, living independently, or traveling for educational or leisure purposes.

Multifamily group (MFG) interventions typically include 5 to 7 families who meet with 2 clinicians on a biweekly basis,[69] following "joining" sessions in which each family meets individually with the clinician to form a relationship and provide information about their family's specific needs. Each MFG session lasts approximately 90 minutes and the content of the sessions map onto 4 treatment stages corresponding to the phases of an episode of psychosis: (1) engagement between client and their family, (2) education about the psychotic disorder, (3) development of strategies, such as stress reduction, to cope with the challenges of psychosis recovery, and (4) social and vocational rehabilitation.[69] Elements of MFG considered to be particularly effective include access to a social network, reduction in perception of stigmatization, availability of mutual aid, and the opportunity to hear similar experiences and solutions.[69] Although there can be some initial challenges with establishing a critical mass of families willing to attend a group, MFG is cost-effective[70] and has been demonstrated to increase perception of ability to cope with a relative's psychosis,[71] and reduce FEP program dropout rates.[72]

CLINICAL CHALLENGES

Individuals with FEP vary tremendously from one another in terms of the severity of positive symptoms, negative symptoms, and cognitive and social functioning. The most significant challenges in therapy with individuals with FEP arise from the need to adapt the treatment to each individual's specific symptom presentation and understanding of his or her problems. Problematic substance use[73] and history of trauma or posttraumatic stress disorder[74] also add complexity to the treatment of some individuals. Furthermore, significant stressors beyond coping with FEP (eg, limited income, transportation barriers, homelessness) can interfere with the feasibility of delivering treatment and, thus, should be considered when trying to engage and maintain persons in therapy. In these instances, mobile teams and/or case management supports (eg, transportation paid for by health insurance or access to disability payments[75]) are essential ingredients to involve the individual and family in care and reduce strain on poorer families.

Negative symptoms, cognitive deficits, and impaired social and occupational functioning tend to co-occur in primary psychotic disorders and are defining features of FEP. Clinicians may struggle to engage individuals with negative symptoms and families may blame these individuals for being "lazy" or "unmotivated," which can amplify familial stress and impede recovery. Education about negative symptoms, spending more time getting to know the individual (eg, befriending techniques[76,77]), and slowing down the pace of therapy as well as breaking goals into small steps can be useful. An important part of the educational process involves dispelling the myth that negative symptoms indicate a lack of distress, because in fact, individuals with negative symptoms are often bothered by these symptoms and this is related to poor quality of life.[78] Therefore, recognizing and labeling this distress can serve as a rationale to build coping skills for these symptoms. Another important discovery has been the identification of common dysfunctional beliefs expressed by individuals with negative symptoms,[79,80] such as beliefs about self-efficacy (eg, "I don't have enough energy or I don't have anything to say") and anticipatory pleasure (eg, "I won't have a good time"), which are thought to impair effortful responding and can be addressed through cognitive restructuring and behavioral experiments.[81,82] Further, given the variability in cognitive functioning among persons with FEP (eg, due to age, effects of medication/electroconvulsive therapy, symptoms), psychosocial interventions should be appropriately tailored to the cognitive capacity of each individual.

Another challenge when working with persons with FEP and their families is sensitively and effectively addressing the role of trauma in therapy. Many persons with FEP have had traumatic experiences in their lives,[83] which may have been associated with the experience of psychosis and psychiatric treatment (eg, involuntary hospitalization, coercive treatment, use of restraints, and/or police involvement).[84] IRT includes a module called "processing the episode," which aims to help individuals integrate, process and understand the trauma of experiencing psychosis, and interventions designed to facilitate cognitive processing of traumatic experience in FEP have shown positive outcomes.[85]

Cultural and religious factors can also impact the willingness of clients and families to engage in treatment. For example, individuals of some cultural and religious backgrounds may not believe that psychological or psychiatric medication approaches to treatment are appropriate and may seek out alternative options (eg, shaman, exorcism, religious practices). Therapists should try to work within the cultural context of the given client and family to best support the recovery of the person with FEP. Therapists should use a curious attitude about these alternative approaches and better understand how they fit within the cultural context of the family and, importantly, assess any potential risk for the person. However, people may also be open to alternative explanations of their experience, especially when they are less distressing or more helpful. Therapists may also offer an "open door" policy so that individuals and families know that they are welcome to reconnect in the future.

SUMMARY

CSC programs provide team-based, comprehensive, evidence-based care, education, and support across 2 to 3 years to individuals experiencing their first episode of psychosis and their families. A collaborative clinical approach within CSCs are important. Individual, group, and family therapies represent critical aspects of CSC as they are aimed at helping individuals with FEP and their families navigate the distressing experience of psychosis and to promote recovery and well-being. Several individual (eg, CBT-p, IRT), group (eg, SST, SCIT, CET), and family (eg, family psychoeducation) therapies have demonstrated benefits for this population and are guided by the individual's goals and long-term vision of recovery. However, there are many clinical challenges that often accompany FEP therapy delivery that warrant significant attention. Therapists should be aware of these challenges and develop strategies to engage and maintain clients and their families in therapy. It is through awareness of challenges, prioritization of the therapeutic alliance, and effective delivery of evidence-based therapies that therapists can help clients and their families work toward recovery.

REFERENCES

1. Heinssen RK, Goldstein AB, Azrin ST. Evidence-Based Treatments for First Episode Psychosis: Components of Coordinated Specialty Care. NIMH White Pap. 2014.
2. Breitborde NJK, Moe AM. Early intervention in psychosis in the United States. Policy Insights Behav Brain Sci 2017;4(1):79–87.
3. National Institute for Health and Care Excellence. Implementing the early intervention in psychosis access and waiting time standard: guidance, vol. 57, 2016. Available at: https://www.england.nhs.uk/mentalhealth/wp-content/uploads/sites/29/2016/04/eip-guidance.pdf. Accessed April 30, 2019.
4. Correll CU, Galling B, Pawar A, et al. Comparison of early intervention services vs treatment as usual for early-phase psychosis. JAMA Psychiatry 2018;75(6):555.
5. Bertolote J, McGorry P. Early intervention and recovery for young people with early psychosis: consensus statement. Br J Psychiatry 2005;187(Suppl.48): s116–9.
6. Marshall M, Rathbone J. Early intervention for psychosis. Schizophr Bull 2011; 37(6):1111–4.
7. Kane JM, Robinson DG, Schooler NR, et al. Comprehensive versus usual community care for first episode psychosis: two-year outcomes from the NIMH RAISE early treatment program. Am J Geriatr Psychiatry 2016;173(4):362–72.

8. Malla AK, Norman RMG, Manchanda R, et al. One year outcome in first episode psychosis: influence of DUP and other predictors. Schizophr Res 2002;54(3): 231–42. Available at: http://www.ncbi.nlm.nih.gov/pubmed/11950548.

9. McGorry PD, Killackey E, Yung AR. Early intervention in psychotic disorders: detection and treatment of the first episode and the critical early stages. Med J Aust 2007;187(7 Suppl):S8–10. Available at: http://www.ncbi.nlm.nih.gov/pubmed/17908033.

10. Rosenheck R, Leslie D, Sint K, et al. Cost-effectiveness of comprehensive, integrated care for first episode psychosis in the NIMH raise early treatment program. Schizophr Bull 2016;42(4):896–906.

11. Dixon LB, Goldman H, Bennett M, et al. Implementing coordinated specialty care for early psychosis: the RAISE connection program. Psychiatr Serv 2015;66(7): 691–8.

12. Kane JM, Robinson DG, Schooler NR, et al. Comprehensive versus usual community care for first-episode psychosis: 2-year outcomes from the NIMH RAISE early treatment program. Am J Psychiatry 2015;173(4):362–72.

13. Srihari VH, Tek C, Kucukgoncu S, et al. First-episode services for psychotic disorders in the U.S. public sector: a pragmatic randomized controlled trial. Psychiatr Serv 2015;66:705–12.

14. Srihari VH, Tek C, Kucukgoncu S, et al. First-episode services for psychotic disorders in the U.S. Public sector: a pragmatic randomized controlled trial. Psychiatr Serv 2015;66(7):705–12.

15. Valmaggia LR, Byrne M, Day F, et al. Duration of untreated psychosis and need for admission in patients who engage with mental health services in the prodromal phase. Br J Psychiatry 2015;207(2):130–4.

16. Bird V, Premkumar P, Kendall T, et al. Early intervention services, cognitive-behavioural therapy and family intervention in early psychosis: systematic review. Br J Psychiatry 2010;197(5):350–6.

17. Thorup A, Petersen L, Jeppesen P, et al. Integrated treatment ameliorates negative symptoms in first episode psychosis-results from the Danish OPUS trial. Schizophr Res 2005;79(1):95–105.

18. Bertelsen M, Jeppesen P, Petersen L, et al. Five-year follow-up of a randomized multicenter trial of intensive early intervention vs standard treatment for patients with a first episode of psychotic illness. Arch Gen Psychiatry 2008;65(7):762–71.

19. Chen EYH, Honer WG, Yew CWS, et al. Three-year outcome of phase-specific early intervention for first-episode psychosis: a cohort study in Hong Kong. Early Interv Psychiatry 2011;5(4):315–23.

20. Mihalopoulos C, Harris M, Henry L, et al. Is early intervention in psychosis cost-effective over the long term? Schizophr Bull 2009;35(5):909–18.

21. Hardy KV, Landa Y, Meyer-Kalos P, et al. Psychotherapeutic interventions for early psychosis. In: Hardy KV, Ballon JS, Noordsy DL, et al, editors. Intervening early in psychosis: a team approach. Washington, DC: American Psychiatric Publishing; 2019. p. 211–39.

22. Gleeson JF, Cotton SM, Alvarez-Jimenez M, et al. Family outcomes from a randomized control trial of relapse prevention therapy in first-episode psychosis. J Clin Psychiatry 2010;71:475–83.

23. Becker D, Swanson S, Drake R, et al. Supported Education for persons experiencing a first episode of psychosis. In: In Issue Brief: Technical Assistance Material Developed for SAMHSA/CMHS under Contract Reference: HHSS283201200002I/ Task Order No. HHSS28342002T. 2015:1-15.

24. Rosenheck R, Mueser KT, Sint K, et al. Supported employment and education in comprehensive, integrated care for first episode psychosis: effects on work, school, and disability income. Schizophr Res 2017;182:120–8.

25. Addington DE, McKenzie E, Norman R, et al. Essential evidence-based components of first-episode psychosis services. Psychiatr Serv 2013;64(5):452–7.

26. Bertelsen M, Jeppesen P, Petersen L, et al. Five-year follow-up of a randomized multicenter trial of intensive early intervention vs standard treatment for patients with a first episode of psychotic illness: the OPUS trial. Arch Gen Psychiatry 2008;65(7):762–71.

27. Norman RMG, Manchanda R, Malla AK, et al. Symptom and functional outcomes for a 5-year early intervention program for psychoses. Schizophr Res 2011; 129(2–3):111–5.

28. Mueser KT, Penn DL, Addington J, et al. The NAVIGATE program for first-episode psychosis: rationale, overview, and description of psychosocial components. Psychiatr Serv 2015;66(7):680–90.

29. Modini M, Tan L, Brinchmann B, et al. Supported employment for people with severe mental illness: systematic review and meta-analysis of the international evidence. Br J Psychiatry 2016;209(1):14–22.

30. Albert N, Melau M, Jensen H, et al. Five years of specialised early intervention versus two years of specialised early intervention followed by three years of standard treatment for patients with a first episode psychosis: randomised, superiority, parallel group trial in Denmark (OPUS II). BMJ 2017;356:1–14.

31. Shepherd G, Boardman J, Slade M. Making recovery a reality. Scottish Recover Netw 2008;1–23.

32. Mueser KT, Penn DL, Addington J, et al. The NAVIGATE program for first-episode psychosis: rationale, overview, and description of psychosocial components. Psychiatr Serv 2015;66(7):680–90.

33. Shattock L, Berry K, Degnan A, et al. Therapeutic alliance in psychological therapy for people with schizophrenia and related psychoses: a systematic review. Clin Psychol Psychother 2018;25(1):e60–85.

34. Browne J, Nagendra A, Kurtz M, et al. The relationship between the therapeutic alliance and client variables in individual treatment for schizophrenia spectrum disorders and early psychosis: narrative review. Clin Psychol Rev 2019;71:51–62.

35. Browne J, Bass E, Mueser KT, et al. Client predictors of the therapeutic alliance in individual resiliency training for first episode psychosis. Schizophr Res 2019;204: 375–80.

36. Browne J, Mueser KT, Meyer-Kalos P, et al. The therapeutic alliance in individual resiliency training for first episode psychosis: relationship with treatment outcomes and therapy participation. J Consult Clin Psychol 2019;87(8):734–44.

37. Bordin ES. The generalizability of the psychoanalytic concept of the working alliance. Psychol Psychother Theor Res Pract 1979;16(3):252–60.

38. Kreyenbuhl J, Nossel IR, Dixon LB. Disengagement from mental health treatment among individuals with schizophrenia and strategies for facilitating connections to care: a review of the literature. Schizophr Bull 2009;35(4):696–703.

39. Turkington D, Kingdon D, Weiden PJ. Reviews and overviews cognitive behavior therapy for schizophrenia. Am J Psychiatry 2006;163:365–73. Available at: https://ajp.psychiatryonline.org/doi/pdf/10.1176/appi.ajp.163.3.365.

40. Wykes T, Steel C, Everitt B, et al. Cognitive behavior therapy for schizophrenia: effect sizes, clinical models, and methodological rigor. Schizophr Bull 2008; 34(3):523–37.

41. Gumley A, O'Grady M, McNay L, et al. Early intervention for relapse in schizophrenia: results of a 12-month randomized controlled trial of cognitive behavioural therapy. Psychol Med 2003;33(3):419–31.
42. Burns AMN, Erickson DH, Brenner CA. Cognitive-behavioral therapy for medication-resistant psychosis: a meta-analytic review. Psychiatr Serv 2014; 65(7):874–80.
43. Turkington D, Kingdon D, Weiden PJ. Reviews and overviews cognitive behavior therapy for schizophrenia. Am J Psychiatry 2006;163:365–73.
44. Lecomte T, Leclerc C, Corbière M, et al. Group cognitive behavior therapy or social skills training for individuals with a recent onset of psychosis? Results of a randomized controlled trial. J Nerv Ment Dis 2008;196(12):866–75.
45. Saksa JR, Cohen SJ, Srihari VH, et al. Cognitive behavior therapy for early psychosis: a comprehensive review of individual vs. group treatment studies. Int J Group Psychother 2009;59(3):357–83.
46. Zubin J, Spring B. Vulnerability: a new view of schizophrenia. J Abnorm Psychol 1977;86(2):103–26.
47. Fowler D, Garety P, Kuipers E. Cognitive behavior therapy for psychosis. Theory and Practice 1995;25.
48. Meyer PS, Gottlieb JD, Penn D, et al. Individual resiliency training: an early intervention approach to enhance well-being in people with first-episode psychosis. Psychiatr Ann 2015;45(11):554–60.
49. Gingerich S, Mueser KT. Illness management and recovery: personalized skills and strategies for those with mental illness. 3rd edition. Center City (MN): Hazelden; 2011.
50. Penn DL, Uzenoff SR, Perkins D, et al. A pilot investigation of the Graduated Recovery Intervention Program (GRIP) for first episode psychosis. Schizophr Res 2011;125(2–3):247–56.
51. Kurtz MM, Gagen E, Rocha NBF, et al. Comprehensive treatments for social cognitive deficits in schizophrenia: a critical review and effect-size analysis of controlled studies. Clin Psychol Rev 2016;43:80–9.
52. Kurtz MM, Mueser KT. A meta-analysis of controlled research on social skills training for schizophrenia. J Consult Clin Psychol 2008;76(3):491–504.
53. Turner DT, McGlanaghy E, Cuijpers P, et al. A meta-analysis of social skills training and related interventions for psychosis. Schizophr Bull 2018;44(3): 475–91.
54. Lecomte T, Leclerc C, Wykes T. Group CBT for early psychosis—are there still benefits one year later? Int J Group Psychother 2012;62(2):309–21.
55. Lecomte T, Leclerc C, Wykes T, et al. Understanding process in group cognitive behaviour therapy for psychosis. Psychol Psychother 2015;88(2):163–77.
56. Healey KM, Bartholomeusz CF, Penn DL. Deficits in social cognition in first episode psychosis: a review of the literature. Clin Psychol Rev 2016;50:108–37.
57. Bellack A, Mueser KT, Gingerich S, et al. Social skills training for schizophrenia: a step-by-step guide. New York: The Guilford Press; 2013.
58. Hogarty GE, Greenwald DP. Cognitive enhancement therapy: the training manual. University of Pittsburgh Medical Center. Available at: www.CognitiveEnhancementTherapy.com. Accessed April 30, 2019.
59. Keshavan MS, Eack SM. Cognitive enhancement in schizophrenia and related disorders. Cambridge (United Kingdom): Cambridge University Press.; 2019.
60. Hogarty GE, Flesher S, Ulrich R, et al. Cognitive enhancement therapy for schizophrenia. Effects of a 2-year randomized trial on cognition and behavior. Arch Gen Psychiatry 2004;364(9452):2163–5.

61. Eack S, Greenwalf D, Hodgarty S, et al. Cognitive enhancement therapy for early-course schizophrenia: effects of a two-year randomized controlled trial. Psychiatr Serv 2009;60(11):1468–76.

62. Kurtz M, Richardson C. Social cognitive training for schizophrenia: a meta-analytic investigation of controlled research. Schizophr Bull 2012;38(5):1092–104.

63. Bartholomeusz CF, Allott K, Killackey E, et al. Social cognition training as an intervention for improving functional outcome in first-episode psychosis: a feasibility study. Early Interv Psychiatry 2013;7(4):421–6.

64. Penn PD, Roberts DL, Combs D, et al. Best practices: the development of the social cognition and interaction training program for schizophrenia spectrum disorders. Psychiatr Serv 2007;58(4):3–5.

65. Glynn SM. Family interventions in schizophrenia: promise and pitfalls over 30 years. Curr Psychiatry Rep 2012;14(3):237–43.

66. Pharoah F., Mari J., Steiner D. Family interventions for schizophrenia (Cochrane systematic reviews). Cochrane Library. Available at: www.cochranelibrary.com. Accessed September 19, 2019.

67. Pilling B, Kuipers G, Kuipers E, et al. Psychological treatments in schizophrenia: I. Meta-analysis of family intervention and cognitive behaviour therapy. Psychol Med 2002;32(5):763–82. Available at: http://ovidsp.ovid.com/ovidweb.cgi?T=JS&PAGE=reference&D=emed5&NEWS=N&AN=2002271676.

68. Camacho-Gomez M, Castellvi P. Effectiveness of family intervention for preventing relapse in first-episode psychosis until 24 months of follow-up: a systematic review with meta-analysis of randomized controlled trials. Schizophr Bull 2019 [pii:sbz038] [Epub ahead of print].

69. McFarlane WR. Family intervention in first episode psychosis. J Fam Psychother 2005;16(3):85–104.

70. Breitborde NJK, Woods SW, Srihari VH. Multifamily psychoeducation for first-episode psychosis: a cost-effectiveness analysis. Psychiatr Serv 2009;23(20):1–10.

71. Regina R, Cabral F, Chaves AC. Multi-family group intervention in a programme for patients with first-episode psychosis: a Brazilian experience. Int J Soc Psychiatry 2010;56(5):527–32.

72. Rossberg JI, Johannessen JO, Klungsoyr O, et al. Are multi family groups appropriate for patients with first episode psychosis? A 5-year naturalistic follow-up study. Acta Psychiatr Scand 2010;122(5):384–94.

73. Weibell MA, Hegelstad WTV, Auestad B, et al. The effect of substance use on 10-year outcome in first-episode psychosis. Schizophr Bull 2017;43(4):843–51.

74. Neria Y, Bromet EJ, Sievers S, et al. Trauma exposure and posttraumatic stress disorder in psychosis: findings from a first-admission cohort. J Consult Clin Psychol 2002;70(1):246–51.

75. Rosenheck RA, Estroff SE, Sint K, et al. Incomes and outcomes: Social Security disability benefits in first-episode psychosis. Am J Psychiatry 2017;174(9):886–94.

76. Penn DL, Mueser KT, Tarrier N, et al. Supportive therapy for schizophrenia: possible mechanisms and implications for adjunctive psychosocial treatments. Schizophr Bull 2004;30(1):101–12.

77. Samarasekera N, Kingdon D, Siddle R, et al. Befriending patients with medication-resistant schizophrenia: can psychotic symptoms predict treatment response? Psychol Psychother 2007;80(1):97–106.

78. Mueser KT, Douglas MS, Bellack AS, et al. Assessment of enduring deficit and negative symptom subtypes in schizophrenia. Schizophr Bull 1991;17(4):565–82.

79. Rector NA, Beck AT, Stolar N. The negative symptoms of schizophrenia: a cognitive perspective. Can J Psychiatry 2005;50(5):247–57.

80. Beck AT, Grant PM, Huh GA, et al. Dysfunctional attitudes and expectancies in deficit syndrome schizophrenia. Schizophr Bull 2013;39(1):43–51.

81. Staring ABP, Ter Huurne MAB, Van Der Gaag M. Cognitive Behavioral Therapy for negative symptoms (CBT-n) in psychotic disorders: a pilot study. J Behav Ther Exp Psychiatry 2013;44(3):300–6.

82. Perivoliotis D, Cather C. Cognitive behavioral therapy of negative symptoms. J Clin Psychol 2010;66(4):430–41.

83. Grubaugh AL, Zinzow HM, Paul L, et al. Trauma exposure and posttraumatic stress disorder in adults with severe mental illness: a critical review. Clin Psychol Rev 2011;31(6):883–99.

84. Mueser KT, Lu W, Rosenberg SD, et al. The trauma of psychosis: posttraumatic stress disorder and recent onset psychosis. Schizophr Res 2010;116(2–3): 217–27.

85. Jackson C, Trower P, Reid I, et al. Improving psychological adjustment following a first episode of psychosis: a randomised controlled trial of cognitive therapy to reduce post psychotic trauma symptoms. Behav Res Ther 2009;47(6):454–62.

Community Rehabilitation for Youth with Psychosis Spectrum Disorders

Pamela Rakhshan Rouhakhtar, MA, Jason Schiffman, PhD*

KEYWORDS

- Psychosis • Youth • Community rehabilitation • Recovery • Care coordination
- Cognitive rehabilitation • Supported education and employment • Peer support

KEY POINTS

- Similar to individuals with chronic psychosis, youth and young adults with early psychosis often experience poor functional outcomes.
- Community rehabilitation programs for psychosis, including care coordination, cognitive rehabilitation, supported education and employment, and peer support, are effective complementary interventions for youth with psychosis.
- Some community rehabilitation programs, including supported education and employment, for youth with psychosis are empirically supported and should be integrated into standard care, whereas others appear promising, but require further evidence to demonstrate feasibility, efficacy, and relevance for youth.

INTRODUCTION

With the aspiration of integrating care within the community, the deinstitutionalization of mental health care for people with psychotic disorders was one of the catalysts of the development of what is now broadly referred to as community rehabilitation.[1–4] The guiding philosophy behind this approach to treatment is that individuals with serious mental health concerns receive care that is person-centered, striving toward both symptomatic and functional recovery, with care embedded *within* their

Disclosure Statement: This work was supported by the National Institute of Mental Health (grants R01MH112612 and R34MH110506 to J. Schiffman), the Maryland Department of Health and Mental Hygiene, Behavioral Health Administration through the Center for Excellence on Early Intervention for Serious Mental Illness (OPASS# 14-13717G/M00B4400241 to J. Schiffman), and the Substance Abuse and Mental Health Services Administration (Community Intervention for those at Clinical High Risk for Psychosis, vis à vis the Maryland State Department of Health, SM081092-01).

Department of Psychology, University of Maryland, Baltimore County, 1000 Hilltop Circle, Baltimore, MD 21250, USA
* Corresponding author.
E-mail address: schiffma@umbc.edu

Child Adolesc Psychiatric Clin N Am 29 (2020) 225–239
https://doi.org/10.1016/j.chc.2019.08.012
1056-4993/20/© 2019 Elsevier Inc. All rights reserved.

childpsych.theclinics.com

community. Putting this philosophy into practice has yielded a collection of interventions designed to help people with psychosis and related concerns develop skills that assist in daily living, moving beyond approaches that limit attention to clinical symptoms. With its origins firmly rooted in an effort to provide care in the contexts in which clients carry out their lives, community rehabilitation emphasizes functional recovery in domains such as school and work, interpersonal relationships, and tasks of basic daily living.[1,5] At the same time, functional recovery is supported by a concurrent focus on symptomatic functioning through an integration of targeted therapy and pharmacologic methods.

Across all domains of intervention, a recovery-oriented approach to treatment is taken in community rehabilitation interventions, promoting active engagement, autonomy, and respectful collaboration between clients and providers.[6] This is not unique to community rehabilitation programs, but reflects the broader move toward recovery-oriented care for individuals with psychosis across the life span.[7,8] Individuals experiencing the early phases of psychosis endorse autonomy and empowerment as important aspects of the recovery process,[9] highlighting the importance of recovery-oriented, person-centered approaches in early interventions for psychosis spectrum disorders.

Although community rehabilitation provides significant incremental value to individuals at all stages of development, there may be specific advantages for young people who often experience the onset of psychosis spectrum disorders during critical periods of development. Gold-standard, evidence-based intervention models for people in the early stages of psychosis therefore include developmentally tailored rehabilitation components, with clients showing greater functional and symptomatic improvement, better engagement in treatment, and higher quality of life than peers in typical care.[10,11] Important improvements in functional domains like school and work seem to be linked directly to provision of community rehabilitation interventions.[12] Although the scope of community rehabilitation for early psychosis is vast, this article focuses on 4 specific interventions within community rehabilitation: care coordination, cognitive rehabilitation, supportive employment and education, and peer mentoring.

CARE COORDINATION
Challenges

Ample and concerning evidence suggests that many individuals who have been hospitalized for a psychotic illness are discharged without connections to mental health services, and as a result, often enter a "revolving door" of discharge to readmission.[13,14] In a review of the supportive care needs of individuals experiencing their first episode of psychosis, practical needs, or the need for active assistance with the tasks of daily life, were found to be both endorsed and unmet among youth across studies.[15] Although it is an almost universal challenge for adolescents and young adults to gain competence and independence in daily life tasks as they transition to adulthood, research indicates that youth with psychosis experience significantly greater difficulties as compared with their peers without mental health concerns, particularly in the domains of housing, financial independence, educational attainment, and social functioning.[16] Thus, rehabilitation interventions that provide practical support to youth with psychosis are vital to promote not only engagement in care, but also in life and work within the community.

Current Interventions

Having a mental health professional work alongside clients in the early phases of psychosis to facilitate connection to services and identify and address unmet needs is at the core of all comprehensive community rehabilitation efforts. Several terms exist in the literature to describe this clinical intervention strategy and care partnership, including "case management" (perhaps the most commonly used), "care management," or "care coordination."[17] Despite the widespread use of the term "case management" in the health care field, we use the term "care coordination" (CC), as have others in the field,[18] given the illness-centric etymology of the word "case" (originally a medical term referring to the clinical state or symptomatic presentation of an ill or diseased person[19]), as well as its connection to stigmatizing terminology for those who experience mental health concerns (eg, "nut *case*" or "head *case*"[20]). Similarly, style guides for both the American Medical Association and the American Psychological Association suggest careful use of the word "case," cautioning against dehumanizing conflation between a person and a manifestation of illness.[21,22] Regardless of the label, the role of care coordinators (CCs) is to create a partnership with clients toward the goal of improving the well-being and quality of life of the client, often through the enhancement of care, including care continuity, availability, and efficiency, often across treatment domains and teams.[23]

Practices within CC can be diverse and broad in scope. Gold-standard CC provision is flexible, focused, and client-centered.[23] Best practice suggests limiting the number of clients on a coordinator's care roster so that the appropriate amount of personalized time and attention can be dedicated to each individual. Strategies for engagement tend to take a strengths-based approach, and are both centered on and driven by clients. Techniques or approaches used in CC can include brokering of care with other providers; limited provision of psychotherapy, skills training, and psychoeducation; strengths-based assessment and treatment planning; outreach and community-based care; and peer-based care.[18] Aspects of cognitive-behavioral therapy also have been integrated into the role of CCs, and can include specific strategies for engagement, stigma reduction, problem identification, problem solving, and monitoring symptoms and functioning.[24] CCs strive to connect clients to appropriate specialty care intended to support successful reintegration into the community, often requiring CCs to provide their services in the community and as frequently as needed, rather than the typical weekly 45-minute clinical hour delivered in an outpatient setting.

Despite its ubiquity in clinical care, CC has not received unmitigated support from empirical investigation. Compelling evidence does suggest that intensive, flexible care programs that integrate aspects of CC (such as assertive community treatment [ACT]) are typically effective in improving service engagement and utilization, clinical and functional outcomes for individuals with later-stage psychosis, whereas CC interventions alone (eg, intensive case management) are generally thought to be effective in improving factors such as role functioning, emergency service use, and quality of life.[18,25–27] The impact of CC on social functioning or hospitalization reduction, however, as well as the direct contribution of CC on outcomes seen in multicomponent intervention research is less clear.

Similar to the broader literature on adults with more long-standing illness, CC is considered an essential ingredient in gold-standard practices within interventions for youth at risk for or in early stages of psychosis, despite lack of extensive evidence of *unique* contributions of its specific role on outcomes.[14,28–32] CC elements, when added to first-episode treatment, may be helpful in improving engagement and connection with outpatient care, reduction in hospitalizations, and improvements in symptoms and functioning.[13,30] Given the manifest differences in the needs of youth as compared with adults, a sensitivity to developmental considerations can enhance efficacy of treatment when CCs are working with transition-aged youth and young adults. Skills in working in areas such as education, employment, peer relationships, and transition to a more autonomous lifestyle are all required attributes particularly when working with people in the early phases of psychosis who tend to fall within this developmental window.[16]

COGNITIVE REHABILITATION
Challenges

Deficits in cognitive functioning are thought to be core features of psychotic illness, resulting in impairments across a broad range of functional domains. Individuals with schizophrenia show both generalized and specific deficits across domains of cognition. Compared with nondiagnosed peers, people with schizophrenia tend to show impairments in memory, language, executive functioning, attention, and global cognitive functioning.[33,34] The first episode and early stages of psychosis also seem to be associated with similar deficits in nature and magnitude to those seen in chronic psychosis.[35–38] Premorbid and longitudinal evidence suggests deficits often emerge in childhood and adolescence.[39–41] As it pertains to community rehabilitation, cognitive deficits experienced by individuals with psychosis in high-risk, early-course, and chronic phases of illness are related to impairments in key domains of functioning in the community, including social and vocational outcomes, quality of life, and general daily living skills.[42–47]

Current Interventions

The intervention strategies within the field of cognitive rehabilitation for psychosis may be categorized into 2 separate traditions: cognitive enhancement, or interventions that seek to ameliorate cognitive deficits, and compensatory approaches, or programs that aim to address functional impairments caused by cognitive deficits.[48,49]

Cognitive enhancement

Cognitive enhancement interventions seek to improve cognition of individuals, with the underlying goal of eliminating or reducing targeted deficits.[50] Cognitive remediation therapy (CRT), perhaps the most well-known and studied cognitive enhancement intervention, targets cognitive capacity and processing, knowledge and cognitive schemas, motivation, and metacognition.[51] Other enhancement interventions include cognitive enhancement therapy (addressing social and nonsocial cognitive deficits[52]), attention shaping (which uses operant learning principles to address neurocognitive deficits[53]), and integrated psychological therapy for schizophrenia (a group-based, manualized cognitive-behavioral therapy program combining neurocognitive interventions with other psychosocial treatments, including social cognition, communication, social skills, and problem solving[54]). Empirical studies evaluating the feasibility and efficacy of cognitive enhancement interventions for individuals with schizophrenia suggest that such programs are generally feasible and effective in improving cognitive outcomes; however, positive *functional* outcomes are generally seen only in those interventions that are combined with other rehabilitation or psychosocial interventions like vocational skills training or psychotherapy.[52,54–56]

Similar to the established literature on adults with schizophrenia, cognitive enhancement interventions for youth experiencing early/first-episode psychosis are generally associated with improvements in cognition compared with control conditions, although effects are somewhat smaller when compared with those seen in individuals with schizophrenia, potentially due to higher baseline cognitive performance in those with first-episode psychosis.[57] Additional research has indicated CRT is effective compared with control treatments in improving specific outcomes like social functioning and negative symptoms for youth with first-episode psychosis.[58] Despite some promising findings, it is unclear whether these effects are due to adjunctive psychosocial interventions (eg, social skills training). Regardless, similar to the literature for later-stage illness, cognitive enhancement programs typically appear more effective and linked to more functional improvement when paired with other psychosocial rehabilitation interventions.[57]

Recent years have seen an interest in cognitive enhancement interventions for youth in prodromal or psychosis-risk phases of illness. Early results hold promise for feasibility of treatment, and suggest some reasons for optimism regarding efficacy; however, no work to date has demonstrated a robust link between enhancement intervention and improvement in functional domains independent of other psychosocial rehabilitation programs.[59–64]

Cognitive adaptation

Unlike enhancement strategies, cognitive adaptation or compensation programs for individuals with psychosis *do not* seek to improve cognitive deficits per se, but rather promote pragmatic strategies and interventions that assist clients in engaging and succeeding in functional domains.[49] Examples of these interventions include cognitive adaptation training (uses comprehensive assessment and implementation of adaptive strategies like using checklists, organization methods, and other environmental supports) and errorless learning interventions (breakdown of tasks into small components ordered by complexity, with training and aids given to prevent errors and promote automation in task completion).[49] Cognitive adaptation interventions for individuals with schizophrenia are associated with improvements in symptomatic and functional outcomes including community functioning, task or work performance, negative symptoms, social functioning, life satisfaction, decreases in caregiver burden, and improved treatment adherence.[65–72]

Despite promising findings for interventions targeted toward individuals in later stages of illness, the literature on compensatory cognitive interventions for youth with psychosis is relatively small. Although Hansen and colleagues[73] did not find that cognitive adaptation training provided additional benefit when combined with ACT in a multicenter study for individuals with first-episode psychosis, some recent work has documented feasibility of adaptive interventions, as well as improvements in global, occupational, and life quality domains in pre-posttest comparison.[74,75] Other research working with individuals in their first episode of psychosis has indicated that compensatory cognitive interventions are superior to treatment-as-usual in improving cognition, but not functional outcomes.[76] Although the results from research on adaptive cognitive interventions detailed previously, as well as additional preliminary work,[77–79] show promise for both feasibility and efficacy of adaptive cognitive interventions for youth in the early stages of psychosis, a great deal more work is needed to establish the incremental value of this rehabilitative intervention above current evidence-based practices.

Enhancement versus adaptive strategies

More work is needed to definitively identify which intervention strategies are best practice for youth with psychosis; however, current clinical thinking posits that cognitive enhancement interventions are particularly relevant for youth in earlier stages of psychosis relative to individuals with chronic illness. From a prevention perspective, cognitive enhancement techniques are thought to be indicated in early stages of psychosis with the hopes of preemptively staving off progressive cognitive deficits, while cognition is still relatively intact. In contrast, adaptive interventions are theoretically considered appropriate for deficits or functional impairments that are long-standing or intractable.[80,81] Whether either approach, when implemented early, is actually able to prevent the cognitive deficits and consequential functional impairments often seen in individuals with chronic psychosis is as of yet unclear.

Empirical work consistently demonstrates that effects of enhancement and adaptation programs are strongest when paired with other psychosocial rehabilitation intervention strategies.[57] Reflecting this, many current cognitive remediation programs combine both restorative exercises as well as adaptive strategies to promote functioning.[52,77,82] Thus, the distinction between enhancement versus adaptive strategies may be less meaningful, as most approaches integrate some of both. Nonetheless, future mechanism studies may provide important insights regarding which cognitive interventions and strategies are the most effective forms of care for youth in early stages of psychosis.

SUPPORTIVE EDUCATION AND EMPLOYMENT
Challenges

Youth with developmental and psychiatric disabilities often experience significant challenges in the domains of education and employment.[83] Work and educational experiences of youth with psychosis generally follow this trend, with such individuals experiencing significant difficulty in academic functioning, completion of degree programs, employment security, and financial stability.[16,39,84–88] Beyond the direct impact that cognitive deficits and other illness-related factors associated with psychosis may have on work and school, the onset of psychosis often occurs during periods critical for educational and vocational success, and can disrupt the trajectories of young people in these domains. The vicious cycle of symptom and effect, if not addressed via targeted interventions, may therefore have lasting or even irreversible negative implications for youth.

Current Interventions

Given the deficits associated with early psychosis in the domains of school and work, as well as the stigma and barriers experienced by individuals with psychosis,[89] supportive education and employment (SEE) rehabilitation programs are vital elements of early intervention for youth with psychosis. SEE programs typically provide aid and support to individuals in the domain of education with the goal of facilitating completion of educational programs or training. Common elements within these models include CC, educational skills development, and client advocacy.[90] Similarly, SEE programs targeting employment seek to facilitate a pathway from training to acquisition of jobs by promoting client choice, competitive employment, work incentives, supported job search, skills training, and individualized job supports when engaged in work.[91]

One of the most widely studied supported employment interventions is Individual Placement and Support (IPS). IPS increases participation and engagement in work among individuals with severe mental illness,[91] as well as employment rates in youth in the early stages of psychosis.[92,93] Other treatment models, such as the SEE program integrated into the NAVIGATE care program for first-episode psychosis,[94] or other modified IPS intervention models,[95] have adapted the principles and methods of IPS to integrate educational as well as vocational components, with promising results for both work and school engagement.

As compared with those receiving typical treatment, youth engaged in evidence-based, supported education/employment programs show superior involvement in work and/or school.[12] SEE programs, particularly those focusing on vocational interventions, show high levels of empirical support across the field, with a review by Addington and colleagues[96] indicating that among early psychosis treatment modalities, supported employment programs represented one of the few interventions that demonstrates an "A" level of evidence regarding efficacy. Although educational outcomes in IPS and other supported education/employment programs are not as robust when compared with vocational,[92] evidence seems to suggest that provision of educational and employment support is feasible and effective when delivered in one unified program.[95]

Despite the promising evidence regarding efficacy of supported education and employment interventions for youth with psychosis, a number of issues still exist regarding the long-term success in these domains for youth. For instance, there are mixed findings with respect to equal access and engagement in these services between minority and majority groups, with some findings suggesting worse outcomes for people who identify as ethnic minorities.[97,98] In addition, those with the best vocational outcomes in first-episode psychosis treatment programs are individuals with higher premorbid cognition and functioning, fewer concurrent symptoms, and previous work history or educational attainment.[44,98] Thus, future clinical and investigative work is needed to identify for whom SEE programs are *not* working, and what adaptations or modifications may be effective in promoting universal benefit of this rehabilitative program.

PEER SUPPORT
Challenges

Similar to those with more chronic forms of illness,[99] many people in their first episode of psychosis report limited social support networks and high levels of loneliness.[100] Stigma is an additional barrier for individuals with psychosis experience across a myriad of domains, with significant implications for care engagement and pursuit of goals.[101–103] In addition, youth in early stages of illness report the need to connect with and receive information from peers with similar lived experience.[15] Peer support interventions represent an accessible form of care that can address these concerns, with peer advocates lending value and perspective to mental health treatment teams in their efforts to engage and aid youth in the early stages of psychosis.

Current Interventions

Having faced and overcome similar challenges as the clients with whom they work, peer workers often serve as role models and advocates for people less far along on their illness trajectory. Peer work tends to be relationship based, focusing on connection; recognizing strengths; and creating a sense of partnership, mutuality, and respect. Although there may be variability in how to approach their role with clients, it is thought that a peer's self-disclosure of his or her lived experience conveys empathy, and ultimately increases self-efficacy of the client.[104,105] Peers can provide services in many forms and formats, including services unique to their role (eg, peer education, empathic support from the perspective of a peer, peer mentoring), or services considered more consistent with those provided by a traditional mental health professional (eg, care management, psychoeducation, traditional therapy).[18] Given the broad nature of the services they deliver, peer workers can fall along a continuum of nonpaid peer support to professional peer.[106]

The published research in this area provides a wide range of goals and processes used by peer workers. Strategies could include, but are not limited to, attempts to increase service engagement, self-disclosure to motivate change, the provision of skills training, and empowering their client/peer to be stronger advocates within their own treatment team.[104] Peer services are delivered in group as well as individual formats, with the frequency and duration varying without clear guidelines.[107] The variability in modality and process makes it difficult to generalize conclusions about a more single construct of "peer support," nonetheless, the theme that some number of services are being provided to clients by others who have similar lived experience is a unifying thread.

Despite the clear need for such services, the evidence for effectiveness of peer support interventions remains controversial. A well-cited review in 2014 by Lloyd-Evans and colleagues[107] concluded that the evidence did not support the efficacy of peer-led interventions for people with psychosis. The investigators highlighted a variety of methodological considerations, however, that likely impede a clear view of the true state of affairs with respect to the impact of peer-to-peer support. Issues such as recruitment strategies, the nature of samples, the content/delivery of the supports, the type of peer support provided (eg, peer-delivered mental health services vs mutual support), and the quality and completeness of outcome data all likely confounded findings. Recent reviews indicate this pattern still holds regarding efficacy of peer support in later-stage psychosis,[108] reflecting a broader trend in the literature on efficacy of peer support programs for mental health concerns.[106,109] Unsurprisingly, there is a similar lack of consensus or dearth of work regarding the efficacy of peer interventions for youth in early stages of psychosis. Given the promising nature of initial intervention trials for young people with other mental health concerns,[110] as well as qualitative work demonstrating the importance of peer support programs for families and youth,[111] this field seems promising. Alvarez-Jimenez and colleagues[112] recently completed a randomized clinical trial comparing an online intervention for youth with early psychosis to treatment-as-usual, with the intervention including peer-to-peer online social networking and peer moderation, in addition to interactive online therapy and expert moderation. Findings from this and other work on peer support for youth in early stages of psychosis will shed light on the efficacy of peer support interventions for young people, as well as the specific adaptations required for individuals in earlier stages of illness.

As peer involvement in care continues to evolve and becomes more mainstream in care, a variety of issues remain that will have implications for this area. One issue that requires awareness is the notion of roles. In particular, at what point does someone who is salaried and credentialed shift from the role of a peer to that of a professional in the eyes of his or her client, and how does that impact their relationship and efficacy? In addition, traditional program development and evaluation (and research) tend to be driven by professionals. Creating room for more active and equal peer collaboration from the ground up at every level of activity will have implications for the impact of peers for clients. A further consideration for work with youth where there is no existing guidance is potential age/generational differences between peers, and how these differences may impact services.

The existing research in the area of peer workers is as varied as the provision of support by peers. Issues including the definition of a "peer"; role of peers in care; frequency, duration, and intensity of peer services; fidelity to a model; reliability across studies; inclusion of specific outcome measures; use of both qualitative and quantitative approaches in harmony; and appropriate conducting and reporting of randomized controlled trials all contribute to confusion in this area. Of additional note, no compelling research in this area provides particular guidance with respect to differential effects of peer services for youth versus adults. These issues and more await future research.

SUMMARY

Community rehabilitation programs reflect the broader trends in mental health care toward recovery-oriented, outcomes-focused services. Interventions for youth with psychosis share this approach, attempting to reduce long-term disability and improve functioning through preventive, multi-modal, client-centered treatment. Since the model of early intervention in psychosis was first introduced, there has been a rapid expansion in policy, research, and clinical advances to aid the ultimate goal of reducing or even avoiding the disability often associated with chronic psychosis. Community rehabilitation is an important component of this intervention movement.

The current article reviewed 4 community rehabilitation interventions for youth in early stages of psychosis: CC, cognitive rehabilitation, supported education and employment, and peer support. Within each intervention domain, the evidence suggests that current rehabilitation programs are generally feasible and have the potential to aid in functional recovery and care engagement among youth in early stages of psychosis. Some interventions, however, such as supported education and employment, seem to be associated with greater quantity and quality of empirical support compared with other intervention domains requiring further work to establish feasibility and specific efficacy among youth, such as cognitive rehabilitation strategies.

More work is needed to establish the mechanisms behind successful findings. Understanding mechanisms will also contribute to more personalized approaches to the implementation of these interventions, as the field becomes more sophisticated in addressing questions related to what strategies, and at what intensity, work for whom. In particular, generalizability of rehabilitative interventions to diverse settings and populations, as well as the adaptations needed for success of such programs across contexts and individuals, remain a priority. Despite a need for continued work, the existing evidence suggests the essential nature of community rehabilitation efforts to support youth with early stages of psychosis. CC, cognitive remediation, supported education/employment, and peer support all represent crucial elements of care within a successful recovery-oriented approach to working with young people with psychosis.

REFERENCES

1. Killackey E, Alvarez-Jimenez M, Allott K, et al. Community rehabilitation and psychosocial interventions for psychotic disorders in youth. Child Adolesc Psychiatr Clin N Am 2013;22(4):745–58.
2. Killaspy H. Contemporary mental health rehabilitation. East Asian Arch Psychiatry 2014;24(3):89.
3. van der Meer L, Wunderink C. Contemporary approaches in mental health rehabilitation. Epidemiol Psychiatr Sci 2019;28(1):9–14.
4. Wykes T, Holloway F. Community rehabilitation: past failures and future prospects. Int Rev Psychiatry 2000;12(3):197–205.
5. Lloyd C, Bassett J, Samra P. Rehabilitation programmes for early psychosis. Br J Occup Ther 2000;63(2):76–82.
6. Corrigan PW, Mueser KT, Bond GR, et al. What is psychiatric rehabilitation. In: Principles and practice of psychiatric rehabilitation: an empirical approach. 2nd edition. New York: Guilford Press; 2016. p. 47–65.
7. Silverstein SM, Bellack AS. A scientific agenda for the concept of recovery as it applies to schizophrenia. Clin Psychol Rev 2008;28(7):1108–24.
8. Lieberman JA, Dixon LB, Goldman HH. Early detection and intervention in schizophrenia: a new therapeutic model. JAMA 2013;310(7):689–90.

9. Temesgen WA, Chien WT, Bressington D. Conceptualizations of subjective recovery from recent onset psychosis and its associated factors: a systematic review. Early Interv Psychiatry 2019;13(2):181–93.

10. Kane JM, Robinson DG, Schooler NR, et al. Comprehensive versus usual community care for first-episode psychosis: 2-year outcomes from the NIMH RAISE early treatment program. Am J Psychiatry 2016;173(4):362–72.

11. Chan V. Schizophrenia and psychosis: diagnosis, current research trends, and model treatment approaches with implications for transitional age youth. Child Adolesc Psychiatr Clin N Am 2017;26(2):341–66.

12. Correll CU, Galling B, Pawar A, et al. Comparison of early intervention services vs treatment as usual for early-phase psychosis: a systematic review, meta-analysis, and meta-regression. JAMA Psychiatry 2018;75(6):555–65.

13. Anderson D, Choden T, Sandseth T, et al. NYC START: a new model for securing community services for individuals hospitalized for first-episode psychosis. Psychiatr Serv 2019;70(8):644–9.

14. Baumann PS, Crespi S, Marion-Veyron R, et al. Treatment and early intervention in psychosis program (TIPP-Lausanne): implementation of an early intervention programme for psychosis in Switzerland. Early Interv Psychiatry 2013;7(3):322–8.

15. Davies EL, Gordon AL, Pelentsov LJ, et al. The supportive care needs of individuals recovering from first episode psychosis: a scoping review. Perspect Psychiatr Care 2019;55(1):6–14.

16. Roy L, Rousseau J, Fortier P, et al. Transitions to adulthood in first-episode psychosis: a comparative study. Early Interv Psychiatry 2013;7(2):162–9.

17. Watson AC. Finding common ground in case management: new titles and terminology along the health care continuum. Prof Case Manag 2011;16(2):52–4.

18. Corrigan PW, Mueser KT. Principles and practice of psychiatric rehabilitation. In: An empirical approach. 2nd edition. New York: Guilford Publications; 2016. p. 151–62.

19. Oxford English Dictionary. Case, n.1. Oxford University Press. Available at: http://www.oed.com/view/Entry/28393. Accessed September 19, 2019.

20. Rose D, Thornicroft G, Pinfold V, et al. 250 labels used to stigmatise people with mental illness. BMC Health Serv Res 2007;7:97.

21. Iverson C. AMA manual of style. A guide for authors and editors, 10th edition. Oxford, New York: Oxford University Press; 2009.

22. American Psychological Association, Publication manual of the American Psychological Association, 6th edition. Washington, DC: American Psychological Association; 2010.

23. Intagliata J. Improving the quality of community care for the chronically mentally disabled: the role of case management. Schizophr Bull 1982;8(4):655–74.

24. Montesano VL, Sivec HJ, Munetz MR, et al. Adapting cognitive behavioral therapy for psychosis for case managers: increasing access to services in a community mental health agency. Psychiatr Rehabil J 2014;37(1):11–6.

25. Scott JE, Dixon LB. Assertive community treatment and case management for schizophrenia. Schizophr Bull 1995;21(4):657–68.

26. Aberg-Wistedt A, Cressell T, Lidberg Y, et al. Two-year outcome of team-based intensive case management for patients with schizophrenia. Psychiatr Serv 1995;46(12):1263–6.

27. Mueser KT, Bond GR, Drake RE, et al. Models of community care for severe mental illness: a review of research on case management. Schizophr Bull 1998;24(1):37–74.

28. Lecardeur L, Meunier-Cussac S, Dollfus S. Mobile intensive care unit: a case management team dedicated to early psychosis in France. Early Interv Psychiatry 2018;12(5):995–9.

29. McGorry PD, Edwards J, Mihalopoulos C, et al. EPPIC: an evolving system of early detection and optimal management. Schizophr Bull 1996;22(2):305–26.

30. Brewer WJ, Lambert TJ, Witt K, et al. Intensive case management for high-risk patients with first-episode psychosis: service model and outcomes. Lancet Psychiatry 2015;2(1):29–37.

31. Malla AK, Norman RMG, Manchanda R, et al. Status of patients with first-episode psychosis after one year of phase-specific community-oriented treatment. Psychiatr Serv 2002;53(4):458–63.

32. McGlashan TH, Addington J, Cannon T, et al. Recruitment and treatment practices for help-seeking "prodromal" patients. Schizophr Bull 2007;33(3):715–26.

33. Heinrichs RW, Zakzanis KK. Neurocognitive deficit in schizophrenia: a quantitative review of the evidence. Neuropsychology 1998;12(3):426–45.

34. Fioravanti M, Bianchi V, Cinti ME. Cognitive deficits in schizophrenia: an updated metanalysis of the scientific evidence. BMC Psychiatry 2012;12(1):64.

35. Mesholam-Gately RI, Giuliano AJ, Goff KP, et al. Neurocognition in first-episode schizophrenia: a meta-analytic review. Neuropsychology 2009;23(3):315–36.

36. Riley EM, McGovern D, Mockler D, et al. Neuropsychological functioning in first-episode psychosis–evidence of specific deficits. Schizophr Res 2000;43(1):47–55.

37. Fusar-Poli P, Deste G, Smieskova R, et al. Cognitive functioning in prodromal psychosis: a meta-analysis. Arch Gen Psychiatry 2012;69(6):562–71.

38. Lencz T, Smith CW, McLaughlin D, et al. Generalized and specific neurocognitive deficits in prodromal schizophrenia. Biol Psychiatry 2006;59(9):863–71.

39. Fuller R, Nopoulos P, Arndt S, et al. Longitudinal assessment of premorbid cognitive functioning in patients with schizophrenia through examination of standardized scholastic test performance. Am J Psychiatry 2002;159(7):1183–9.

40. Reichenberg A, Caspi A, Harrington H, et al. Static and dynamic cognitive deficits in childhood preceding adult schizophrenia: a 30-year study. Am J Psychiatry 2010;167(2):160–9.

41. Bora E, Murray RM. Meta-analysis of cognitive deficits in ultra-high risk to psychosis and first-episode psychosis: do the cognitive deficits progress over, or after, the onset of psychosis? Schizophr Bull 2014;40(4):744–55.

42. Green MF, Kern RS, Braff DL, et al. Neurocognitive deficits and functional outcome in schizophrenia: are we measuring the "right stuff"? Schizophr Bull 2000;26(1):119–36.

43. Green MF, Kern RS, Heaton RK. Longitudinal studies of cognition and functional outcome in schizophrenia: implications for MATRICS. Schizophr Res 2004;72(1):41–51.

44. Humensky JL, Essock SM, Dixon LB. Characteristics associated with the pursuit of work and school among participants in a treatment program for first episode of psychosis. Psychiatr Rehabil J 2017;40(1):108–12.

45. Fu S, Czajkowski N, Rund BR, et al. The relationship between level of cognitive impairments and functional outcome trajectories in first-episode schizophrenia. Schizophr Res 2017;190:144–9.

46. Carrion RE, McLaughlin D, Goldberg TE, et al. Prediction of functional outcome in individuals at clinical high risk for psychosis. JAMA Psychiatry 2013;70(11):1133–42.

47. Haining K, Matrunola C, Mitchell L, et al. Neuropsychological deficits in participants at clinical high risk for psychosis recruited from the community: relationships to functioning and clinical symptoms. Psychol Med 2019;1–9 [Epub ahead of print].

48. Corrigan PW. Psychosis and cognitive challenges. In: Principles and practice of psychiatric rehabilitation: an empirical approach. 2nd edition. New York: Guilford Press; 2016. p. 222–44.

49. Velligan DI, Kern RS, Gold JM. Cognitive rehabilitation for schizophrenia and the putative role of motivation and expectancies. Schizophr Bull 2006;32(3):474–85.

50. Tomás P, Durá I, Roder V, et al. Cognitive rehabilitation programs in schizophrenia: current status and perspectives. Rev Int Psicol Ter Psicol 2010;10(2): 191–204.

51. Wykes T, Reeder C. Cognitive remediation therapy for schizophrenia: theory and practice. New York: Taylor and Francis Inc; 2005.

52. Eack SM, Greenwald DP, Hogarty SS, et al. Cognitive enhancement therapy for early-course schizophrenia: effects of a two-year randomized controlled trial. Psychiatr Serv 2009;60(11):1468–76.

53. Silverstein SM, Menditto AA, Stuve P. Shaping attention span: an operant conditioning procedure to improve neurocognition and functioning in schizophrenia. Schizophr Bull 2001;27(2):247–57.

54. Roder V, Mueller DR, Schmidt SJ. Effectiveness of integrated psychological therapy (IPT) for schizophrenia patients: a research update. Schizophr Bull 2011; 37(suppl_2):S71–9.

55. McGurk SR, Mueser KT, Watkins MA, et al. The feasibility of implementing cognitive remediation for work in community based psychiatric rehabilitation programs. Psychiatr Rehabil J 2017;40(1):79–86.

56. Medalia A, Saperstein AM. Does cognitive remediation for schizophrenia improve functional outcomes? Curr Opin Psychiatry 2013;26(2):151–7.

57. Revell ER, Neill JC, Harte M, et al. A systematic review and meta-analysis of cognitive remediation in early schizophrenia. Schizophr Res 2015;168(1): 213–22.

58. Ventura J, Subotnik KL, Gretchen-Doorly D, et al. Cognitive remediation can improve negative symptoms and social functioning in first-episode schizophrenia: a randomized controlled trial. Schizophr Res 2019;203:24–31.

59. Piskulic D, Romanowska S, Addington J. Pilot study of cognitive remediation and motivational interviewing in youth at risk of serious mental illness. Early Interv Psychiatry 2018;12(6):1193–7.

60. Mullen MG, Thompson JL, Murphy AA, et al. Evaluation of a cognitive remediation intervention for college students with psychiatric conditions. Psychiatr Rehabil J 2017;40(1):103–7.

61. Bechdolf A, Wagner M, Ruhrmann S, et al. Preventing progression to first-episode psychosis in early initial prodromal states. Br J Psychiatry 2012; 200(1):22–9.

62. Piskulic D, Barbato M, Liu L, et al. Pilot study of cognitive remediation therapy on cognition in young people at clinical high risk of psychosis. Psychiatry Res 2015;225(1–2):93–8.

63. Holzer L, Urben S, Passini CM, et al. A randomized controlled trial of the effectiveness of computer-assisted cognitive remediation (CACR) in adolescents with psychosis or at high risk of psychosis. Behav Cogn Psychother 2014;42(4): 421–34.

64. Loewy R, Fisher M, Schlosser DA, et al. Intensive auditory cognitive training improves verbal memory in adolescents and young adults at clinical high risk for psychosis. Schizophr Bull 2016;42(suppl_1):S118–26.

65. Kidd SA, Kerman N, Ernest D, et al. A pilot study of a family cognitive adaptation training guide for individuals with schizophrenia. Psychiatr Rehabil J 2018;41(2): 109–17.

66. Velligan DI, Tai S, Roberts DL, et al. A randomized controlled trial comparing cognitive behavior therapy, cognitive adaptation training, their combination and treatment as usual in chronic schizophrenia. Schizophr Bull 2014;41(3): 597–603.

67. Kern RS, Liberman RP, Kopelowicz A, et al. Applications of errorless learning for improving work performance in persons with schizophrenia. Am J Psychiatry 2002;159(11):1921–6.

68. Pijnenborg GHM, Withaar FK, Brouwer WH, et al. The efficacy of SMS text messages to compensate for the effects of cognitive impairments in schizophrenia. Br J Clin Psychol 2010;49(2):259–74.

69. Mahmood Z, Clark JMR, Twamley EW. Compensatory cognitive training for psychosis: effects on negative symptom subdomains. Schizophr Res 2019;204: 397–400.

70. Lutgens D, Gariepy G, Malla A. Psychological and psychosocial interventions for negative symptoms in psychosis: systematic review and meta-analysis. Br J Psychiatry 2017;210(5):324–32.

71. Kern RS, Zarate R, Glynn SM, et al. Improving work outcome in supported employment for serious mental illness: results from 2 independent studies of errorless learning. Schizophr Bull 2017;44(1):38–45.

72. Garrido G, Penadés R, Barrios M, et al. Computer-assisted cognitive remediation therapy in schizophrenia: durability of the effects and cost-utility analysis. Psychiatry Res 2017;254:198–204.

73. Hansen JP, Østergaard B, Nordentoft M, et al. Cognitive adaptation training combined with assertive community treatment: a randomised longitudinal trial. Schizophr Res 2012;135(1):105–11.

74. Allott KA, Killackey E, Sun P, et al. Improving vocational outcomes in first-episode psychosis by addressing cognitive impairments using cognitive adaptation training. Work 2017;56(4):581–9.

75. Allott KA, Killackey E, Sun P, et al. Feasibility and acceptability of cognitive adaptation training for first-episode psychosis. Early Interv Psychiatry 2016; 10(6):476–84.

76. Mendella PD, Burton CZ, Tasca GA, et al. Compensatory cognitive training for people with first-episode schizophrenia: results from a pilot randomized controlled trial. Schizophr Res 2015;162(1):108–11.

77. Vidarsdottir OG, Magnusdottir BB, Roberts D, et al. A randomized, controlled trial on integrated cognitive remediation for early psychosis: effectiveness and factors associated with treatment response. Paper presented at: Early Intervention in Psychiatry 2018;12(S1):74.

78. Robles-Guerrero C, Twamley EW, Cadenhead K. Compensatory cognitive training in the prodrome and first episode psychosis. 8th International Conference on Early Psychosis. San Francisco, October 11, 2012.

79. Deyoe J, Kelsven S, Robles-Guerrero C, et al. SA103. Compensatory cognitive training in high-risk Latino youth. Schizophr Bull 2017;43(suppl_1):S150.

80. Pantelis C, Wannan C, Bartholomeusz CF, et al. Cognitive intervention in early psychosis — preserving abilities versus remediating deficits. Curr Opin Behav Sci 2015;4:63–72.

81. Corbera S, Wexler BE, Poltorak A, et al. Cognitive remediation for adults with schizophrenia: does age matter? Psychiatry Res 2017;247:21–7.

82. Vidarsdottir OG, Roberts DL, Twamley EW, et al. Integrative cognitive remediation for early psychosis: results from a randomized controlled trial. Psychiatry Res 2019;273:690–8.

83. Noel VA, Oulvey E, Drake RE, et al. Barriers to employment for transition-age youth with developmental and psychiatric disabilities. Adm Policy Ment Health 2017;44(3):354–8.

84. Bowman S, McKinstry C, McGorry P. Youth mental ill health and secondary school completion in Australia: time to act. Early Interv Psychiatry 2017;11(4):277–89.

85. Carr VJ, Waghorn G. To love and to work: the next major mental health reform goals. Aust N Z J Psychiatry 2013;47(8):696–8.

86. Rinaldi M, Killackey E, Smith J, et al. First episode psychosis and employment: a review. Int Rev Psychiatry 2010;22(2):148–62.

87. Marwaha S, Johnson S. Schizophrenia and employment: a review. Soc Psychiatry Psychiatr Epidemiol 2004;39(5):337–49.

88. Strauss GP, Allen DN, Miski P, et al. Differential patterns of premorbid social and academic deterioration in deficit and nondeficit schizophrenia. Schizophr Res 2012;135(1):134–8.

89. Bassett J, Lloyd C, Bassett H. Work issues for young people with psychosis: barriers to employment. Br J Occup Ther 2001;64(2):66–72.

90. Mueser KT, Cook JA. Supported employment, supported education, and career development. Psychiatr Rehabil J 2012;35(6):417–20.

91. Luciano A, Drake RE, Bond GR, et al. Evidence-based supported employment for people with severe mental illness: past, current, and future research. J Vocat Rehabil 2014;40(1):1–13.

92. Bond GR, Drake RE, Luciano A. Employment and educational outcomes in early intervention programmes for early psychosis: a systematic review. Epidemiol Psychiatr Sci 2015;24(5):446–57.

93. Bond GR, Drake RE, Campbell K. Effectiveness of individual placement and support supported employment for young adults. Early Interv Psychiatry 2016;10(4):300–7.

94. Rosenheck R, Mueser KT, Sint K, et al. Supported employment and education in comprehensive, integrated care for first episode psychosis: effects on work, school, and disability income. Schizophr Res 2017;182:120–8.

95. Nuechterlein KH, Subotnik KL, Turner LR, et al. Individual placement and support for individuals with recent-onset schizophrenia: integrating supported education and supported employment. Psychiatr Rehabil J 2008;31(4):340–9.

96. Addington DE, McKenzie E, Norman R, et al. Essential evidence-based components of first-episode psychosis services. Psychiatr Serv 2013;64(5):452–7.

97. Kam SM, Singh SP, Upthegrove R. What needs to follow early intervention? Predictors of relapse and functional recovery following first-episode psychosis. Early Interv Psychiatry 2015;9(4):279–83.

98. Tapfumaneyi A, Johnson S, Joyce J, et al. Predictors of vocational activity over the first year in inner-city early intervention in psychosis services. Early Interv Psychiatry 2015;9(6):447–58.

99. Eglit GML, Palmer BW, Martin AS, et al. Loneliness in schizophrenia: construct clarification, measurement, and clinical relevance. PLoS One 2018;13(3): e0194021.

100. Sundermann O, Onwumere J, Kane F, et al. Social networks and support in first-episode psychosis: exploring the role of loneliness and anxiety. Soc Psychiatry Psychiatr Epidemiol 2014;49(3):359–66.

101. Gronholm PC, Thornicroft G, Laurens KR, et al. Mental health-related stigma and pathways to care for people at risk of psychotic disorders or experiencing first-episode psychosis: a systematic review. Psychol Med 2017;47(11):1867–79.

102. Gerlinger G, Hauser M, De Hert M, et al. Personal stigma in schizophrenia spectrum disorders: a systematic review of prevalence rates, correlates, impact and interventions. World Psychiatry 2013;12(2):155–64.

103. Corrigan PW, Larson JE, RÜSch N. Self-stigma and the "why try" effect: impact on life goals and evidence-based practices. World Psychiatry 2009;8(2):75–81.

104. Mahlke CI, Kramer UM, Becker T, et al. Peer support in mental health services. Curr Opin Psychiatry 2014;27(4):276–81.

105. Mead S, Hilton D, Curtis L. Peer support: a theoretical perspective. Psychiatr Rehabil J 2001;25(2):134–41.

106. King AJ, Simmons MB. A systematic review of the attributes and outcomes of peer work and guidelines for reporting studies of peer interventions. Psychiatr Serv 2018;69(9):961–77.

107. Lloyd-Evans B, Mayo-Wilson E, Harrison B, et al. A systematic review and meta-analysis of randomised controlled trials of peer support for people with severe mental illness. BMC Psychiatry 2014;14(1):39.

108. Chien WT, Clifton AV, Zhao S, et al. Peer support for people with schizophrenia or other serious mental illness. Cochrane Database Syst Rev 2019;(4):CD010880.

109. Cabassa LJ, Camacho D, Vélez-Grau CM, et al. Peer-based health interventions for people with serious mental illness: a systematic literature review. J Psychiatr Res 2017;84:80–9.

110. Gleeson J, Lederman R, Koval P, et al. Moderated online social therapy: a model for reducing stress in carers of young people diagnosed with mental health disorders. Front Psychol 2017;8:485.

111. Leggatt M, Woodhead G. Family peer support work in an early intervention youth mental health service. Early Interv Psychiatry 2016;10(5):446–51.

112. Alvarez-Jimenez M, Bendall S, Koval P, et al. HORYZONS trial: protocol for a randomised controlled trial of a moderated online social therapy to maintain treatment effects from first-episode psychosis services. BMJ Open 2019;9(2): e024104.

School-Based Approaches in Youth with Psychosis

Samantha Hines, BA, Drew C. Coman, PhD*

KEYWORDS

- Psychosis • Schizophrenia • Education • Special education • School-based
- Youth

KEY POINTS

- A major recovery milestone for most youth affected by psychosis is the reintegration back into a school setting.
- Gold standard practice for psychosis comprises supportive educational services that are focused on successful academic reintegration and achievement.
- Providers can guide educational institutions via comprehensive assessment procedures in the delineation of key educational programming that can help youth reintegrate back into school and achieve academic success.

INTRODUCTION

A major recovery milestone for most youth affected by psychosis is the reintegration back into a school setting. Although this is not always an easy achievement, and it is a period commonly fraught with many uncertainties for all parties involved, school reintegration is an important and attainable treatment goal. Indeed, this time point is often a barometer of sorts for the individuals affected and their families. It assists them in calibrating what the next appropriate steps are in getting their lives back. It is also a critical juncture because if it goes well, it is a beacon of hope that highlights that experiencing psychosis does not have to dictate someone's future or put a ceiling on their long-term goals, and usually elicits substantial momentum in the recovery process. On the contrary, if the reintegration goes unfavorably, the resulting setbacks are counterproductive to recovery. Given the bearing that these two courses can have, it is not surprising that the gold standard practice in first-episode psychosis (FEP) clinical care comprises comprehensive supportive educational services that are explicitly focused on one critical functional outcome for youth impacted by psychosis: successful academic reintegration and achievement.

This specialized wraparound clinical practice for individuals experiencing FEP, which is commonly referred to as coordinated specialty care (CSC), is vital to recovery.

Disclosure Statement: The authors have nothing to disclose.
Department of Psychiatry, Massachusetts General Hospital, Harvard Medical School, 1 Bowdoin Square, Seventh Floor, Boston, MA 02114, USA
* Corresponding author.
E-mail address: dcoman@mgh.harvard.edu

Child Adolesc Psychiatric Clin N Am 29 (2020) 241–252
https://doi.org/10.1016/j.chc.2019.08.014
1056-4993/20/© 2019 Elsevier Inc. All rights reserved.

childpsych.theclinics.com

CSC programs comprise a multidisciplinary treatment team delivering a synchronized effort of individualized psychopharmacology, psychosocial treatment, family psycho-education, employment assistance, and the previously mentioned supported educational services. The evidence for the importance of CSC in FEP has been established for some time because these early intervention services have been implemented and evaluated for effectiveness across the globe for more than two decades.[1] Indeed, a recent systematic review and meta-analysis identified 10 separate randomized clinical trials of early intervention services for FEP, conducted across seven different countries (United Kingdom, China, Denmark, United States, Italy, Norway, and Mexico), and highlighted their superiority to "treatment as usual" for an array of measurable outcomes.[2] Fortunately, these clinics have proliferated across the United States, are becoming more accessible to those affected, and more youth are able to successfully reintegrate back into school after a psychotic episode.

Thus, the collaboration between CSC teams and educational institutions, spanning across public and private primary and secondary schools, colleges, and professional schools, is integral to youth impacted by psychosis. Schools are not only well-positioned to be on the front lines of identification of psychosis in youth, but they are also vital to an individual's treatment and recovery. To assist with this important collaboration between clinical practitioners (eg, psychiatrists, psychologists, social workers, supported educational specialists) and their patients' educational institutions, and in an overall effort to further promote positive recovery patterns in youth with psychosis, provided here is a review of some of the key school-based approaches to support affected youth.

GUIDING THE IDENTIFICATION PROCESS

Educational settings are on the front lines of the identification process. More than 3 out of 100 individuals experience psychosis in their lifetime making it more common than diabetes. In addition, the onset typically occurs during the early to mid-20s for men and in the late 20s for women with childhood onset of psychosis (usually after age 7, and before age 13) existing at lower base rates.[3–5] Therefore, it is highly probable that most schools will interface with the management of this condition at some point. Having training on early detection is important for educational settings because they can play an essential role in treatment outcomes. Specifically, schools can greatly reduce the duration of untreated symptoms, termed the duration of untreated psychosis. Lengthier duration of untreated psychosis has been associated with increased severity of symptoms, decreased quality of life, and overall more unfavorable functional outcomes.[6–9] It is therefore important for personnel within educational institutions to be knowledgeable in the detection of early warning signs and symptoms of psychosis. Broadly, psychotic symptoms may comprise a permutation of hallucinations, delusions, atypical behaviors, and a decline in someone's baseline level of functioning. **Table 1** provides some of the earlier indications and signs of psychosis for schools to be vigilant of, although this is not an exhaustive list, because psychosis presents differently for everyone. It is also important to note that the behaviors listed are not diagnostic and may be indications of a myriad of other experiences (eg, depression, substance use) or events (eg, relational issues) that are occurring for a young person.

PSYCHOSIS EFFECTS ON FUNCTIONING

A person's educational level exerts the strongest influence on their health.[10] It has been found that young people with diagnoses of serious mental health conditions (SMHC), such as psychosis, have compromised educational attainment. One national

Table 1
Signs and indications of psychosis within educational contexts

Decline in grades or performances in coursework	Isolative behaviors or a marked change in socialization (eg, not attending class, leaving their dorm room)	Language that is nonsensical
Changes in day-to-day activities, such as eating or sleeping patterns and/or hygiene and self-care	Behaviors that are discrepant from baseline that are odd or bizarre in nature (eg, laughing at inappropriate times or to self with no stimuli, wearing a winter coat to class during the early fall semester when temperatures are warm)	A student noting a high level of suspiciousness of others, feeling persecuted, or feeling that others might be out to harm them (or their reputation) or others[a]
Displays of extreme discomfort in innocuous situations, or difficulties attending class		A student reporting that others can read their thoughts, that they are not in control of them, or that someone or something is inserting or stealing their ideas or thoughts[a]
Changes in a student's ability to pay attention in class, recall information from lessons/lectures	A student reporting they are hearing, seeing, feeling, smelling, or tasting things that are not there[a]	
An emergence of repetitive narrowed interests being observed in a student's work; preoccupations (eg, focused on the number 11, or another student/professor)	Aggression and/or irritability	Reports from a student that they are getting messages from their environment (eg, assigned reading materials are about their life)[a]
	Distracted or heightened sensitivities to stimuli	
	Odd beliefs, such as believing they have special abilities, or have completed a remarkable academic feat or otherwise, which is not aligned with others' perceptions[a]	
Reported experiences of not being themselves, "out of body" phenomena, or a feeling of watching themselves in a movie		

[a] Indicates a clear symptom of psychosis.

survey found that by age 19, for those in special education because of an SMHC, the high school completion rate is only 56%. Correspondingly, it found that few students with SMHC, that were diagnosed by high school age, go on to attend postsecondary education programs; those who do continue do not complete such programs, studies suggest.[11] In another study by Goulding and colleagues[12] it was found that in a sample of adolescents hospitalized for FEP 44% had dropped out of high school, much higher than the average reported high school dropout rates of 12.8% to 17.8%. Youth experiencing FEP are also more likely to need to take one or multiple leaves of absence from school to focus on treatment. This can prolong or derail the process of educational attainment for many, especially during postsecondary education.

Cognitive deficits are a core feature of psychotic disorders, and they are present in the prodromal period before the onset of psychosis and are stable throughout the course of the illness in most individuals.[13] These deficits are associated with functional outcomes and are thought to be potential functional prognostic markers, especially for longer-term outcomes. Onset of psychosis can also cause substantial distress for an adolescent by disrupting fulfilment of their educational and vocational goals, social relationships, and identity formation.[14] For youth experiencing psychosis, their developmental stage may play a mediating role in the relationship between functional outcomes and cognitive deficits.[15] Additionally, evidence suggests that cognitive deficits in psychotic disorders are apparent before the FEP. The prodromal period preceding FEP 3 to 4 years has been associated with cognitive deficits in the domains of general intelligence, verbal fluency, verbal and visual memory, and working memory.[16]

When individuals experience FEP, their cognitive deficits become more established and pervasive. The severity of impairment varies among the multiple domains.[17] The domains that are often affected in the FEP are: speed of processing, visual memory, verbal memory, problem solving and reasoning, social cognition, attention and vigilance, and working memory.[18] The most marked deficits are seen in the domains of information processing speed and verbal and visual memory.[17] These domains are assessed by the administration of several neuropsychological measures (described later), although the Measurement and Treatment Research to Improve Cognition in Schizophrenia Consensus Cognitive Battery is one of the most validated and widely used tools.[19,20]

NEUROPSYCHOLOGICAL AND EDUCATIONAL TESTING

The emergence of psychosis often results in either an onset or exacerbation of prior neurocognitive and learning challenges. One of the more helpful initial procedures to support a student who is considering reintegrating back into the school setting, often after a medical leave of absence, is to obtain neuropsychological and educational testing. These testing procedures can delineate an individual's profile of neurocognitive and learning strengths and weaknesses. Ideally, this should occur once their clinical team is in support of this next step in their recovery. Such evaluations are typically not as informative or assistive when an individual is experiencing an acute level of psychotic symptoms. Stability, to a sufficient degree, should be achieved before testing. At an appropriate stage of stability, evaluations are assistive in developing a better understanding and insight for the student, their family, the school, and their clinical team. For the student specifically, having an idea of what comes easy to them versus more difficult from a thinking and learning standpoint is helpful in calibrating their readiness for reintegration and the kind of school-related tasks and expectations they are prepared to manage. Moreover, a delineation of a student's profile of strengths and vulnerabilities by way of testing is enlightening (and is usually required from an administrative standpoint) as to what types and level of specialized educational programming would be supportive, including but not limited to direct services, accommodations, and placement (eg, full inclusion settings vs therapeutic placements).

There are ranges of evaluations in terms of depth that can be conducted. Unfortunately, there are no written rules as to which is best. Practices invariably differ among clinics and evaluators. Given the far-reaching effects on an individual's functioning, most agree that it is best clinical practice for most individuals to receive a comprehensive neurocognitive and academic work-up. Alternative options may include focused academic evaluations or using the Measurement and Treatment Research to Improve Cognition in Schizophrenia Consensus Cognitive Battery. Testing should broadly comprise a detailed clinical interview, observations, standardized assessments, and rating scales. As with any evaluation, the overarching methodology of the assessment, including test battery selection, is dictated by several factors (eg, chronologic age, areas of concern). A clinician's goal during the assessment process should be to determine whether abilities fall within age-appropriate expectations across the following: cognition, language, academic skills, memory, attention and other executive functions, socioemotional (eg, anxiety, social cognition), behavioral functioning (eg, self-regulation), and adaptive functioning. **Fig. 1** further illustrates many of the global areas along with some common subsidiary abilities to be potentially assessed.

SECTION 504 PLANS, INDIVIDUALIZED EDUCATION PROGRAMS, AND THE LEGALITY

Fortunately, federal laws, such as the Americans with Disabilities Act, Section 504 of the Rehabilitation Act of 1973 (Section 504), and numerous state laws cover students with psychiatric disabilities, such as youth with FEP. The US Department of Education enforces Section 504 in programs and activities that receive funds from the Department of Education. Recipients of these funds include public school districts, institutions of higher education, and other state and local education agencies.[21] Under Section 504, this is free and appropriate public education. This ensures that special education and related services for children ages 3 to 21 must be provided at public expense for those eligible. The Individuals with Disabilities Education Act (IDEA) was first passed by Congress in 1990. This act defined the disabilities eligible for special services in public schools and outlined the process by which special education services are provided for students with disabilities. Under this law, each eligible student (from age 3 through high school) is provided an individualized education program (IEP) that is tailored to their unique educational needs. IDEA guarantees all children with disabilities free and appropriate public education. Youth with FEP fall under the category of "emotional disturbance" in the IDEA classified disabilities, which is defined as "an inability to learn, build or maintain satisfactory interpersonal relationships, inappropriate behaviors or feelings, pervasive mood of unhappiness or depression, over a longer period of marked time."[22]

Both IEPs and Section 504 plans support students with disabilities, but are different entities. They are covered by two separate laws: IEPs are covered by special education law (IDEA), whereas Section 504 plans fall under federal disability law. Almost all students that are covered by IDEA are also covered by Section 504, but not vice versa.[23] For youth with FEP and no comorbid learning disorders, a Section 504 plan may be suitable for their learning needs. Section 504 plans are formal plans that schools develop to give students with disabilities support and remove barriers from their consumption of the curriculum. Under Section 504, a person with a disability is defined as: a person who is regarded to, has a record of such, or has a mental or physical disability that substantially limits one or more of the person's major life activities (eg, self-care, performing manual tasks, learning, or working). Under that definition, most youth with FEP meet the criteria for a disability. Even if a student is effectively treated with medication, this is not a mitigating measure and should not make a student ineligible because of the Americans with Disabilities Act (ADA) 2008 amendment.[23]

Section 504 plans and IEPs do not transfer over from high school to college. They can, however, inform the accommodations students can receive in college. Colleges have to provide accommodations to students under Section 504. The process of obtaining these accommodations and how they are implemented differ from grade school. Accommodations can be set up before the start of the college semester through the office of disability or accessibility services. Self-advocacy tends to be stressed by colleges for transition-age youth throughout this process. It typically involves the student making an appointment with a disabilities counselor to discuss setting up accommodations. Every college is different in their requirement for documentation: some require a confirmation of diagnosis, others ask for specific documentation with questions for providers and even students, and sometimes a copy of previous IEPs, Section 504 plans, or neuropsychological testing is requested. How the accommodations are delivered to the professors differs from college to college. It is usually up to the student to decide what they would like to disclose to their professors and they must be sure to continue working with disability services each year to continue to receive their accommodations.

REINTEGRATION PROCEDURES, DIRECT SERVICES, AND ACCOMMODATIONS

With the data in hand post an evaluation, the next step is for the student, their family, and clinical team to design a blueprint for successful reintegration and subsequent

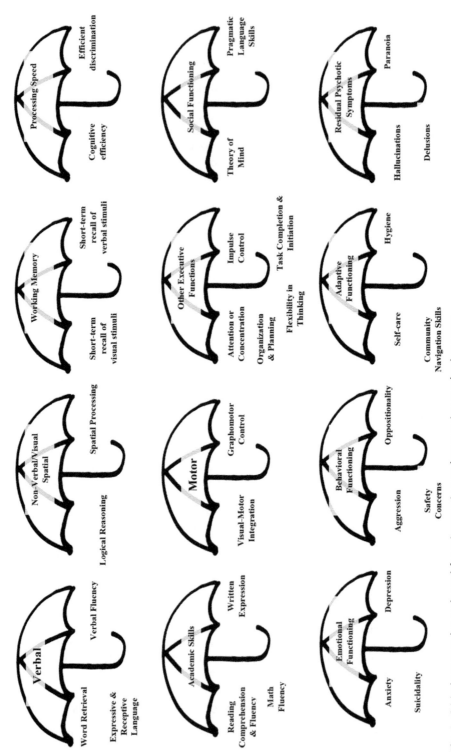

Fig. 1. Critical areas to be evaluated for reintegration and supporting academic success.

academic success. To this end, specialized educational programming, which is available across all grade levels via different avenues as described previously (ie, IEP in middle school vs services from an office of disability in college), can greatly increase the probability of success. Discussed next are general principles to consider, along with accommodations, direct services, and placements if necessary. Other excellent resources for these procedures are available in the back-to-school toolkits provided by Schiffman and coworkers[24] and Jones and coworkers.[25]

There are several general principles that are important to consider. First, all parties involved ought to be mindful that this stage should be viewed as a calibration period; that is, this will be the "truest" measure of an individual's readiness for school reintegration because no standardized assessment protocol or clinical opinion can infallibly predict the outcome. Moreover, if reintegration is unsuccessful, it is important for the individual and their team to not peg this as any sort of failure on anyone's behalf. On the contrary, this should more accurately be viewed as not the appropriate time for this step and all should understand that this could be revisited at a more stable time. A priori discussions around this point are often useful. One overarching approach to reintegration planning that some may find beneficial is infusing the evidence-based guidelines of multifamily group treatment.[26] **Box 1** lists these general principles along with applications to educational planning.

With these general guidelines at the helm, it is then important for the student and their team to consider eligibility for accommodations and services. There is an eligibility determination process within most educational settings and these could be delivered via an IEP, Section 504 plan, or through a postsecondary institution's office of disability. Broadly, it is essential that the accommodations and services are highly individualized and have targeted goals. An extensive level of communication between the student/family, school administrators, teachers/professors, special education support or office of disability staff, and the community treatment providers is also vital. For students who are enrolled into primary and secondary school with significant challenges and/or multiple unsuccessful attempts at reintegration into their previous school, they may require a substantially separate therapeutic educational placement. **Table 2** lists the key components of this type of specialized placement, along with commonly helpful accommodations and direct services for students in elementary school to high school. An essential component to educational programming for students in secondary schooling is to also ensure that there is ongoing transition planning. **Table 3** offers various beneficial accommodations and direct services for students within a college setting.

SUPPORTED EDUCATION WITHIN COORDINATED SPECIALTY CARE

Treaters and care teams can play an important role as advocates for educational services for their patients. FEP CSC programs can assist patients and families with navigating educational obstacles by having a supported education and employment (SEE) specialist on the team. A SEE specialist helps people with a psychiatric disorder achieve their vocational and educational goals by working with clients to identify their personal preferences regarding educational goals and then provides the necessary supports to help the person achieve those goals as defined in the NAVIGATE SEE specialist manual.[27] Some components of SEE services can include, although are not limited to, school searching, course selection, problem solving around symptoms and school impact, corresponding with the school, assisting with services, and collecting proper documentation from the treatment team. It is important that there is a respect for patient preferences and a positive collaborative relationship between the SEE specialist and patient. One recent study by Humensky and colleagues[28] found

---

Box 1
General principles to consider (multifamily group treatment family guidelines)

- Go slow
  - Schools are not going anywhere—individuals should allow themselves appropriate time for recovery, focus on their well-being, and take their time reintegrating. Recovery takes longer than most want.
  - Consider taking an incremental approach: start taking an online course, then a course at a local college from home, then two courses.

- Keep it cool
  - Avoid taking on too much at once.
  - Consider taking a longer leave of absence from school.

- Pick-up on early warning signs
  - Develop an explicit relapse prevention plan with clinicians and family to assist in identifying early warning signs and triggers.

- Lower expectations, temporarily
  - Progress is progress. Celebrate small steps and achievement of goals. Do not put pressures to make leaps in recovery.

- Give each other space
  - Caregivers should allow for space, extra time for decision-making, and avoid hovering.

- Observe limits
  - Keep important, established family rules intact. Observe these rules.

- Ignore what you cannot change
  - Students may have academic desires discrepant from the family or treatment team (eg, desires to go back into school taking all honors/AP courses). This is part of the calibration process.
  - Do not ruminate over disagreements around the school plan.

- Keep it simple
  - Communicate about school desires and plans. When communicating, do this in a clear, calm, and positive manner.

- Carry on business as usual
  - Consider reaching out to friends at school, re-establish family routines and get-togethers, schedule social events. This will all help with the calibration process.

- Consider using medications and avoiding substances or alcohol
  - Continue to support one's well-being with medication, and abstinence or reductions in substances can assist with the success of the reintegration process.

- Solve problems step by step
  - Focus on one thing at a time and make changes in increments.

Adaped from McFarlane WR. Multifamily Groups in the Treatment of Severe Psychiatric Disorders. New York & London: Guilford Press; 2002; with permission.

---

that participants in FEP programs that emphasized school had high rates of educational participation, engaging early, often simultaneously in school and work. Similar findings were reflected in the study by Rosenheck and colleagues.[29] This study examined the implementation of the NAVIGATE model in CSC FEP programs and found that individuals recovering from FEP received far more SEE services and showed significantly greater increases in school participation over 2-years compared with those who received standard community care. Patients who began school or work tended to do so within the first year of treatment. There are ample data to support that, despite the common belief that people with FEP cannot withstand the pressures of competitive work or school as they are recovering, with appropriate supports success in these

Table 2
Direct services, accommodations, and key components of therapeutic placements for primary and secondary school

Accommodations and Additional Supports	Direct Services	Key Components of a Therapeutic Placement
Extended time on all tasks, tests, and standardized testing	Counseling services	Full-day, year-round, placement that is substantially separate and therapeutic
Access to school nurse for medication administration	1:1 or small group academic tutoring	A small student-to-teacher ratio
Access to "quiet" or "cool down" spaces	Social skills training	Similar peers
Have a "point person" to assist in identifying symptoms or someone to offer support	Executive functioning tutoring	Frequent access to 1:1 assistance from a certified special education teacher, highly experienced clinical/mental health staff, and an in-house consulting psychiatric care team
Frequent 1:1 access to special education personnel within the classroom	Assistive technology (eg, speech-to-text devices)	A high level of structure, with a predictable routine that entails frequent monitoring and assessment of progress
Planner support, and guidance with ensuring student has all the necessary materials for a lesson	Extended school year services	Offers specialized socioemotional and behavioral interventions across the day
Advanced notice for larger assignments	Occupational therapy	Supports and interventions rooted in evidenced-based treatment, such as cognitive-behavioral therapy for psychosis
Consultations with specialists: speech and language pathologist, certified behavioral analyst (ie, Board Certified Behavior Analyst), or other providers	Speech and language	Coping tools should be taught and reinforced across the day
Provide a slower pace to lessons	Self-help/life skills training	
Provide a written checklist of steps for a task or a template	In-home tutoring or therapeutic supports to address school refusal or support access to curriculum on leave of absence	
Graphic organizers	Vocational training	
Use of headphones	Transition planning into college or workforce	
Use of fidget objects	1:1 aide	
The use of a "standing" desk		
Books (and textbooks) on tape		
Breaks across tasks and provide outlets for energy and physical activity on a needed basis		
Modified workloads, or formats to testing (eg, eligibility to oral examinations)		
Flexible deadlines for assignments		
Eligibility for test make-ups		
Advanced warnings for changes to routine		
Breaking assignments into smaller tasks; taking step-by-step approaches		
Presenting information in a multisensory format		
Preferential seating		

Table 3
Direct services and accommodations for college settings

Accommodations and Additional Supports	Direct Services
On-campus counseling and psychiatric services; or referrals to nearby clinics	On-campus counseling and psychiatric services; or referrals to nearby clinics
Tutoring services	Tutoring services
Access to class notes that are either provided by professors or a service via the office of disability (eg, other students serving as scribes and/or note-takers for students)	Access to class notes that are either provided by professors or a service via the office of disability (eg, other students serving as scribes and/or note-takers for students)
Access to a single dorm or a setting that is of most comfort	Access to a single dorm or a setting that is of most comfort
Extended-time to complete all assignments and tests, including on all standardized testing	
Allowed to take examinations and standardized tests in a separate setting	
Eligibility for extra breaks between sections and exempt from any test portions that are not required (eg, experimental test sections)	
Permitting part-time registration for courses as full-time to avoid issues with financial services or scholarships	
Allow for student to retrospectively complete missed work that was not completed because of illness	
Eligibility for pass/fail	
Flexibility with deadlines and policies and reduction of penalties	
Flexible deadlines for assignments	
Eligible for test make-ups when missed or test redos when performances are unfavorable (eg, retaking an examination for partial credit)	
Ability to work closely with an academic advisor to choose a balanced course load across academic years	
Eligibility for an alternate schedule for prerequisites	
Eligibility for priority (or early) class registration each semester	
Access to books on tape or similar assistive technology services	
Permitted to tape record lectures	
Not penalized for taking breaks during lectures	
Excused absences	
Limit penalties for lack of classroom participation	
Student should not be required to take more than 1 examination or final in a day; or more than 2 examinations in a week	
Permitted to use a notecard or classroom notes during an examination	

areas is possible and the support from a SEE specialist and a CSC team helps increase the likelihood.[27,30]

SUMMARY

One of the most important recovery milestones for youth affected by psychosis is the reintegration back into a school setting. This is, for many reasons, not an easy achievement for the affected individual and their family, but it is nonetheless an important and attainable treatment goal for most. Obtaining neuropsychological and educational testing along with the acquisition of specialized educational programming, perhaps under the care of a supported educational specialist, is highly supportive in the functional goal of academic reintegration and success. Therefore, efforts should continue to be made to further establish educational support services, with a focus on successful academic reintegration and achievement, as not only the gold standard practice, but more simply the sole standard practice in first-episode clinical care.

REFERENCES

1. Dixon LB, Goldman HH, Srihari VH, et al. Transforming the treatment of schizophrenia in the United States: the RAISE initiative. Annu Rev Clin Psychol 2018; 14:237–58.
2. Correll CU, Galling B, Pawar A, et al. Comparison of early intervention services vs treatment as usual for early-phase psychosis: a systematic review, meta-analysis, and meta-regression effectiveness of early intervention services for early-phase psychosis effectiveness of early intervention services for early-phase psychosis. JAMA Psychiatry 2018;75(6):555–65. Available at: https://doi.org/10.1001/jamapsychiatry.2018.0623.
3. American Psychiatric Association (APA). Diagnostic and statistical manual of mental disorders: Dsm-5 (5th ed.). Arlington, VA: APA. 2013.
4. Gejman PV, Sanders AR, Duan J. The role of genetics in the etiology of schizophrenia. Psychiatr Clin North Am 33(1) 2010;35–66.
5. WHO Schizophrenia. 2014, November 21. Available at: https://www.who.int/topics/schizophrenia/en/. Accessed June 1, 2019.
6. Kane JM, Robinson DG, Schooler NR, et al. Comprehensive versus usual community care for first-episode psychosis: 2-year outcomes From the NIMH RAISE Early Treatment Program. American Journal of Psychiatry 2016;173(4):362–72.
7. Larsen TK. Poor social and interpersonal functioning prior to diagnosis predicts poor outcome for people with first episode psychosis. Evidence-Based Mental Health 2006;9:5.
8. Marshall M, Lewis S, Lockwood A, et al. Association between duration of untreated psychosis and outcome in cohorts of first-episode patients. Archives of General Psychiatry 2005;62(9):975.
9. Perkins DO, Gu H, Boteva K, et al. Relationship between duration of untreated psychosis and outcome in first-episode schizophrenia: A critical review and meta-analysis. American Journal of Psychiatry 2005;162(10):1785–804.
10. Lund I. Dropping out of school as a meaningful action for adolescents with social, emotional and behavioural difficulties. J Res Spec Educ Needs 2013;14(2): 96–104.
11. Ellison ML, Klodnick VV, Bond GR, et al. Adapting supported employment for emerging adults with serious mental health conditions. J Behav Health Serv Res 2014;42(2):206–22.
12. Goulding SM, Chien VH, Compton MT. Prevalence and correlates of school dropout prior to initial treatment of nonaffective psychosis: further evidence suggesting a need for supported education. Schizophr Res 2010;116(2–3):228–33.
13. Bowie CR, Harvey PD. Cognitive deficits and functional outcome in schizophrenia. Neuropsychiatr Dis Treat 2006;2(4):531–6.

14. Cotton SM, Lambert M, Schimmelmann BG, et al. Predictors of functional status at service entry and discharge among young people with first episode psychosis. Soc Psychiatry Psychiatr Epidemiol 2017;52(5):575–85.
15. Allott K, Liu P, Proffitt T, et al. Cognition at illness onset as a predictor of later functional outcome in early psychosis: systematic review and methodological critique. Schizophr Res 2010;125(2–3):221–35.
16. Fusar-Poli P, Deste G, Smieskova R, et al. Cognitive functioning in prodromal psychosis. Arch Gen Psychiatry 2012;69(6). https://doi.org/10.1001/archgen psychiatry.2011.1592.
17. Rajji TK, Miranda D, Mulsant BH. Cognition, function, and disability in patients with schizophrenia: a review of longitudinal studies. Can J Psychiatry 2014; 59(1):13–7.
18. Townsend LA, Norman RM. Course of cognitive functioning in first episode schizophrenia spectrum disorders. Expert Rev Neurother 2004;4(1):61–8.
19. Kern RS, Nuechterlein KH, Green MF, et al. The MATRICS Consensus cognitive battery, Part 2: co-norming and standardization. Am J Psychiatry 2008;165: 214–20.
20. Kern RS, Gold JM, Dickinson D, et al. The MCCB impairment profile for schizophrenia outpatients: results from the MATRICS psychometric and standardization study. Schizophr Res 2011;126(1–3):124–31.
21. Free Appropriate Public Education under Section 504. (n.d.). Available at: https://www2.ed.gov/about/offices/list/ocr/docs/edlite-FAPE504.html. Accessed July 4, 2019.
22. Altshuler SJ, Kopels S. Advocating in schools for children with disabilities: what's new with IDEA? Soc Work 2003;48(3):320–9.
23. Gallant M. Section 504 in Massachusetts [PESI, Inc. Presentation]. Taunton, MA, November 03, 2017.
24. Schiffman J, Hoover S, Redman S, et al. Engaging with schools to support your child with psychosis. Alexandria, VA: National Association of State Mental Health Program Directors; 2018.
25. Jones N, Bower K, Furuzawa A. Back to school: Toolkits to support the full inclusion of students with early psychosis in higher education. Alexandria, VA: National Association of State Mental Health Program Directors; 2018.
26. McFarlane WR. Multifamily groups in the treatment of severe psychiatric disorders. New York: Guilford Press; 2002.
27. Lynde, D. W., Gingerich, S., McGurk, S. R., et al (2014). NAVIGATE supported employment and education (SEE) manual. 1-286. Available at: http://www.raiseetp.org/StudyManuals/SEE%20Complete%20Manual.pdf. Accessed July 3, 2019.
28. Humensky JL, Essock SM, Dixon LB. Characteristics associated with the pursuit of work and school among participants in a treatment program for first episode of psychosis. Psychiatr Rehabil J 2017;40(1):108–12.
29. Rosenheck R, Mueser KT, Sint K, et al. Supported employment and education in comprehensive, integrated care for first episode psychosis: effects on work, school, and disability income. Schizophr Res 2016;182:120–8.
30. Killackey E, Jackson HJ, McGorry PD. Vocational intervention in first-episode psychosis: individual placement and support v. treatment as usual. Br J Psychiatry 2008;193(2):114–20.

Moving?

Make sure your subscription moves with you!

To notify us of your new address, find your **Clinics Account Number** (located on your mailing label above your name), and contact customer service at:

Email: journalscustomerservice-usa@elsevier.com

800-654-2452 (subscribers in the U.S. & Canada)
314-447-8871 (subscribers outside of the U.S. & Canada)

Fax number: 314-447-8029

Elsevier Health Sciences Division
Subscription Customer Service
3251 Riverport Lane
Maryland Heights, MO 63043

*To ensure uninterrupted delivery of your subscription, please notify us at least 4 weeks in advance of move.

Printed and bound by CPI Group (UK) Ltd, Croydon, CR0 4YY

03/10/2024

01040400-0004